# Medical Writing in Early Modern English

Medical writing tells us a great deal about how the language of science has developed in constructing and communicating knowledge in English. This volume provides a new perspective on the evolution of the special language of medicine, based on the electronic corpus of *Early Modern English Medical Texts*, containing over 2 million words of medical writing from 1500 to 1700. The book presents results from large-scale empirical research on the new materials and provides a more detailed and diversified picture of domain-specific developments than any previous book. Three introductory chapters provide the sociohistorical, disciplinary and textual frame for nine empirical studies, which address a range of key issues in a wide variety of medical genres from fresh angles. The book is useful for researchers and students within several fields, including the development of special languages, genre and register analysis, (historical) corpus linguistics, historical pragmatics, and medical and cultural history.

IRMA TAAVITSAINEN is Professor of English Philology in the Department of Modern Languages at the University of Helsinki.

PÄIVI PAHTA is Professor of English Philology in the School of Modern Languages and Translation Studies at the University of Tampere.

STUDIES IN ENGLISH LANGUAGE



The aim of this series is to provide a framework for original studies of English, both present-day and past. All books are based securely on empirical research and represent theoretical and descriptive contributions to our knowledge of national and international varieties of English, both written and spoken. The series covers a broad range of topics and approaches, including syntax, phonology, grammar, vocabulary, discourse, pragmatics and sociolinguistics, and is aimed at an international readership.

**Already published in this series:**

Charles F. Meyer: *Apposition in Contemporary English*
Jan Firbas: *Functional Sentence Perspective in Written and Spoken Communication*
Izchak M. Schlesinger: *Cognitive Space and Linguistic Case*
Katie Wales: *Personal Pronouns in Present-Day English*
Laura Wright: *The Development of Standard English, 1300–1800: Theories, Descriptions, Conflicts*
Charles F. Meyer: *English Corpus Linguistics: Theory and Practice*
Stephen J. Nagle and Sara L. Sanders (eds.): *English in the Southern United States*
Anne Curzan: *Gender Shifts in the History of English*
Kingsley Bolton: *Chinese Englishes*
Irma Taavitsainen and Päivi Pahta (eds.): *Medical and Scientific Writing in Late Medieval English*
Elizabeth Gordon, Lyle Campbell, Jennifer Hay, Margaret Maclagan, Andrea Sudbury and Peter Trudgill : *New Zealand English: Its Origins and Evolution*
Raymond Hickey (ed.): *Legacies of Colonial English*
Merja Kytö, Mats Rydén and Erik Smitterberg (eds.): *Nineteenth Century English: Stability and Change*
John Algeo: *British or American English? A Handbook of Word and Grammar Patterns*
Christian Mair: *Twentieth-Century English: History, Variation and Standardization*
Evelien Keizer: *The English Noun Phrase: The Nature of Linguistic Categorization*
Raymond Hickey: *Irish English: History and Present-Day Forms*
Günter Rohdenburg and Julia Schlüter (eds.): *One Language, Two Grammars? Differences between British and American English*
Laurel J. Brinton: *The Comment Clause in English*
Lieselotte Anderwald: *The Morphology of English Dialects: Verb Formation in Non-standard English*

Geoffrey Leech, Marianne Hundt, Christian Mair and Nicholas Smith: *Change in Contemporary English: A Grammatical Study*
Jonathan Culpeper and Merja Kytö: *Early Modern English Dialogues: Spoken Interaction as Writing*
Daniel Schreier, Peter Trudgill, Edgar Schneider and Jeffrey Williams: *The Lesser-Known Varieties of English: An Introduction*
Hilde Hasselgård: *Adjunct Adverbials in English*
Raymond Hickey: *Eighteenth-Century English: Ideology and Change*
Charles Boberg: *The English Language in Canada: Status, History and Comparative Analysis*
Thomas Hoffmann: *Preposition Placement in English: A Usage-Based Approach*
Claudia Claridge: *Hyperbole in English: A Corpus-Based Study of Exaggeration*
Päivi Pahta and Andreas H. Jucker (eds.): *Communicating Early English Manuscripts*

# Medical Writing in Early Modern English

*Edited by*
IRMA TAAVITSAINEN
*University of Helsinki*
and
PÄIVI PAHTA
*University of Tampere*

CAMBRIDGE
UNIVERSITY PRESS

CAMBRIDGE UNIVERSITY PRESS
Cambridge, New York, Melbourne, Madrid, Cape Town, Singapore,
São Paulo, Delhi, Dubai, Tokyo, Mexico City

Cambridge University Press
The Edinburgh Building, Cambridge CB2 8RU, UK

Published in the United States of America by Cambridge University Press, New York

www.cambridge.org
Information on this title: www.cambridge.org/9780521117661



First published 2011

Printed in the United Kingdom at the University Press, Cambridge

*A catalogue record for this publication is available from the British Library*

*Library of Congress Cataloguing in Publication data*
Medical Writing in Early Modern English / [edited by] Irma Taavitsainen, Päivi Pahta.
p. cm. – (Studies in English Language)
ISBN 978-0-521-11766-1
1. Medical writing–Great Britain–History–16th century. 2. Medical writing–Great Britain–History–17th century. 3. Literature and medicine–Great Britain–History–16th century. 4. Literature and medicine–Great Britain–History–17th century. 5. English literature–Early modern, 1500-1700–History and criticism. I. Taavitsainen, Irma, 1946– II. Pahta, Päivi, 1959– III. Title. IV. Series.
R119.M444 2011
808′.06661–dc22
2010045746

ISBN 978-0-521-11766-1 Hardback

# Contents

*List of plates* *page* ix
*List of figures* x
*List of tables* xii
*Notes on contributors* xiv
*Preface* xvii
*List of abbreviations* xix

1 An interdisciplinary approach to medical writing in Early Modern English PÄIVI PAHTA AND IRMA TAAVITSAINEN 1

2 Medical texts in 1500–1700 and the corpus of *Early Modern English Medical Texts* IRMA TAAVITSAINEN, PETER MURRAY JONES, PÄIVI PAHTA, TURO HILTUNEN, VILLE MARTTILA, MAURA RATIA, CARLA SUHR AND JUKKA TYRKKÖ 9

3 Medical literacies and medical culture in early modern England PETER MURRAY JONES 30

4 Verbs of knowing: discursive practices in early modern vernacular medicine TURO HILTUNEN AND JUKKA TYRKKÖ 44

5 Defining in Early Modern English medical texts ROD McCONCHIE AND ANNE CURZAN 74

6 Dissemination and appropriation of medical knowledge: humoral theory in Early Modern English medical writing and lay texts IRMA TAAVITSAINEN 94

7 Code-switching in Early Modern English medical writing PÄIVI PAHTA 115

8 New arguments for new audiences: a corpus-based analysis of interpersonal strategies in Early Modern English medical recipes VILLE MARTTILA 135

9 Efficacy phrases in Early Modern English medical recipes MARTTI MÄKINEN 158

10 Medical pamphlets: controversy and advertising MAURA RATIA AND CARLA SUHR 180

11 The development of specialized discourse in the *Philosophical Transactions* MAURIZIO GOTTI 204

12 The expression of stance in early (1665–1712) publications of the *Philosophical Transactions* and other contemporary medical prose: innovations in a pioneering discourse BETHANY GRAY, DOUGLAS BIBER AND TURO HILTUNEN 221

*Appendix A: Raw data tables corresponding to Figures 4.3–4.14* 248
*Appendix B: Raw data tables corresponding to Figures 8.1–8.4* 252
*Appendix C: Stance markers used in the analysis in Chapter 12* 255
*Appendix D: Preliminary list of texts in the corpus of* Early Modern English Medical Texts *(EMEMT)* 258

*Bibliography* 264
*Index* 294

# Plates


1 Title page, with owner signature and scribblings in the margin, of *The Castel of Helth* by Sir Thomas Elyot, 1534 *page* 26
2 William Clowes, *A Briefe and Necessarie Treatise, Touching the Cure of the Disease Called Morbus Gallicus*, 1585 27
3 Page providing almanac lore and depicting a zodiac man from Frende, *A New Almanacke and Prognostication*, 1593 28
4 Frontispiece and title page, *The Christians Refuge*; *or, Heavenly Antidotes Against the Plague* by W.W., 1665 29
5 Anatomical diagrams of the female body from *The Birth of Mankynde* by Eucharius Rösslin, 1565 92
6 Pages 1 and 2 of the beginning of William Harvey's discussion on the motion of the heart and the circulation of blood in *Anatomical Exercises*, 1653 93
7 Title page of *A Pretious Treasury*: *Or a New Dispensatory. Contayning* 70. *Approved Physicall Rare Receits …* by Salvator Winter, 1649 133
8 Frontispiece portrait and title page of *The Gentlewomans Companion or a Guide to the Female Sex*, 1682 by Hannah Woolley, 1682 134
9 Frontispiece and title page, *The English Physician*; *or, an Astrologo-Physical Discourse of the Vulgar Herbs of This Nation – Being a Compleat Method of Physick* by Nicholas Culpeper, 1652 178
10 Title page of *Elixir Salutis: The Choice Drink of Health* by Anthony Daffy, 1675 179

# Figures


| | | |
|---|---|---|
| 2.1 | Proportions of *EMEMT* text categories | *page* 19 |
| 2.2 | *EMEMT* timeline with background developments | 21 |
| 4.1 | Frequency of knowing-verbs by corpus category | 51 |
| 4.2 | Frequency of knowing-verbs in extracts longer than 2,000 words | 52 |
| 4.3 | Modal auxiliaries and their type by category | 54 |
| 4.4 | Modal auxiliaries and their type on the timeline | 55 |
| 4.5 | Trends in the use of pronominal subjects in the categories | 56 |
| 4.6 | Polarity in relation to category | 58 |
| 4.7 | Polarity in relation to timeline | 58 |
| 4.8 | Changes in the knower class on the timeline | 60 |
| 4.9 | Knower classes of third-person singular subjects in relation to category | 61 |
| 4.10 | Knower classes of third-person plural subjects in relation to category | 62 |
| 4.11 | Topoi in relation to timeline | 68 |
| 4.12 | Sub-topoi of assertive knowledge | 69 |
| 4.13 | Sub-topoi of practical knowledge | 70 |
| 4.14 | Topoi of knowledge in relation to category | 71 |
| 8.1 | Frequency of overt reader reference (per 1,000 words) | 144 |
| 8.2 | Frequency (per 1,000 words) and proportion of references to reader as patient | 146 |
| 8.3 | Frequency (per 1,000 words) and proportion of patient references in second and third person | 146 |
| 8.4 | Frequency of classical terminology (per 1,000 words) | 154 |
| 9.1 | Presence of efficacy phrases in lay texts | 172 |
| 9.2 | Presence of efficacy phrases in learned texts | 173 |
| 9.3 | Efficacy phrase types in lay texts | 173 |
| 9.4 | Efficacy phrase types in learned texts | 174 |
| 9.5 | Distribution of efficacy phrases between Latin and English in lay texts | 175 |
| 12.1 | Distribution of grammatical structures | 232 |
| 12.2 | Distribution of modals | 232 |

12.3 Distribution of stance adverbials 234
12.4 *That*-complement clause types 235
12.5 Non-communication verb-controlled *that*-complement clauses 236
12.6 Communication verb-controlled *that*-complement clauses 236
12.7 Adjective-controlled *that*-complement clauses 240
12.8 Noun-controlled *that*-complement clauses 240

# Tables


| | | |
|---|---|---|
| 4.1 | Classification of knowers | *page* 59 |
| 4.2 | Topoi of knowledge | 64 |
| 6.1 | Frequency of 'humour' in *EMEMT* | 100 |
| 8.1 | Frequency (per 1,000 words) of direct authority reference by type | 152 |
| 9.1 | Texts, their division and the types of efficacy phrases | 166 |
| 10.1 | The frequencies of first- and second-person singular and plural pronouns in two controversies | 186 |
| 10.2 | Frequencies of first- and second-person pronouns in medical pamphlet advertisements | 191 |
| 10.3 | Frequencies of deictic markers in two medical pamphlet controversies | 196 |
| 10.4 | Frequencies of intertextual deictic markers in two medical controversies | 197 |
| 10.5 | Frequencies of deictic markers in medical pamphlet advertisements | 198 |
| 12.1 | Corpus material for this study | 229 |
| 12.2 | Stance categories and example items | 230 |
| 12.3 | Stance patterns in the use of verb-controlled *that*-complement clauses | 242 |
| A1 | Raw frequencies of modal auxiliaries and their type by category (see Figure 4.3) | 248 |
| A2 | Raw frequencies of modal auxiliaries and their type on the timeline (see Figure 4.4) | 248 |
| A3 | Trends in the use of pronominal subjects in the categories (see Figure 4.5) | 248 |
| A4 | Polarity in relation to category (see Figure 4.6) | 249 |
| A5 | Polarity in relation to timeline (Figure 4.7) | 249 |
| A6 | Changes in the knower class on the timeline (see Figure 4.8) | 249 |
| A7 | Knower classes of third-person-singular subjects in relation to category (see Figure 4.9) | 250 |

A8 Knower classes of third-person plural subjects in relation to category (see Figure 4.10) 250
A9 Topoi in relation to timeline (see Figure 4.11) 250
A10 Sub-topoi of assertive knowledge (see Figure 4.12) 250
A11 Sub-topoi of practical knowledge (see Figure 4.13) 251
A12 Topoi of knowledge in relation to category (see Figure 4.14) 251
B1 Raw and normalized frequencies of all overt references to the reader in the texts (see Figure 8.1) 252
B2 Raw and normalized frequencies of references to reader as patient, with percentage of all reader references in each text (see Figure 8.2) 252
B3 Raw and normalized frequencies of references to the patient in the second and third person, with percentage of all patient references in each text (see Figure 8.3) 253
B4 Raw and normalized frequencies of classical terminology by category (see Figure 8.4) 254
C1 Forms used in the analysis of stance 255

# Notes on contributors

DOUGLAS BIBER is Regents' Professor of English (Applied Linguistics) at Northern Arizona University. His research efforts have focused on corpus linguistics, English grammar and register variation (in English and cross-linguistic; synchronic and diachronic). He has written thirteen books and monographs, including academic books published with Cambridge University Press (1988, 1995, 1998, 2009) and the co-authored *Longman Grammar of Spoken and Written English* (1999).

ANNE CURZAN is Associate Professor of English at the University of Michigan. Her research focuses primarily on the history of English, lexicography, language and gender and historical corpus linguistics. In addition to numerous articles and book chapters, she is the author of *Gender Shifts in the History of English* (Cambridge University Press, 2003) and co-author of *How English Works: A Linguistic Introduction* (2nd edn, 2009).

MAURIZIO GOTTI is Professor of English Language and Translation at the University of Bergamo. His main research areas are English syntax, English lexicology and lexicography and the features and origins of specialized discourse, both in a synchronic and diachronic perspective. He is the editor of *English Diachronic Syntax* (1993), co-author of *Variation in Central Modals* (2002) and author of *The Language of Thieves and Vagabonds* (1999), *Robert Boyle and the Language of Science* (1996) and *Investigating Specialized Discourse* (2nd edn, 2008). He is a member of the editorial board of several national and international journals and edits the Linguistic Insights series for Peter Lang.

BETHANY GRAY is a Ph.D. candidate in applied linguistics at Northern Arizona University. Her research investigates register variation using corpus linguistics methodologies, with a focus on documenting variation across written academic registers and disciplines. She has published in the *Journal of English for Academic Purposes*.

TURO HILTUNEN'S Ph.D. thesis (2010) deals with disciplinary differences in present-day English academic writing. He is a member of the Scientific Thought-Styles project at the Research Unit for Variation, Contacts and

Change in English, University of Helsinki. His research interests include corpus linguistics, English for academic purposes, history of scientific and medical writing and historical pragmatics.

ROD McCONCHIE Ph.D. is a senior lecturer and researcher at the University of Helsinki. He has published on medical terminology and lexicography (*Lexicography and Physicke*, 1997) and, more recently, articles on the prefix *dis-* in Middle English, and on sixteenth- and seventeenth-century English lexicographers. He has also edited and co-edited volumes of essays and conference proceedings. He has an ongoing interest in book history, and his most recent research is on the earliest English medical dictionaries.

MARTTI MÄKINEN is a senior lecturer at Hanken School of Economics, Helsinki. His research interests include corpus linguistics, manuscript and genre studies and historical linguistics. His dissertation was on the medieval English herbal genre (University of Helsinki). He was one of the compilers of the corpus of *Middle English Medical Texts* (2005) and is a co-compiler of *The Middle English Grammar Corpus* (2007–).

VILLE MARTTILA MA is a postgraduate researcher at the University of Helsinki, working on his Ph.D. thesis on medieval culinary recipes and their pragmatic features. He is a member of the Scientific Thought-Styles project at the Research Unit for Variation, Contacts and Change in English and also a member of the Digital Editions for Corpus Linguistics project. His research interests include manuscript studies, digital editing, historical pragmatics and the historical development of the recipe genre.

PETER MURRAY JONES is Fellow and Librarian at King's College, Cambridge. He has published *Medieval Medicine in Illuminated Manuscripts* (1998) and studies on medieval and early modern medicine and surgery. He is interested in the circulation of medical books in early modern England and in the relationship of communication in print to oral and manuscript circulation of medical knowledge.

PÄIVI PAHTA is Professor of English Philology at the School of Modern Languages and Translation Studies, University of Tampere. Her research interests include manuscript studies, historical (corpus) linguistics, history of scientific writing, language contact and multilingualism. Her main publications include *Medieval Embryology in the Vernacular* (1998), *Medical and Scientific Writing in Late Medieval English* (co-edited with Irma Taavitsainen, Cambridge University Press, 2004), the corpus of *Middle English Medical Texts* (with Irma Taavitsainen and Martti Mäkinen, 2005), *Social Roles and Language Practices in Late Modern English* (co-edited with Minna Nevala, Arja Nurmi and Minna Palander-Collin, 2010), and *Communicating Early English Manuscripts* (co-edited with Andreas H. Jucker, Cambridge University Press, 2010).

MAURA RATIA MA is a Ph.D. student and member of the Scientific Thought-Styles project at the Research Unit for Variation, Contacts and Change in English, University of Helsinki, working on argumentative strategies in the early modern tobacco controversy in a multidisciplinary frame, combining the study of language and medical history. For her thesis, she has compiled a corpus of tobacco texts of different genres.

CARLA SUHR holds an MA in history and in English philology. She is Assistant at the Department of English, University of Helsinki, and a member of the Scientific Thought-Styles project at the Research Unit for Variation, Contacts and Change in English. She is preparing her Ph.D. dissertation on the evolution of Early Modern English witchcraft pamphlets.

IRMA TAAVITSAINEN is Professor of English Philology and Deputy Director of the Research Unit for Variation, Contacts and Change in English at the University of Helsinki. Her research focuses on the evolution of scientific and medical writing, historical pragmatics, corpus linguistics and stylistics. She has co-edited several books, including *Medical Writing in Late Medieval English* (with Päivi Pahta, Cambridge University Press, 2004), *Diachronic Perspectives on Domain-Specific English* (with Marina Dossena, 2006), *Speech Acts in the History of English* (with Andreas H. Jucker, 2008) and *Methods in Historical Pragmatics* (with Susan Fitzmaurice, 2007), and the handbook *Historical Pragmatics* (with Andreas H. Jucker). She compiled the corpus of *Middle English Medical Texts* (with Päivi Pahta and Martti Mäkinen, 2005). She also co-edits the *Journal of Historical Pragmatics*.

JUKKA TYRKKÖ MA is a postgraduate researcher and member of the Scientific Thought-Styles project at the Research Unit for Variation, Contacts and Change in English, University of Helsinki. His forthcoming Ph.D. thesis studies coherence in hypertext narratives. In addition to textual coherence and text linguistics, his research interests include the history of scientific writing, historical corpus linguistics and the history of the book, with a particular focus on early lexicography.

# Preface

The large field of medical writing in Early Modern English is still a fairly uncharted area from a linguistic point of view, and this is what our book sets out to explore. In language-external developments, the era between 1500 and 1700 is remarkable: the world view gradually changed from Ptolemaic to Copernican, new continents were discovered, and people ceased to believe in received knowledge. Scientific and medical writing became more diversified with the new medium of the printing press, and the position of English, which had begun to emerge as a language of science and medicine from the shadow of Latin during the fourteenth and fifteenth centuries, became stronger. Medieval conventions continued in medical writing well beyond the Late Middle English period as early printed books imitated manuscripts, and it took at least half a century or more for a new print culture to break away from the old. Generic developments were dynamic: during the two centuries, the top genres of old scholasticism declined, lost their position as the spearhead of science and were adapted to writings that dealt with established or inherited knowledge. This process created a vacuum at the top. Institutional developments gave an incentive to further changes, and by the time of the Royal Society the written word in the printed form had achieved a leading role in communicating science. Members of the new, close-knit discourse community made a conscious decision to communicate their scientific findings and opinions by writing in the new *Philosophical Transactions*.

The birth of the scientific journal paved the way to future developments that led to the spearhead position of the new medium. The genres in use by Royal Society members have direct relevance to present-day scientific writing; today, new discoveries and achievements are first reported to the global discourse community in research articles in scientific journals. But there is continuity at the lower end of the scale as well. The aftermath of medieval science lives on in popular adaptations of the *homo signorum* and other astrological doctrines to broad and heterogeneous readerships, even today. This development can be traced to the early modern period and beyond to almanac literature. Between these two means of communicating, *Philosophical Transactions* and the almanac, there is a wide range of publications, including textbooks, treatises, health guides, collections of remedies and pamphlets. The scale is broad and interesting, with different types of new manifestations of commercialism in advertisements, debate conflicts in short tracts and household literature for women in demand with increasing literacy.

The research reported in this book is mostly produced in the frame of the Scientific Thought-Styles project, launched about fifteen years ago at the University of Helsinki. In this book venture, the project team has been complemented by other scholars – visiting fellows, as it were – sharing an interest in scientific discourse and in the history of medicine and medical writing. We would like to thank the Research Unit for Variation, Contacts and Change in English at the University of Helsinki for providing us with the opportunity to organize workshops with some of our visiting fellows to discuss, on the one hand, the interdisciplinary nature of our endeavour with Peter Murray Jones, and, on the other hand, the more technical questions and software solutions of corpus linguistics with Douglas Biber and Raymond Hickey.

The members of the Scientific Thought-Styles project have received funding from various organizations during their work on this book, and we gratefully acknowledge this: the Academy of Finland; the Research Unit for Variation, Contacts and Change in English at the University of Helsinki; the Emil Aaltonen Foundation; the Finnish Cultural Foundation; the Finnish Graduate School in Language Studies; and the School of Modern Languages and Translation Studies at the University of Tampere. We would also like to thank the Department of English at the University of Helsinki for financial aid in editing the book.

We would like to express our thanks to the anonymous reviewers at Cambridge University Press for their helpful comments. We are grateful to Merja Kytö, the series editor of *Studies in English Language*, for recommending the book for publication, and to Helen Barton for all her editorial work. It has been a great pleasure for us to collaborate with them. We are grateful to the Wellcome Library and to Catherine Draycott, for giving us permission to publish pictures from the Wellcome collections, and to Julianne Simmons, for suggesting the interesting range of pictures to us, many of which have not been used as book illustrations before.

Our team deserves our deepest gratitude. We wish to thank the authors – core project members and visiting fellows alike – for their excellent collaboration, enthusiasm and willingness to participate in this exciting joint venture. We thank Jukka Tuominen for his valuable contribution as our editorial assistant, Anu Lehto and Raisa Oinonen for their careful and cheerful assistance in various tasks and Mark Shackleton for polishing our language. Finally, our home teams deserve a special word of thanks for their support and understanding.

# Abbreviations

| | |
|---|---|
| *CED* | *A Corpus of English Dialogues 1560–1760* |
| *EMEMT* | *Early Modern English Medical Texts* |
| EP(s) | efficacy phrase(s) |
| *ESTC* | *English Short-Title Catalogue* |
| KWIC | keyword in context |
| *MEMT* | *Middle English Medical Texts* |
| MS | manuscript |
| *OED* | *Oxford English Dictionary* (Murray et al. 1989–2009) |
| *PCEEC* | *Parsed Corpus of Early English Correspondence* |
| *PT* | *Philosophical Transactions* |
| *STC* | *A Short-Title Catalogue of Books Printed in England, Scotland, & Ireland and of English Books Printed Abroad* 1475–1640 (Pollard et al. 1976–91) |
| VP | verb phrase |

# 1 An interdisciplinary approach to medical writing in Early Modern English

PÄIVI PAHTA AND IRMA TAAVITSAINEN

> Historically, language is an indispensable guide both to theoretical scientific ideas and to real actions. Any language embodies a theory of meaning, a logic, a classification of experience, a conception of perceiver, knower and agent and their objects, and an apprehension of existence in space and time. We need to ask how language conditioned scientific thinking and was in turn altered by it. We may distinguish three levels: those of the structure of a language itself, of general conceptions of the nature of things expressed in it, and of particular theories.
>
> (Crombie 1995: 232–3)

This book examines the connection of language and science in English medical writings in the period 1500–1700. We approach this link through situated analyses of language and texts, paying attention to context in all its multifaceted aspects, from the broad context of culture to situational and cognitive discourse contexts and to the narrow linguistic context. The twelve chapters of the book analyse language use in medical texts in their disciplinary, social and societal embedding. The basic theoretical assumption on which the book relies is the view of language as communication that always takes place in a particular context of discourse, characterized by time and place, between people – speakers and hearers or writers and readers – and for a particular purpose. This communicative situation has an impact on how the speakers or writers formulate their message. In such communicative events, negotiating meaning is a process that needs to be viewed in the multilayered context, but it can be viewed from different perspectives; when the perspective changes, new features of the object of enquiry become visible. In historical texts, the facts of production and reception are often elusive, and in the absence of historical evidence, the communicative situations need to be reconstructed hypothetically, and it is also possible to place the focus on the discourse itself.

The approach adopted in the book presents an interdisciplinary challenge, as a contextualized analysis of medical language requires an understanding of the contemporary history of medicine as an area of special knowledge and practice. The key to meeting this challenge is the collaboration between medical historians and historical linguists, as it is often at the interfaces between various disciplines where innovations are created by fusions of various ways of thinking and methodological triangulation. In this volume, the methods of historical research are represented in taking the background socio-historical developments into account and considering how they influenced textual reality and readership. The politics of medical literacy and book historical details are important for an understanding of the reception of these works by audiences of various social and educational backgrounds and mindsets. Linguistic methodologies to studying the special language of medicine provide various angles. Several chapters adopt the framework of historical pragmatics, understood here in a broad sense as a perspective to language use, including societal aspects and overlapping with sociolinguistics (see Taavitsainen and Jucker 2010). In some chapters, the approach is semantic, and some chapters apply advanced corpus-linguistic methods with statistical tests. All empirical contributions take variation and change of early modern medical writing as their point of departure (see, for example, Milroy 1992). Variability in language use is a key concept here, as variation in linguistic features mirrors the varying underlying language-external parameters, both in micro-level speaker/writer-related factors and at the macro-level of historical and sociocultural context. The studies make use of a new database, the corpus of *Early Modern English Medical Texts* (*EMEMT*), but the ways in which they exploit it for answering their research questions vary. In most chapters, the methods are corpus-aided, i.e. the database has been searched with relevant lexical items for the research task in question, and the located passages have been scrutinized with qualitative assessments. Automatically created word lists have been employed to make the searches as precise as possible, taking, for example, spelling variation into account. Statistical corpus-linguistic methods have been applied in three chapters, one of which relies on co-occurrence patterns of several linguistic features with stance-marking functions.

The book is part of a larger project on the evolution of English as the language of medicine, where the history of science and medicine provides a language-external frame of reference against which linguistic forms and functions are examined. In scientific communication, one of the contextual sociocultural factors influencing the message is the prevailing scientific ideology or thought-style.[1] Scientific thought-styles can be defined as the underlying scientific concepts, objects of enquiry, methods, evaluations and intellectual commitments related to the epistemology of science (Crombie 1994: 5–6). Like any other ideologies, scientific thought-styles are mediated through language and are connected with particular ways of using language.

[1] See http://www.helsinki.fi/varieng/domains/scientific%20thought.html (accessed 17 August 2010).

The styles of thinking within any society or culture endure as long as the underlying commitments and dispositions remain stable, and with changes in the ways of scientific thinking, the ways of communicating science also change (see Taavitsainen and Pahta 1995). But everything does not change: in fact, changes come about in a less conspicuous way than generally assumed, and recent research shows that the great majority of early modern medical writings continue in the old vein, carrying over conventions from previous writing (Taavitsainen 2009c). New knowledge is constructed through questions based on earlier knowledge, and, similarly, innovations in communicating knowledge take place within the existing frame.

What changes in the language and how, and what remains the same, are questions for the linguist to answer. Our general claim is that changes in the underlying scientific ideology as well as in the discourse community can be verified both on the micro-level of individual linguistic features and on the macro-level of argumentative structures and textual organization. Continuities and changes in early English medical writings need to be examined with special reference to materials written in the prevailing institutional language of science, Latin. In our earlier research, we have focused on continuity and change in medieval English medical writing from the fourteenth and fifteenth centuries, the first phase in the vernacularization of science and medicine (see Taavitsainen and Pahta 2004). In this book, we explore the essence of medical writing in the second and third waves of vernacularization in the period between 1500 and 1700, with a focus on the continuities and changes that can be observed in language and text.[2]

The 200-year period in focus in this book is characterized by major sociocultural changes that affected the domain of medicine as an area of knowledge and praxis. This needs to be taken into account in the analysis of writings produced within it. During this period, the scientific paradigm experienced a major epistemological shift: medieval scholastic, logocentric science, relying on knowledge derived from Galen, Hippocrates and other ancient writers, gave way to new ways of constructing knowledge, relying on empirical methods and explanatory principles based on observation and cognition (see Crombie 1994; Taavitsainen and Pahta 1995). Significant advances were made in medical theory. Dissatisfaction with deeply entrenched ancient medical doctrines had begun to increase by the late Middle Ages, and in the course of the sixteenth and seventeenth centuries the new intellectual climate produced several momentous publications, laying the foundations for the new science of medicine. Andreas Vesalius' *De humani corporis fabrica* (1543), based on solid facts observed in careful dissections, was a breakthrough in the field of anatomy. Although the work did not contain startling

[2] The first wave, 1375–1475, and the beginning of the second were dealt with in our previous book (Taavitsainen and Pahta 2004). The first fifty years examined in this book still belong to the second phase. The early modern period, 1550–1700, has not been dealt with from this perspective before.

new discoveries, it induced a shift in intellectual strategy, marking an end to appeals to ancient authority (Porter 1996: 155–7). The growing prestige of anatomical discoveries based on first-hand knowledge also began to change the orientation towards the physiological composition of the body and its mechanisms. Here the breakthrough came a century later than in anatomy: the revolutionary work by William Harvey in *Exercitatio anatomica de motu cordis et sanguinis in animalibus* (1628) marks the beginning of a new phase in physiological inquiry (Siraisi 1990: 190–2; French 1994: 85). The new knowledge was also gradually translated to medical praxis, although old practices in treatment continued by the side of innovation.

The domain of medicine was also undergoing a major language shift. In the course of the late medieval period, English medical writing had slowly begun to emerge from the shadow of Latin in non-institutional contexts (see, for example, Voigts 1989b; Taavitsainen and Pahta 1998; Pahta and Taavitsainen 2004). By 1700, English had challenged Latin as the language of institutional medical science and had become the dominant language of medical writing in England, used as the original medium of communicating new scientific discoveries. The triumph of English is illustrated in the increase of medical books listed in the *English Short-Title Catalogue* (*ESTC*; see Chapter 2). An important milestone in the history of English scientific and medical writing is the foundation of the Royal Society of London in 1662 (M. Hunter 1981: 48). Despite its early international connections, the innovative society decided to publish its *Philosophical Transactions* (*PT*) from the very beginning in 1665 primarily in English, a decision that in the first phases involved extensive translation from other European languages into English (Gotti 2006a).[3]

Furthermore, the newly discovered printing technology caused changes in the dissemination of knowledge by written communication (see, for example, McKitterick 2003). Texts became more widely available in identical multiple copies and accessible to the literate at a relatively cheap price. Medical publishing really took off in the 1640s, and after 1660 over 150 medical books were printed per decade. The first scientific journals and periodicals began to appear towards the end of the seventeenth century. At the same time, medical knowledge continued to circulate in handwritten texts, including letters and notebooks, and oral exchange remained an important means of communicating medical advice (see Chapter 2).

New ideas are always born within the old, and it takes time for the innovations to gain ground. The roots of early modern medicine lie deep in medieval medicine and antiquity, and the first half of the sixteenth century saw little change in medical literature as the new print medium simply replicated old materials that had earlier circulated in manuscripts. Perhaps the most dramatic change is the general shift from anonymous writings to

[3] But see Note 8 in Chapter 2.

texts written by individuals under their own names. The New World had been discovered, but news from beyond the seas was delivered in the old thought-style, and it took several decades for information about new medicines, such as tobacco and coca, to reach European medical literature (see Ratia and Suhr in this volume, Chapter 10). Doubt was raised as to whether ancient authorities were right after all, as observation did not agree with, for example, plant illustrations derived from old books. Changes in the reporting styles of news from the New World took place in the latter half of the sixteenth century (Taavitsainen 2009b). The seventeenth century saw further changes. A more general stylistic change has been attributed to the Royal Society period, with the birth of new genres of experimental essays and book reviews, for instance. This statement needs to be reassessed as well, and with the new extensive corpus of medical texts it will be possible to date the changes and to define the locus of change more precisely than has been done before.

The 'foreign culture of early modern medicine' (Wear 2000: 1) has received increasing attention lately, with new book-length studies on more ephemeral materials, such as almanacs and recipe books (e.g., Curth 2007; Jenner and Wallis 2007; Leong and Pennell 2007). There is a clear shift of interest from more elite professional writing to the literature that reached the heterogeneous 'ordinary' readerships, new women audiences and 'the poor'. With the new knowledge gained from previously unstudied materials, cultural diversity has come to the forefront, and the overall picture of early modern medical writings is changing, as earlier knowledge is challenged by the new perspectives and discoveries. The borderlines between the different periods and different types of writing are not clear-cut, and we can notice an array of varying cultural practices that overlap and are exploited by society at large, by both professional and laypeople, but in somewhat different forms.

Features connected with stance and attitudes to knowledge are relevant for tracing reflections of scientific ideology in texts on the temporal axis. Studies on evaluation and attitude are a major trend in recent synchronic and diachronic linguistic research. In the time period under scrutiny here, 1500–1700, a great deal happened in the style of writing. The attitude to the object of enquiry changed from the absolute certainty of the scholastic thought-style to cautious assumptions of the researcher employing new instruments in laboratory conditions, with peer researchers of heterogeneous backgrounds watching the experiment. Another noticeable line of development is seen in the audience involvement and politeness scale, from respectful address to humiliating remarks addressed to the readership where the educated author places his own knowledge high above the multitude:

First to the Vulgar: Kind souls I am sorry it hath been your hard mishap to have been so long trained in such Egyptian darkness, even darkness which to your sorrows may be felt; the vulgar road of Physick is not my practice, and I am therefore the more unfit to give you advice; ... You must not think (curtaeous People) that I can spend time to give you examples of all Diseases, these are enough to let you see so much light as you without Art are able to receive, If I should set you to look upon the Sun I should dazle your eyes and make you blind. (Culpeper 1652b: 242)

The chapters in this book are organized so that large-scale mappings of linguistic features across the whole *EMEMT* corpus come first, and detailed investigations of individual genres or shorter time periods are placed towards the end of the volume. The first chapter defines our approach and sets the scene of our research. Chapter 2 describes the primary data used in the book, the *EMEMT* corpus, which provides new comprehensive material for studies on the role of language in science and makes it possible to study early modern medical writing with more precision and to probe into the 'medical mindsets as represented in vernacular medical books' (Wear 2000: 2). Chapter 2 places the corpus texts in the broader context of medical books and the dissemination of knowledge in the early modern period. Chapter 3 relates to an essential cultural background feature and describes various literacy practices, turning the spotlight from the texts to the actual readers of medical texts. Literacy is approached as a multilayered analytical concept constituting different levels of practices. Together, these chapters at the beginning of the volume pave the way to the empirical linguistic studies.

Verbs of knowing are investigated by Hiltunen and Tyrkkö in Chapter 4. They scrutinize their distributions along the time axis in periods of fifty years and across the various corpus categories as defined in the description in Chapter 2. The results show variation between the categories. The distinctions are clear and can be related to the sociocultural backgrounds. The study sheds new light on the diachronic development of thought-styles and indicates that a large-scale modelling of the underlying ideologies of the history of written documents is possible.

Medical definitions provide a means of organizing and systematizing medical knowledge. This core feature is the topic of lexicological and lexicographical assessment by McConchie and Curzan in Chapter 5. Their analysis combines an assessment of *EMEMT* materials and early dictionaries. The study shows that medical practitioners with university education were more precise and more innovative than contemporaneous lexicographers in their formulations.

The chapter by Taavitsainen, Chapter 6, examines a key notion of a medical theory: the concept of *humour*. She investigates its appropriation in different types of texts, aimed at professional and lay audiences, but her assessment also extends beyond *EMEMT* to contemporary correspondence and to drama, showing the influence of the humoral theory in early modern culture. By contextual analysis, she demonstrates how different the semantic associations are in these registers of writing.

Multilingualism is in focus in Pahta's chapter, Chapter 7. Her analysis of multilingual practices in *EMEMT* material pays attention to the linguistic and textual forms and functions in which writers of vernacular medical texts made use of other languages. The study reveals a wide repertoire of languages, including Latin, Greek, Arabic and European vernaculars, which the writers use primarily to communicate domain-specific knowledge.

The chapters by Marttila and Mäkinen, Chapters 8 and 9, examine recipes, an important and widely disseminated genre in early modern England. Marttila focuses on authors' strategies, paying special attention to how they take the audience into account. Metatextual passages often emphasize helping 'the poor' as the motivation for writing. Such comments have been dismissed as a social decorum, but Marttila's analysis shows that there is more to these statements as, for example, many recipe books depict the recipient of the advice as the patient. In general, authors strived to get their message across to the uninitiated. The epistemology of knowledge is addressed from a different angle by Mäkinen, who studies the continuity and change of expressions used for confirming the efficacy of recipes, thus persuading the readers to accept the advice provided as being useful.

Ratia and Suhr focus their attention on medical pamphlets in Chapter 10 and examine linguistic structures connected with interpersonal language use. Pamphlets were a new means of distributing knowledge, and the medium was especially well suited for debating, bringing forth viewpoints in controversies and spreading news of efficient medicines to potential consumers. The textual strategies discovered in the analysis include features intended to facilitate reader or listener comprehension, to involve the audience and to influence the early consumers' behaviour.

Chapter 11 by Gotti discusses functional macrostructures of language, focusing on the early phases of the new medium to distribute medical and scientific knowledge, the first long-standing scientific journal in England, the *Philosophical Transactions* (*PT*) of the Royal Society of London. This was the period when specialized discourse was still in its embryonic stages, but the new lines of development leading to present-day conventions can already be discerned.

In the final chapter, Chapter 12, Gray, Biber and Hiltunen examine the qualification of knowledge by the use of various stance markers across three categories within the *PT*, with contemporary material from the other five categories in *EMEMT* for comparison. The analytical grid is dense and provides interesting results both across the whole corpus and within the *PT* genres. In contrast to earlier assumptions, the study shows that book reviews contained the most innovative language use.

In the quotation that opens this chapter, Crombie specifies three levels on which language has conditioned scientific thinking and has in turn been altered by it in the history of science: the structure of a language, the general conceptions of the nature of things and particular scientific theories. The role of language in expressing general conceptions of the nature of things is at the heart of the studies in this volume, examining the knowledge base of medicine, the essence and meaning of knowledge and attitudes towards it, which are all expressed by specific and varying linguistic structures. We have made an attempt to probe into the practices of early modern medical authors and have shed light on the reception of their texts and the use of medical theories in early modern society. The individual studies show that it is possible to achieve new knowledge with more extensive materials structured according to the socio-historical background factors. This book shows what can be done with the new corpus, and we hope that new paths will open up with little-explored materials and new methods developed within corpus linguistics.[4]

[4] *EMEMT* was released for public use in December 2010. In addition to texts that faithfully preserve their original spellings, the corpus includes normalized versions of texts, making new applications of corpus linguistics possible, e.g., keyword and cluster analysis.

# 2 Medical texts in 1500–1700 and the corpus of *Early Modern English Medical Texts*

IRMA TAAVITSAINEN, PETER MURRAY JONES, PÄIVI PAHTA, TURO HILTUNEN, VILLE MARTTILA, MAURA RATIA, CARLA SUHR AND JUKKA TYRKKÖ

## 2.1 Introduction

English medical texts from the period 1500–1700 are a large and heterogeneous group of writings, including texts circulating in print and manuscript forms on a range of medical topics, representing a variety of genres, written by authors with varying educational and professional backgrounds for different types of target audiences. The 200 years in focus here were a period of important changes from the medieval world view to the first stages of empirical science. In this chapter, we shall first discuss the background and the transmission of medical knowledge with different modes, oral and written, and media, printed books and manuscripts. Sections 2.2 and 2.3 give an overview of medical literature throughout the two-century period. Section 2.4 introduces the *Early Modern English Medical Texts* (*EMEMT*), a computer-readable text collection designed to facilitate research on printed medical texts of the period and used as primary material in the studies in this book.

## 2.2 Printing and manuscript circulation

Dissemination of medical knowledge underwent major changes in the early modern period. The advent of printing introduced a new technology that enabled the production of multiple copies of a text more quickly and more cheaply than had been possible with copying by hand. This affected both the more prestigious kinds of text, those produced by learned men, and those texts that were meant to provide basic medical information to laypeople, for instance almanacs that might sell for 2d. Printed books in the period are found in different formats from folio-size display objects with fine illustrations to small pocket-size manuals to be carried around and consulted at the bedside. The almanac gained the widest possible print distribution, and various types were issued with medical concerns, astrological prognostications and useful advice, which sold in hundreds of thousands, or even millions of copies (Capp 1979; Curth 2006). However, the progress of medical printing in England was slow in comparison with Continental Europe. In the late fifteenth and early sixteenth centuries, relatively few editions of printed books on medicine in English appeared. Only after 1550 did the numbers of medical books printed in England begin to increase sharply. In part, the explanation for this relative backwardness may have been the small scale of the local printing industry compared to places such as Paris, Lyon, Venice or Strasbourg, whose own print productions could be readily imported to England. Demand for English-language printing was, in any case, modest compared to that for Latin or other European vernaculars.

Still, the impact of print on the circulation of medical ideas and information was profound, in England as elsewhere. But this impact is best understood not as a displacement or replacement of other more 'primitive' methods of communication, primarily speech and handwriting, but as a process of dynamic interaction with them. Take, for example, the giving of medical advice in this period. Leong and Pennell (2007: 138) write:

Oral exchange was still the primary vehicle for communication of medicinal advice in early modern England. However, the setting down of advice to preserve that exchange (but by no means to fix the information transmitted during it) was not the sole preserve of the prescribing physician or apothecary. Instructions to make medicaments for all sorts of ailments and illnesses were exchanged during social visits, circulated in letters, and were recorded into bound notebooks. Sometimes they were even merely bundled together as batches of paper. The onward circulation of individually inscribed recipes and prescriptions, indeed of entire manuscripts, provided other compilers with an important source for their own collections.

The availability of medical advice in print did not replace these kinds of circulation of information but acted as a new resource, a kind of accelerant of them. Recipes could be copied from a printed book into a manuscript, or collections of recipes in manuscript could find their way into print.

Even where printed medicine was readily available, some kinds of medical texts were still better suited to handwritten production. An obvious instance is the compilation of remedies from various sources which is tailored to the interests and capacities of the individual scribe and user.[1] Second, in an educational or learning environment, the students might want to make notes by hand on lectures they had heard or based on their reading, which would serve their individual needs (Blair 2008). Third, medical practitioners might find it useful to compile by their own hand aides-memoire of useful information or records of treatment they had given to their patients (see P. M. Jones

[1] See the collection of digitized English seventeenth-century recipe books at the Wellcome Library (http://library.wellcome.ac.uk/etexts.html); also microforms in Pennell (2004b).

2008). Examples of all these three categories of medical writing survive in manuscript from the early modern era to the present. We can guess that since the rate of loss over intervening centuries of such personalized writings by hand is likely to be much higher than for those intended for wide circulation, these practices of medical manuscript production may have flourished in ways that the small number of surviving examples tends to conceal.

The relationship between printed books and handwritten works is extremely complicated, and the motivations of an individual who decides to put a particular piece of medical writing into print also vary. Gideon Harvey, a seventeenth-century medical writer, reflects upon his own reasons for printing:

After all, I must tell you, a Self-Interest prevail'd very much with me in the printing of this, which is, that writing an ill hand, and being puzzled sometimes to read it, and the Matter not digested into any sort of order, I might have a more easie resource to my own Thoughts and Sentiments, being expressed in Characters more legible, and so disposed, that I could then more readily turn to them. (G. Harvey 1700: 2)

It is extremely difficult to judge how far the availability of a printed literature of medicine may have made writing medical texts by hand less necessary or desirable. On the one hand, it is likely that the ability to write and the availability of materials for writing (especially affordable paper), both increasing after 1500, encouraged the production of handwritten medical texts; on the other hand, it became increasingly possible to buy printed texts that saved the trouble and expense of hand-copying. Numbers of manuscripts with medical contents in circulation are not available in the same way that we can make estimates using the *English Short-Title Catalogue* (*ESTC*) and Wing's short-title catalogue of numbers of printed medical editions and even surmise average numbers of copies in an edition, so achieving figures for total production of printed copies. The best we can do is to look at significant collections of medical manuscripts such as those formed by Elias Ashmole, Robert Harley or Sir Hans Sloane in the seventeenth century and imagine what hosts of other manuscripts have disappeared.

The interplay of oral, manuscript and print circulations of medicine remains imperfectly understood and in need of investigation. But there is no doubt that none of them can be considered in isolation in this period.

## 2.3 Printed medical books between 1500 and 1700

Information about the development of printed medicine between 1500 and 1700 can be obtained from three principal works. Andrew Wear's *Knowledge and Practice in English Medicine, 1550–1680* (2000) offers a major synthesis of vernacular medical knowledge and practice in England from 1550 to 1680, a period that almost covers the time span of the present volume. History is dealt with in terms of continuity and change. The focus of the book is on vernacular medical texts, on remedies, regimen texts, surgical treatises and other learned tracts. Descriptions of diseases include an extended discussion of plague, but topics such as madness or midwifery, for instance, are not included. Wear (2000) pays attention to popular versions of learned medicine and dissemination of knowledge to ordinary people and presents a view of a shared medical culture. In addition to this book, there are two important studies on patterns of medical publication in this period, the first by Paul Slack (1979) covering 1486 to 1604, and the other by Mary Fissell (2007) covering 1641 to 1740. Between them they cover all but thirty-six years of our period, and the gap is in itself significant as a distinct era in medical publication.

Slack (1979) counted 153 medical titles published before 1605, many of them reprinted again and again, yielding 392 editions of medical works.[2] Medical publication represented a very small part of publishing overall to 1604, perhaps 3 per cent, and the numbers of copies in circulation printed in England were probably swamped by books printed on the Continent and imported to England, mostly in Latin rather than English. The output of English medical titles and editions was spread unevenly over time. The number of medical editions printed in each quinquennium doubled from a previous peak of ten to twenty in 1536–40, and thereafter tended to rise. Significantly new medical titles – as opposed to editions – only began to appear at a rate of more than ten per quinquennium after 1575 and continued at this higher level until 1604. Slack's conclusion is that 'we can scarcely attribute any major social or medical impact to a volume of literature of this size' (1979: 240). On the other hand, he thinks, there were probably enough English medical books available by 1604 for those readers who positively wanted them.

What kinds of medical books were published in the sixteenth century? With language in mind, one-third of the titles published were identified as translations according to Slack's calculations. Some of those that purported to be contemporary medical writings in English were in fact also translations of Latin writings by medieval authors: this is the case with the best-seller among these medical books, Thomas Moulton's *Myrrour or Glasse of Helth* (1539), which went through at least seventeen editions between 1530 and 1580 (Getz 1990: 10–11). Medical publishing in England was highly conservative in the sixteenth century, since printers preferred to produce lots of editions of established texts which had already enjoyed success in Latin in the fifteenth century rather than experimenting with new texts by contemporary authors. Because of this conservatism there

2 Slack's totals can now, with the help of the *Short-Title Catalogue* (Pollard et al. 1976–91), be seen to be underestimates of medical books produced, but the picture he gives of sixteenth-century medical printing is little affected.

is more continuity between the medical writings in circulation in manuscript before 1500 and medical writing in print after 1500 than might be assumed.

Slack points out that for those writings he chose to include in his survey, half of the medical books published in the period can be described as falling in the categories of textbooks of medicine, regimens of health and collections of remedies, as measured by the numbers of editions that appeared.[3] The other categories are works on anatomy and surgery, reflections on theory and practice, herbals, plague tracts, other specific diseases and single or specialized remedies. These are categories that apply to late medieval medical writing just as readily. Most of them are, in effect, long-established 'genres' of medical writing, in which reprinting of long-favoured texts was the norm and novelty rare. Plague tracts tended to appear during or shortly after epidemics of the disease and were not reprinted until the next outbreak. More specialized works on disease or remedy tend to appear in some numbers only after 1575, meaning that medical literature in print after that date was far more varied in content than earlier, as well as surging ahead in numbers of titles and editions published.

In the gap between the end of Slack's period in 1604 and the 1650s, the contours of medical publication change. Although this cannot be measured with precision, as the basic surveying work has not been done, the main outlines have become clearer in recent years. While new editions of the books that fall in the 'genres' identified by Slack continue to appear, there is by comparison with the period between 1575 and 1604 a falling off in the number of new writings on medicine, particularly those in the category of textbooks and collections of remedies. The most likely explanation for this phenomenon is the impact of the agreement between the physicians of London and the apothecaries that led to the formation of the Society of Apothecaries in 1617 (hitherto apothecaries had belonged to the Grocers) and the publication of the *Pharmacopoeia Londinensis* under the aegis of the College of Physicians in 1618. In return for the physicians' support for the creation and continuing establishment of the Society of Apothecaries, and a monopoly given to the apothecaries over the dispensation of medicines, a proclamation required the members of the Society to furnish only those remedies that were published in the *Pharmacopoeia*, and only under the instruction of a physician. The *Pharmacopoeia* continued to be published in Latin in successive editions, and the alliance of the College of Physicians with the Society of Apothecaries, reinforced by the activities of the College as censor of unlicensed medical practice and publications (which might be destroyed at their order), seems successfully to have inhibited the writing of new texts that prescribed remedies. The College also disparaged the use of

[3] The most notable exclusion in Slack's survey is almanacs.

the vernacular in medicine generally, claiming that Latin was the language of learned medicine.[4]

Mary Fissell's database (2007) of all medical works intended for non-practitioners published in English from 1641 to 1740 begins with the decade when medical publishing, like all other publishing, took off. Though the basis for her survey is different to that of Slack, and it measures publication on a much-expanded scale, it bears very useful comparison with Slack's findings on the earlier period.[5] Fissell points out that 'the 1650s represented an extraordinary flowering of vernacular medical publishing' (2007: 113). The publication of books in English had been transformed in 1641 by the closure of the Court of Star Chamber, where violations of censorship had been prosecuted. The number of new publications per year rose sharply in the 1640s, and by the 1650s pamphlet literature consisting of up to four paper sheets had emerged as a new force in the print market. Nevertheless, despite the acceleration in production in absolute numbers from the 1650s to the 1670s, vernacular medical publishing amounted in Fissell's calculations only to 1 or 1.5 per cent of total publications, and this fell back still further from the 1680s onwards to about 0.5 per cent. This still meant that between 150 and 180 vernacular medical books appeared per decade after 1660.

Vernacular medical publication from the 1650s onwards was dominated to an extraordinary degree by the publications associated by name with just one author, Nicholas Culpeper. Between 1649 and 1700, 158 separate editions of his works were published (McCarl 1996). As Fissell (2007: 115) points out, his name is associated with an outstanding 8.5 per cent of all the editions of vernacular medical books produced between 1641 and 1740. This is not to say that he wrote all these titles himself, for his name was in itself a valuable market commodity, defended by his widow against those who sought to profit from it by publishing works that were not his nor even based on his writings. The whole Culpeper phenomenon began with the publication of his English translation of the *Pharmacopoeia Londinensis* as *The London Pharmacopoeia* in 1649. It was a deliberate assault on what Culpeper saw as the monopoly privileges enjoyed by the physicians and apothecaries, and he carried the fight to the monopolists with a series of translations of medical texts from Latin and original writings of his own. Most famous of these was the folio 'Herbal' or *The English Physician* (1652). In 1653, he completed a new translation (*The London Dispensatory*) of the expanded Latin *Pharmacopoeia* as published by the College of Physicians in 1650; the first translation was from 1649. Further editions of his second translation continued up to and well beyond 1700, while the 'Herbal' continues in print today (Sanderson 1999).

[4] These developments are described by Sanderson (1999). The impact on printing of new remedy books is noted by Hunter (1997).

[5] Fissell's survey excludes almanacs and works aimed specifically at medical practitioners but includes some works that fall outside Slack's categories, e.g., cookery books with more than 25 per cent medical recipes.

Recipe books, especially those that could employ the cachet of a royal or noble lady in the title of the book, boomed from the 1650s onwards. Writings such as *The Queen's Closet Opened* or *The Queen-Like Closet* (1655), published by an unknown author known only as 'W.M.', and *A Choice Manual of Rare and Select Secrets* (1653), attributed to Elizabeth Grey, Countess of Kent, enjoyed great success (see Chapters 8 and 9 by Marttila and Mäkinen in this volume). The outbreaks of plague, particularly the Great Plague of London in 1665, led to further bursts of pamphlets giving advice or warning, many of them based on earlier works. Books in English on midwifery did very well in the later seventeenth century, and well-known names such as those of the midwives Jane Sharp and Elizabeth Cellier were used to good effect by publishers.[6] As much as 17 per cent of vernacular medical books were anonymous, as calculated by Fissell, and between 10 and 17 per cent of the total were translations from other languages, chiefly Latin. Just as in Slack's period up to 1604, one has to be wary of assuming that the purported author of a work was in fact the author, or that the work was as new as it claimed to be. Publishers were adept at exploiting the kind of associations with authors or favoured titles that would sell books, and there was little a genuine author could do to protect his name or work against exploitation by others (Feather 1994: Chapters 1–2).

One category of vernacular medical writing that also advanced strongly in the second half of the seventeenth century was that called by Fissell 'proprietary medicine', where the work in question was really a kind of extended advertisement for a commercially available remedy, published in pamphlet form (see Ratia and Suhr in this volume, Chapter 10). Such favourite remedies as 'Daffy's Elixir' or the 'anodyne necklace' obtained widespread currency through publications by rival authors and publishers, each claiming to promote the one true and authorized medicine.[7] Although excluded by Fissell from her database, the 1640s and 1650s were also the golden age of the almanac, built around the success of astrologers such as William Lilly and John Booker. Increasingly, these publications too came to feature advertisements for medical remedies and practitioners, as well as the staple medical information that had been a feature of earlier almanacs (Crawford 1984; Curth 2002; Weber 2003). It has been estimated that some 400,000 almanacs were being produced annually at this time (Curth 2002).

At the very end of the period, we find the first appearance of a medical periodical, *Medicina Curiosa; or, A Variety of New Communications in Physick, Chirurgery, and Anatomy, from the Ingenious of Many Parts of Europe and from Other Parts of the World.* Only two issues appeared in 1684, published by Thomas Basset. It was meant to summarize the contents of

[6] See 'Introductory Note' in Cody (2002) and Jane Sharp's *The Midwives Book; or, the Whole Art of Midwifry Discovered* (Sharp 1671).

[7] For Daffy's Elixir, see Haycock and Wallis (2005).

current medical publications, notably those translated out of other languages by Basset himself (LeFanu 1984; Furdell 2002: 67–8). More important as a place for original medical publications was the *Philosophical Transactions* of the Royal Society of London that first appeared in 1665 (see Gotti, and Gray et al. in this volume, Chapters 11 and 12). Despite its early international connections, the innovative journal was published from the very beginning primarily in English, a decision that in the first phases involved extensive translation. The early issues, however, also contain some texts in Latin.[8]

## 2.4 *Early Modern English Medical Texts*

Primary data for this book comes from a register-specific corpus containing a wide range of medical texts from different traditions and genres of vernacular writing in the period 1500–1700. *EMEMT* is the second component of the *Corpus of Early English Medical Writing*, a three-part corpus of medical texts extending over the period 1375–1800 (see Taavitsainen and Pahta 1998). In the overall corpus design, *EMEMT* succeeds the first component, *Middle English Medical Texts* (*MEMT*), containing texts from the period 1375–1500 (see Taavitsainen et al. 2005, 2006). Together, *MEMT* and *EMEMT* provide an opportunity to trace long-term diachronic shifts and to examine the continuities and patterns of variation in medical writing over several centuries, from the first emergence of the register.

In recent years, a corpus has been understood as a structured computer-readable database of language samples compiled for the purpose of linguistic analysis. In a more general sense, the term 'corpus' is occasionally used in reference to any primary data used in the computer-aided study of language, regardless of whether or not the samples have been systematically collected. However, many linguists argue against this latter, looser definition (see, for example, Tognini-Bonelli 2001: 55) on the grounds that the reliability of a corpus as a representative sample of authentic language can only be achieved through the rigorous application of sampling criteria and an understanding of relevant linguistic and cultural realities.

With slightly over 2 million words of running text, *EMEMT* is a large, principled and systematically collected data pool, covering a period when significant changes were taking place in the status and roles of the languages used in constructing and communicating knowledge. The corpus was designed to be a representative sample of medical texts printed between 1500 and 1700, intended to reflect the development of medical literature during this period. While representativeness and balance are goals in any corpus compilation, in reality these goals are never fully attained (see, for example,

[8] Hall (2004) notes that four volumes of the *PT* appeared in Latin (1666–9), a partial French edition was made for the use of the Académie Royale des Sciences and an Italian edition was published in 1729. For research on the *PT*, see also Atkinson (1999) and Valle (1999).

McEnery et al. 2006). In an article about problems connected with the use of historical corpora, Matti Rissanen writes about 'God's truth fallacy', referring to 'the erroneous impression that [a corpus] gives an accurate reflection of the entire reality of the language it is intended to represent' (1989: 17; 2008). According to Sinclair (2005), the best way to counter this fallacy and ensure that the corpus is as representative as possible is to document carefully each step in the compilation process. To this end, this chapter provides a description of the main characteristics of *EMEMT*.

### *2.4.1 Representativeness and structure*

In corpus linguistics, 'representativeness' is a special term referring to the extent to which a corpus can be reliably taken to represent the text population of which it is a sample (see, for example, Biber 1993; Biber et al. 1998; McEnery et al. 2006; Leech 2007). According to Leech, 'representativeness' means that 'the study of a corpus can stand proxy for the study of some entire language or variety of language' (2007: 135). To this end, it is of paramount importance that the compilers are familiar with the true composition of the population the corpus is intended to represent. To achieve this, it is necessary to have an accurate understanding of how large the population is and of what kinds of material it consists. The knowledge of a larger disciplinary context is also needed if the aim of the research is to trace how advances of medical thought were reflected in the literature and how the traditional ways of thinking continued.

In *EMEMT*, the primary source of information on the composition of the population to be sampled are studies on early modern medical writing in English (see below), bibliographical records, library collections and consultations with medical historians. One of the challenges of producing a representative corpus derives from the criteria used for evaluating representation: is the corpus intended to reflect textual reality, including the proportional distribution of texts across different types of writing, at a given point in time, or to cover as broad a range as possible of different types of texts available to contemporary readers? The answer to this question also relates to the research problems the corpus is designed to answer. For example, it is common corpus linguistic knowledge that lexical studies, dealing with items that often have relatively low frequencies, require large sample sizes and a broad range of texts, while research into high-frequency grammatical features can generally be carried out with smaller samples. The examination of stylistic or discourse patterns also typically requires large data sets. The extracts selected for *EMEMT* are generally 10,000 words in length, allowing for the analysis of syntactical features as well as high- to mid-frequency lexical phenomena. The extracts are exclusively from the main text of the printed book; prefatory material is not included. Original spelling is retained, and all texts have been verified from original copies at scholarly libraries.

In the period covered by the corpus, text population is scanty during the earliest years but increases rapidly after that; thus, the representativeness in *EMEMT* in relation to the textual reality of medical writing changes in character over the time span from 1500 to 1700. The corpus contains samples from approximately two-thirds of all medical titles printed in English in the sixteenth century, while only a small fraction of titles produced after 1650 could be included. This difference is accounted for by the massive expansion in vernacular medical publishing after 1650, compared with the very slow beginnings in the sixteenth century.

Perhaps the most important source of information about printed books in the vernacular used in the compilation of *EMEMT* was provided by Andrew Wear's aforementioned survey (2000) (see also section 2.3). It contains rich bibliographical information on primary sources in the collections of the Wellcome Institute for the History of Medicine Library and acted as a guideline to our corpus compilation work. These notes provided an invaluable source of information for finding relevant corpus texts. In addition, library catalogues and lists of special texts provided help for finding relevant material. Almanacs are a case in point here, as both Cambridge University Library and Huntington Library resources proved valuable for locating relevant material.[9]

A crucial issue related to representativeness and balance is the corpus structure. The guiding principle in corpus compilation is to create text categories on the basis of language-external criteria (see Biber et al. 1998). In historical corpora, the primary principle used for textual categorization varies. For example, genre or text type can be the main ordering principle, as in the Helsinki Corpus of English Texts (see Rissanen et al. 1993). In *EMEMT*, the structure of the corpus is defined in another way. It is structured to provide evidence for continuity of *MEMT* categories (surgical texts, specialized treatises and remedy books), but at the same time we wanted to do justice to innovation, emerging topics, changing emphases and new media. The corpus consists of six text categories (see below), reflecting the textual environment of the early modern period, taking into account persisting textual types as well as new developments in the theory and practice of medicine.

Most of the ground-breaking scientific work was first published in Latin, as was the case with William Harvey's discovery of the circulation of the blood and the consequential work of the Oxford physiologists (Frank 1980). Famous authors such as Robert Boyle and Thomas Sydenham wrote originally in English and had others translate their writings into Latin for

[9] Taavitsainen spent Michlemas term in 2001 at Cambridge selecting materials and visited Huntington in January–February 2008. We are grateful to Professor Paul Monod for drawing our attention to late-seventeenth-century medical almanacs with medical advertisements and other relevant material.

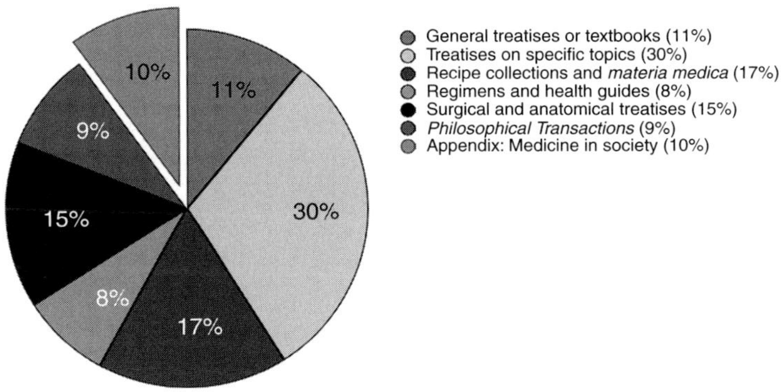


Figure 2.1 Proportions of *EMEMT* text categories.

publication. But new concepts, techniques and remedies were also described first in English, as with the surgeons who championed chemical remedies in the 1580s, or with the English Helmontians of the 1650s who attacked blood-letting and purging and espoused gentler medicines (Webster 1979; Wear 2000). New avenues of communication were opened by the printing press when, for example, bills of mortality or plague orders were published. The categories used in the corpus include texts written for lay readers as well as those intended for an educated audience, and texts within some categories are heterogeneous (see Taavitsainen in this volume, Chapter 6). The six core categories are also supplemented by an appendix of peripheral texts that do not deal with medical science as such but with its relationship to society at large. The text categories are presented in Figure 2.1, which also shows the proportional size of the categories in the corpus structure. The categories are described in more detail in Section 4.4.

### 2.4.2 *Authors and authorities*

While relatively little is known about the writers and production circumstances of English medical texts in the medieval period (see Pahta and Taavitsainen 2004), the situation in early modern England is quite different. Although there are anonymous tracts in *EMEMT*, particularly in the early part of the corpus, most corpus texts are written by named authors about whom something at least is known, and in some cases a great deal of socio-historical information about the authors and contexts of production is available. This is partly related to the professionalization and institutionalization of medicine. Institutionalization of the medical profession had already started in the late medieval period with guilds of barber-surgeons and continued in the sixteenth and seventeenth centuries: the College of Physicians was founded in 1518, and it exerted a monopoly to supervise and license physicians in the City of London within a seven-mile radius (Thomas 1980: 11). The development culminated with the founding of the Royal Society, 'the institutional embodiment of the new science' (M. Hunter 1981: 48) in 1662. Authorities licensing practitioners were the Church and the universities, and the College of Physicians kept the number of practising physicians small in London (see Jones, pp. 39–40). Surgeons were more numerous; for example, in 1514, seventy-two surgeons practised in London. The numbers of qualified country physicians varied: some towns were relatively well supplied while others remained without a resident physician, but this was rare by the end of the seventeenth century (Thomas 1980: 12–13). The tasks of various classes of medical practitioners were not strictly defined in this period. Until 1704, it was common that apothecaries, besides supplying medicine, made the diagnoses and prescribed the medicine. The lower reaches of the population continued to rely on empirics, herbalists, wise women or others of the great multitude of people in the trade. The Parliament had denounced their practice in 1512, but another Act (1542–3) allowed anyone with the necessary knowledge to treat external cases (Thomas 1980: 14). Throughout the period, the most important locus for medical care was the home, and women were the principal providers of remedies. Hospitals were for the poor and were few in number.[10]

The authors of *EMEMT* range from university-trained physicians of the highest level of learning to surgeons and practically trained medical men (see the *EMEMT* catalogue in Appendix D for details). The great majority of texts are by learned men. Women writers of the period are represented by Jane Sharp, a seventeenth-century midwife, whose *Midwives Book* (1671) was the first published English book on midwifery written by a woman (Sharp 1671), and Hannah Woolley, whose works include *The Compleat Servant-Maid*, a handbook for female servants including medical instructions. Also, many recipe collections were attributed to prominent ladies such as Elizabeth Grey, Countess of Kent, whose manual of 'rare and select secrets' in physic and surgery was first published in 1653. Some of the authors were prolific writers, like Nicholas Culpeper (see Section 2.3), and several works may be included by one author. Some authors specialize in giving general overviews, for example Christopher Langton, whose two comprehensive works are included from the first half of the sixteenth century. Some authors wrote with a more general audience in mind; these include John Caius, one of the most learned sixteenth-century physicians, whose only English work, dealing with the sweating sickness for the benefit of the general public, was published in 1552.

### 2.4.3 *Time period*

The timeline of *EMEMT* extends over two centuries, as presented in Figure 2.2. The starting point, 1500, which is also the end point of *MEMT*, is defined by the traditional shift in the periodization of the English language from

[10] London had two hospitals at the end of the seventeenth century (St Barthelomew's and St Thomas's Hospitals), and there were few elsewhere.

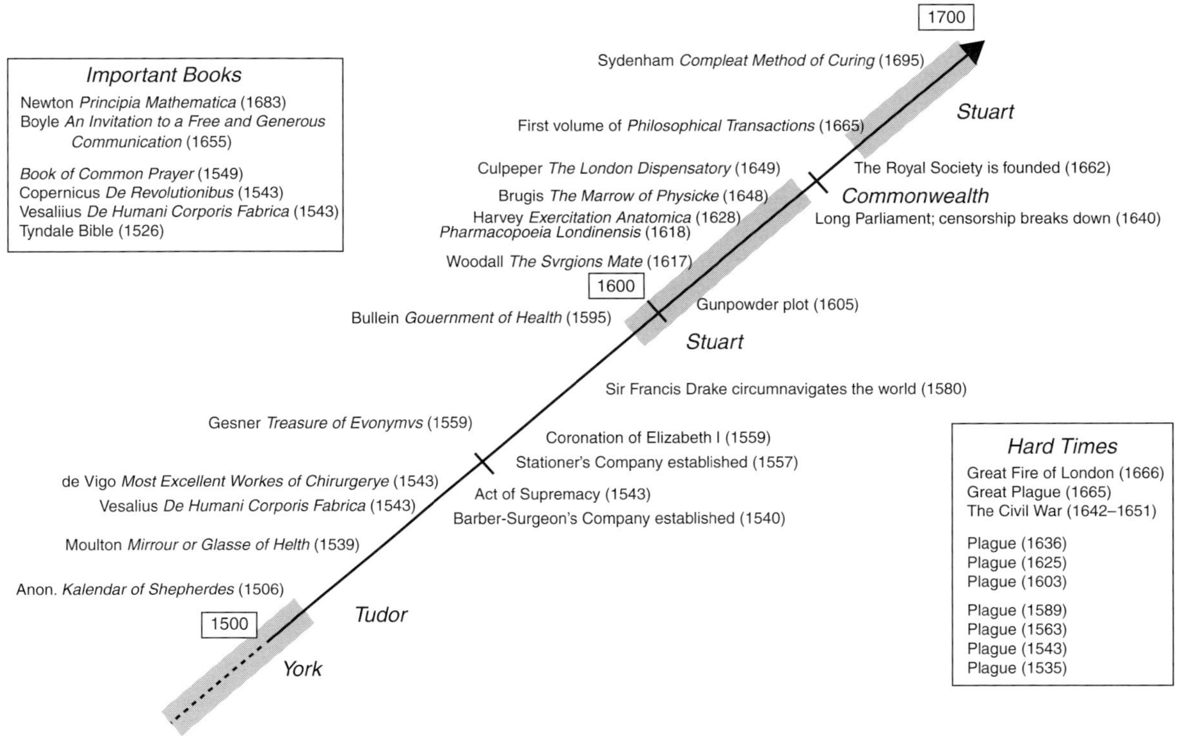


Figure 2.2 *EMEMT* timeline with background developments.

Middle English to Early Modern English. The end of the timeline, 1700, is defined by 'the decline of the old medical regime' (Cook 1986), when the London College of Physicians tried and failed in judicial test cases to exert institutional and intellectual control of medicine. By 1700, developments in medical thought-styles that had begun in the revolutionary ferment of the 1650s had taken successful root in new institutions of the Restoration (e.g., the Royal Society and the Society of Chemical Physicians, founded in 1664/5) and circuits of intellectual exchange (Webster 1979). The year 1700 may also be taken as an appropriate marker for the shift in balance towards English and away from Latin as a linguistic vehicle for communication and practical instruction in medicine. It should not be assumed, however, that this was a steady and inevitable progress: in 1665/6, 48 per cent of articles in the *Philosophical Transactions* (*PT*) employed English, 35 per cent Latin; in 1700/1, the ratios were 29 per cent English, 60 per cent Latin (Allen et al. 1994: 300, Table 5). By 1700, the *PT*, which from its beginnings had carried articles on medical curiosities, dissections and observations, had survived interruptions in publication following the death of its first editor Henry Oldenburg in 1677 and had embarked on its long course as the first and most important scientific journal in England. These critical early decades of its existence as a home for medical articles are represented in our corpus (see Section 2.4.4 below).

### 2.4.4 *EMEMT categories*

The texts included in the *EMEMT* are drawn from the printed vernacular output of the period and are divided into six categories and an appendix. The proportional distribution of texts (see Figure 2.1) reflects the combined effects of perceived significance and availability of texts (cf. Biber 1993; Leech 2007). Comprehensive treatises appear to be scarce especially from the sixteenth century, while specialized treatises and surgical texts are readily available for almost the entire period covered by the corpus. With extracts from approximately two-thirds of all English medical titles printed in the sixteenth century, the corpus is unequivocally representative for that time period. During the seventeenth century, the total volume of printed titles increased, and thus the relative representativeness of *EMEMT* naturally decreases. However, from a corpus linguistic perspective, the corpus does nevertheless maintain its representativeness throughout the whole of its 200-year span.

#### 2.4.4.1 *General treatises or textbooks*

Texts assigned to Category 1 are texts that claim to include 'all physicke' or are intended to give a systematic account of the whole field of medicine. Importantly, the inclusion of a text in this category is not based on the actual comprehensiveness or theoretical complexity of the work in question. There are no equivalents in English to the kind of systematic Latin exposition of medicine to be found in, for example, Jean Fernel's *Universa medicina*, comprising three parts: the *Physiologia*, the *Pathologia* and the *Therapeutice*. Nor do certain genres of medical literature, often used in teaching, such as *consilia* or *observationes*, find translators or publishers in English. General treatises range from the most learned and authoritative textbooks to popular all-in-one books intended to cater to all medical needs of an ordinary family. Texts in this category are targeted at very different audiences ranging from specialist practitioners to laypeople, and some are written specially for women. This category appears to be relatively sparse prior to 1600, and the corpus only includes a few texts published between 1530 and 1596 (see Figure 2.1). In the tripartite categorization of *MEMT*, the predecessors of these texts were included in the 'Specialized texts' category.

#### 2.4.4.2 *Treatises on specific topics*

Texts in this category represent the bulk of early printed books on medicine. They cover a wide range of topics in a wide variety of styles, the common denominator being a focus on an individual disease, method or therapeutic substance. For this reason, the category has been divided into five subcategories based on the nature of the focus:

(a) texts on specific diseases (e.g., struma, ague, fevers, pox);
(b) texts on specific methods of diagnosis or treatment (e.g., urinoscopy, astrology, phlebotomy);
(c) texts on specific therapeutic substances (e.g., gold, mithridatum, nitre);
(d) texts on midwifery and children's diseases;
(e) texts on plague.

This category bears a close relation to Category 1, the differentiating factor being the scope of the text. Although the extracts taken from extensive Category 1 texts are often very similar to individual Category 2 texts, the difference lies in the surrounding context. While the extracts in Category 1 are always parts of a larger general treatise on medicine as a whole, Category 2 texts are self-contained and independent treatises on a specific aspect of medicine. The target audiences range from academic specialists to the widest popular readership; for example, the most popular sex guide for centuries, the anonymous *Aristoteles Master-Piece*, is included in Category 2d alongside top treatises for experts in obstetrics. In *MEMT*, earlier versions of these kinds of specialized texts made up the bulk of the 'specialized texts' category.

#### 2.4.4.3 *Recipe collections and* materia medica

Category 3 contains texts instructing on the preparation of medicines or listing the therapeutic properties of substances. It covers a wide spectrum of material from popular texts bordering on magic and folklore to highly sophisticated and formalized pharmacopoeias. In addition to proper recipe collections, this category also includes herbals and lapidaries as well as instructions for the preparation of miscellaneous therapeutic substances such as waters, oils and cordials. Texts that focus solely on the properties and preparation of individual substances or medicaments are included in Category 2c. This category represents the principal continuation of the 'remedies and *materia medica*' category of *MEMT*.

#### 2.4.4.4 *Regimens and health guides*

The fourth category comprises texts that focus on preventative medicine, which provide guidelines for living a good life and for the preservation of health. Texts in this category provide advice not only on diet (including food and drink) but also on various other 'non-natural' influences such as exercise, sleep and habitat. This category of texts has long roots already in the medieval tradition, going back to Latin *regimina sanitatis* surviving from the ninth century onwards. In the tripartite categorization of the *MEMT* corpus, the representatives of this category were included in the 'Remedies and *materia medica*' category.

#### 2.4.4.5 *Surgical and anatomical treatises*

Texts in Category 5 are defined by topic: all surgical and anatomical works belong to this category regardless of their scope or level of complexity. In addition to descriptions of surgical cures and treatments for wounds, ulcers and fistulas, this category also includes descriptions of human anatomy and observations of physiological processes. Surgical treatises may also contain recipes for ointments and plasters, and remedies for external ailments, but surgeons trespassed freely on medical territory as well. Much of military medicine focused on external trauma, and also falls under this category. This category is the direct descendant of the 'surgical texts' category of *MEMT*.

#### 2.4.4.6 Philosophical Transactions

This final category is a novelty of the early modern period and emerges only during the latter part of the seventeenth century. It also differs from the other categories in that its texts are defined primarily by the format and context of their publication. This category consists exclusively of medical texts published as letters or articles in the *PT* of the Royal Society, the earliest scientific journal in English. The texts published in this journal can be considered to represent the emerging empirical approach to science. The subject matter of these brief texts covers topics such as physiology and anatomy, the nature of various medical substances, accounts of medical experiments and discoveries and reviews of medical books.

#### 2.4.4.7 *Appendix: Medicine in society*

This is a heterogeneous group that does not aim at representativeness. Instead, the idea is to display a spectrum of texts at the fringes of medical writing, representing the fuzzy edges. Texts in this category view medicine from religious, legal, polemical and literary standpoints and illustrate the wider social context of medical writing proper. As a rule, medicine in these texts is treated as a social phenomenon, from a different point of view from analysing and treating diseases. To illustrate the importance of medicine in society, this category also includes social commentaries on various medical treatments and the prevalence of various ailments among the poor, ethical rules of medicine as a profession and religious and moral texts pertaining to medicine and its practitioners.

## 2.5 Conclusion

This survey of the complex history of Early Modern English medical writing has shed light on some of the key challenges facing the historical linguist. The 200 years covered by the *EMEMT* corpus witness not only profound new developments in the transmission of medical texts but also the continuing vitality of several established conventions of writing. The overall volume of medical titles increased significantly, and, due to printing, more of it became available also to the general reading public. The use of the vernacular in learned medical writing, first seen at the end of the Middle English period, became fully accepted. As the communities of writers grew and became more established, so did their styles of discourse.

The *EMEMT* corpus is intended to serve as a representative collection of the language of printed medicine during this period of social and intellectual change. As the chapters of this book demonstrate, the corpus enables the study of medical language from a variety of perspectives. Read in the socio-historical context, these linguistic phenomena increase our understanding of the evolution of medical thought and academic discourse.

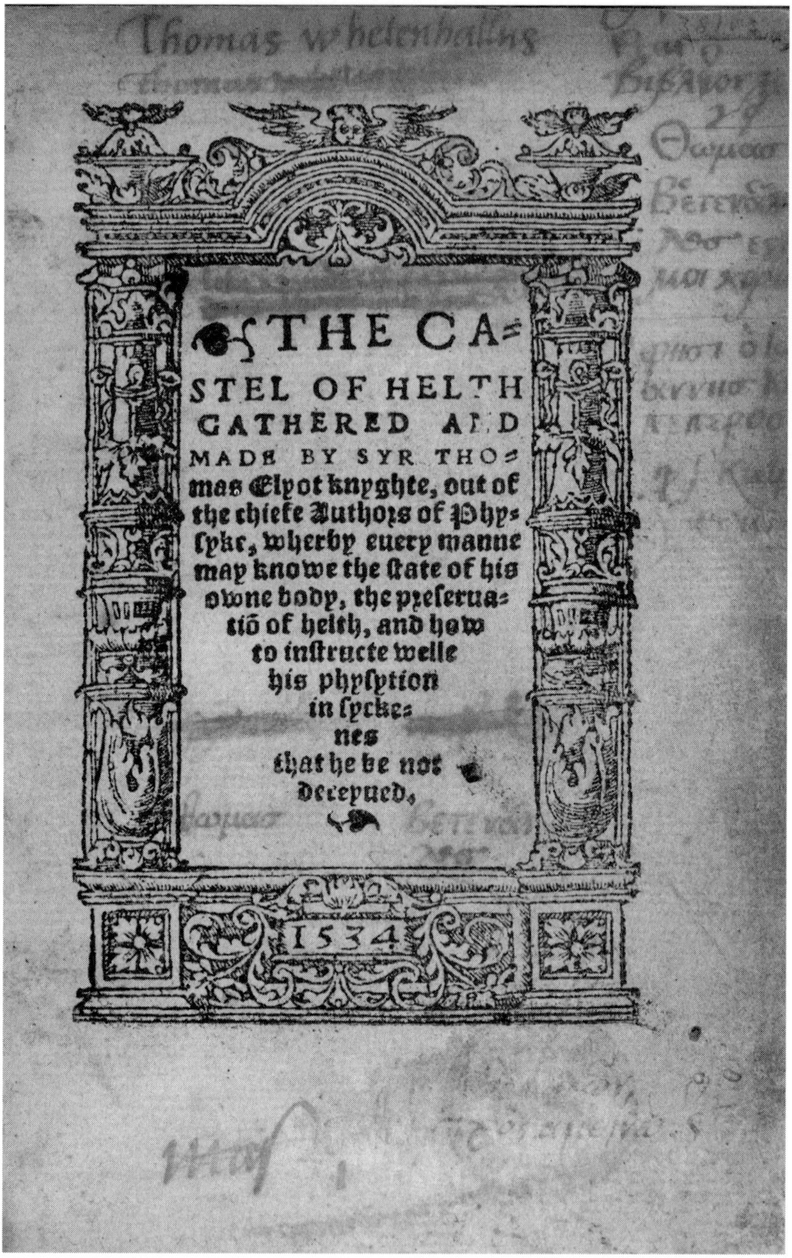


Plate 1 Title page, with owner signature and scribblings in the margin, of *The Castel of Helth* by Sir Thomas Elyot, 1534

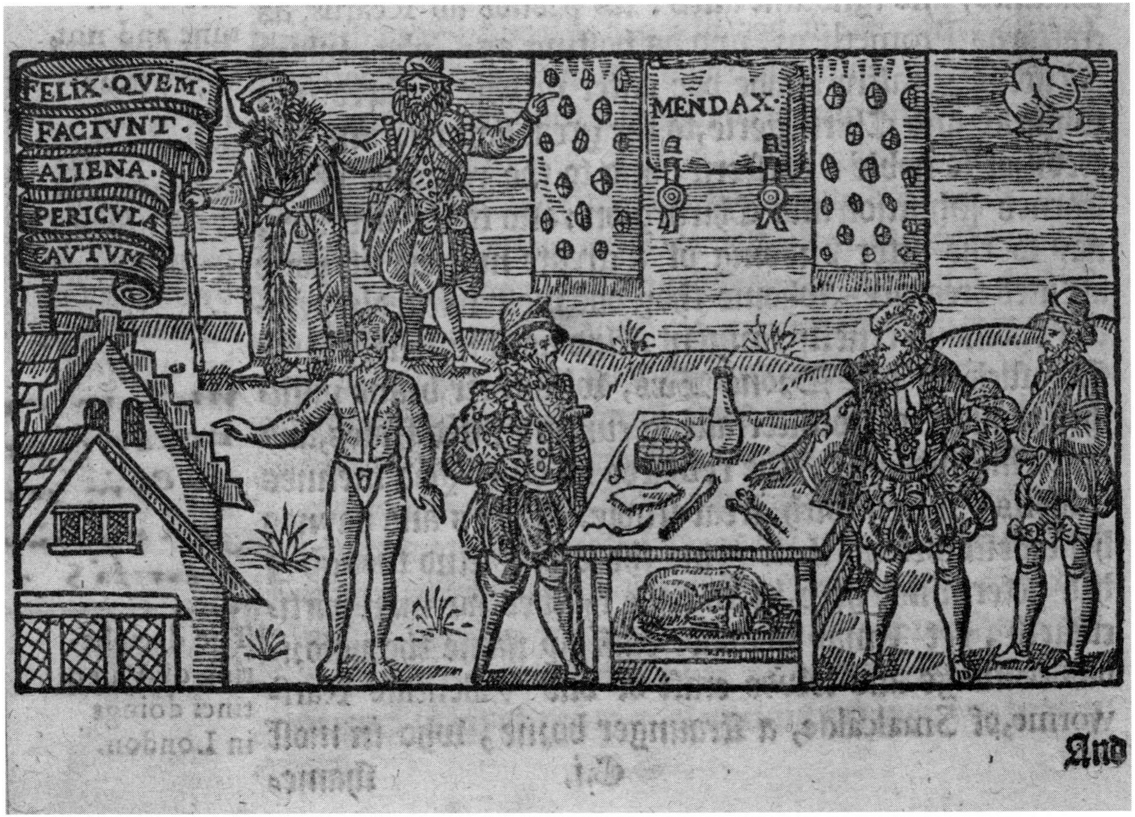


Plate 2 William Clowes, *A Briefe and Necessarie Treatise, Touching the Cure of the Disease Called Morbus Gallicus*, 1585

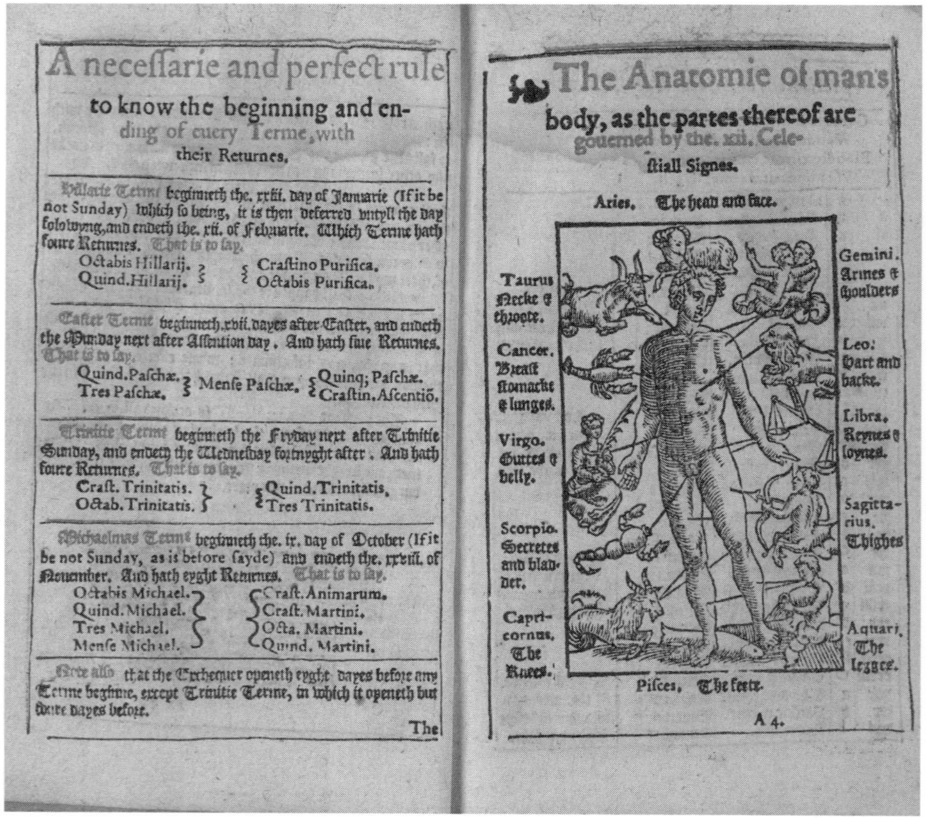


Plate 3 Page providing almanac lore and depicting a zodiac man from Frende, *A New Almanacke and Prognostication*, 1593

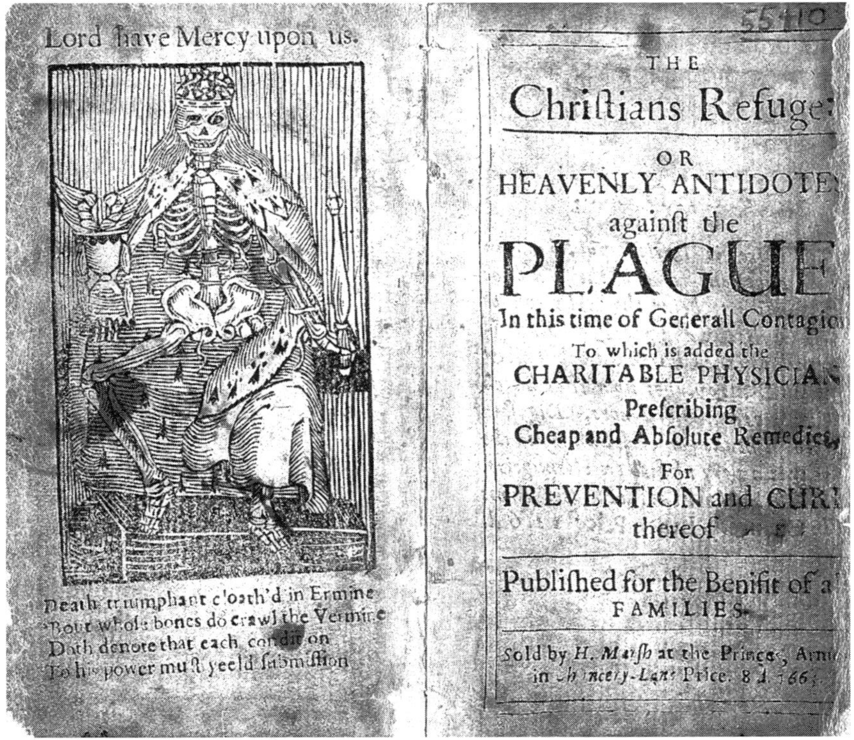


Plate 4 Frontispiece and title page, *The Christians Refuge; or, Heavenly Antidotes Against the Plague* by W.W., 1665

# 3 Medical literacies and medical culture in early modern England

PETER MURRAY JONES

## 3.1 Measuring medical literacy

Who read the medical texts gathered in the corpus of *Early Modern English Medical Texts* (*EMEMT*) between 1500 and 1700, and, equally interesting and important, who did not? These are questions not only about competence and the ability to read but also about ability to gain access to books and other vehicles of print publication, and about the interests and purposes of the potential consumers of print. Questions of competence, the first kind of question, bring us to the problem of literacy. The degree to which the population of early modern England was literate has been keenly debated by historians, and there has been a lot of frustration expressed in that debate with the imperfections involved in trying to measure literacy statistically. Reading itself leaves few marks or none at all for historians to record and interpret, and it has proved impossible to find a useful statistical measure of ability to read in the period 1500–1700. We are left with measures of the ability to sign one's name, which has an uncertain and unquantifiable correlation with the ability to read. However, writing is at least susceptible of statistical measure since the signing of documents for various purposes was required of large numbers of people. Using signatures to documents as a measure, it has been calculated from the subscriptions to the Protestation Oath of 1642 that 70 per cent of adult English men and 90 per cent of English women were illiterate, that is, unable to sign their names as opposed to making marks on documents (Cressy 1980: 176–7). On the face of it, if we took this measure of subscriptional literacy to indicate ability to read, the medical texts in *EMEMT* would have been within the grasp of less than a third of males at this time, and a mere tenth of females. The ability to sign one's name was also highly correlated through this measure of subscriptional literacy with one's position within society, confining reading competence (as measured by signing) to those who had the time and the resources to spend on its acquisition and the practice of the skill once acquired. Whereas among clergy and the professions in rural England all could write (and read) in the seventeenth century, a third of yeomen could not, and three-quarters of carpenters were illiterate. Of labourers, 85 per cent could not sign; probably high numbers of servants were unable to acquire the basic competence that would open up the world of medical writing to them (Cressy 2003: 315). There were significant geographical variations in the ability to sign one's name too. In East Anglia, for example, literacy was considerably in advance of that in Cumbria, for all except the gentry and the professions. Differences in standards of literacy between country and town were of course pronounced, with London being in advance of any other town or region. Thus, in London, only 22 per cent of men were measured as illiterate, while in Nottinghamshire over 75 per cent were.

However, problems with this measure of subscriptional competence have been widely acknowledged. Depositions in ecclesiastical courts form the basis for the quantitative assessment of subscriptional literacy, and they severely under-represent women as deponents and, indeed, labourers and servants too. These groups simply did not make depositions, and literacy was not in itself the issue. It is no surprise in consequence that signatures of people in these groups are so scarce in such documents. A second problem involves readers who did not write. Since we know that reading was taught before writing in the context of formal schooling during this period, we must assume that many may have learned to read, at least at a basic level, but never went on to learn how to sign their names. They might then have been competent readers but only able to make their mark rather than to write their signatures on the documents used for assessing literacy. To compound this problem, a person who makes a mark on such a document may in fact choose to do so while perfectly competent to sign. There are some instances of marking where this is known to have happened. As a result of these problems with the measure of subscriptional literacy, many scholars have been moved to argue that this method seriously underestimates the numbers of readers in early modern England.

In assessing competence to read medical writings, we will need to pay attention to the kind of functional literacy that is required for the purpose, qualifying still further the controversial measures that apply to literacy in general. But before moving on to this question of functional literacy, it will be helpful to remind ourselves of what commands much more general agreement among historians, that is the *progress* in literacy over time between 1500 and 1700. David Cressy's measure suggests that male illiteracy declined from perhaps 90 per cent in 1500 overall to 55 per cent in 1714 (Cressy 1980: 176–7). For women, he argues that 99 per cent illiteracy in 1500 became 75 per cent illiteracy in 1714. Levels of occupational or class literacy also changed markedly over the two centuries, with some groups progressing much faster than others. By 1600, Cressy considers the gentry and professional classes to be almost wholly literate. The trends summarized in these measures of change need to be taken into account. They chart the increasing competence of different social groups in reading medical texts from 1500 to 1700, and they also help to explain the remarkable acceleration in the printing of English medicine after 1575 (see Chapter 2 in this volume).

So far we have considered literacy as something either possessed, or not possessed, by classes or groups of people in early modern England. Yet there are different kinds and degrees of literacy. Some have distinguished so-called 'functional' literacy, the acquisition of skills that enable the individual to achieve basic goals that are suited to a particular way of life or occupation, and 'cultural' literacy, which enables the possessor to read books for religious or literary edification (Ford 1993). Functional literacy, if this distinction is maintained, is something that might potentially be of benefit to anybody, whereas cultural literacy might be restricted to those with leisure and educational attainment sufficient to make its exercise feasible – that is to say, to certain groups of people (gentry, clergy, merchants, etc.) rather than others (husbandmen, labourers and servants, for example). The reading of medical texts in English would seem most obviously to belong to the category of functional literacy, since the acquisition of medical information was of direct help to those trying to maintain or restore the health of members of any household, rich or poor. Yet many medical books in English seem to be designed not for this essentially functional purpose but to appeal to those who wished to exercise their judgement and taste in ways appropriate to their station in life. We might take as an example of the kind of medical book aimed at these kinds of people Sir Thomas Elyot's *Castel of Helth* (1534) (see Plate 1, p. 26). For books apparently targeted at those interested in the functionality of medical literature we might be tempted to cite the cheapest, the almanacs and prognostications typically on sale for 2d each annually, which contain as well as the ephemerides some very basic kinds of medical information about the signs of the zodiac, bloodletting and the days of the moon. However, almanacs and prognostications are good examples of books that might appeal to the gentleman as well as the poor householder, as we see in the buying habits of Samuel Pepys, for example, who bought jest-books, ballads and almanacs as well as 'serious' literature.

In fact, we can identify particular features of the printed output of medicine itself that reveal something of the kind of literacy required to access it. Some kinds of medical text are distinguished by their use of black-letter typesetting, for example, as opposed to the roman fonts that are more familiar to us today. In early modern England, by contrast to today, those least fluent in reading would have been more familiar with black-letter typography. In acquiring the ability to read, the ABCs, hornbooks and primers that they were exposed to by their teachers were first and foremost books set in black-letter type. Many readers seem never to have progressed beyond black-letter to a familiarity with roman type (Brayman Hackel 2004). Black-letter was used for the type of proclamations and other documents designed for public display or for reading out loud to audiences gathered in public places. Such common medical documents of this public type as bills of mortality or plague orders would be in black-letter, so would the vast majority of almanacs and prognostications. These last were not public documents but were targeted at those who may never have progressed beyond black-letter but who could afford the 2d annually required to purchase such useful information. We can assume (as with almanacs and prognostications) that medical texts of this type might have been read easily enough by those who had gone beyond the acquisition of black-letter literacy and who could also master roman type. But the ability to read black-letter did not entail conversely that the reader could also read roman type (Thomas 1986: 99–100). Furthermore, there is reason to suppose that many of those who had acquired black-letter literacy would not have been able to read any kind of handwritten document. The characteristic secretary hands of the period are hard enough to read for present-day students and must have posed a huge problem to those who had acquired their literacy from primers or equivalent black-letter teaching aids. It makes more sense then to think of a gradient of different forms of literacy, running from the black-letter or 'abecederian' to the ability to read roman type and the ability to decipher handwriting, right up to the kind of 'cultural' literacy to which those who read Sir Thomas Elyot aspired. Medical texts were expressed in forms that might correspond to different points on this gradient, with those at the 'higher' points being more exclusive in their readership than those at the lower points. This point about typography as a marker of degrees of literacy might also be extended to other features of early medical books, the presence and technical sophistication of illustrations, or the physical dimensions of the book, for example.

Competence in reading is one of the important factors we must bear in mind when assessing access to the medical texts contained in *EMEMT*. Yet not having achieved that competence, at whatever level, was not the same as being denied access to medical texts. There were ways in which the illiterate might still achieve that access. We have already seen that some kinds of medical text, most obviously proclamations, plague orders or bills of mortality, were designed to be read aloud in public places or to pass on news to a public. If one individual was available to read these documents to others who could not read, he or she could act as the means of transmitting the information contained in the document to others. We must imagine a scenario in which reading aloud was a kind of broadcasting of medical information contained in medical texts of this kind. In times of public emergency, when there was an outbreak of epidemic disease imminent or already present in the community, this kind of broadcasting took on an urgency and an importance, and the weight of the early modern state might be deployed to get the message across, not just by publicizing it but by enforcing various decrees and orders in the interest of public health (a well-known example is the issuing of plague orders that restricted the movements of people and goods). This scenario may be imagined as taking place in the market square or on the streets of English towns, where proclamations and orders could be displayed and read aloud. Sometimes perhaps they might have happened in the local church, where the boundary between the orders for the better regulation of the national church and for those for national welfare in the sense of public health would have been hard to observe. But even within the private household, large or small, the presence of one reader might make it possible for others to be kept informed. Certain kinds of medical text, especially those expressed in dialogue form, or as verse, or as readily memorized sayings or proverbs, were clearly meant to be spoken aloud to others as well as read privately (as, for instance, is the case with the dialogues in Bullein 1888). Reading aloud was much more common in early modern England than it is today, and some medical texts were often clearly meant to be read aloud, in just the same way as chapbooks with ballads, tales and jests.

## 3.2 Locations of medical literacy

This point of intersection between reading and oral circulation suggests that to understand the operation of medical literacy better we need to consider the locations in which it is found. One of these, as we have seen in the case of the proclamation of medical edicts and important information about disease, is in the market square or on the street. This is also the principal site for direct selling of medicines during this period. Those advertising their services or their nostrums made a pitch on the street, often posting bills on doorposts to get public attention. The mountebanks who are constantly referred to in plays such as Ben Jonson's *Volpone*, or pictured amid the criers and hawkers of London, made use of advertisements to bring patrons to their show. Once they mounted the stage they would also distribute printed testimonials to their successful cures and sell printed recipes as well as potions and pills (Matthews 1964; Porter 2000; Gentilcore 2006; Katritzky 2007). Not all of those who advertised their services were humble artisans. One of the few printed advertisements to survive extolled the skills of the surgeon Nicholas Bowden, licensed to practise by the University of Cambridge in 1602. He was the son of a gentleman but also a cutter for the stone and oculist, whose single-sheet notice ended, 'Those which shall have need of me, shall have me …', with the rest of the paper left blank for him to fill in whatever address he was using at the time.[1] We know that such 'bills' were ubiquitous on the streets of London, drawing the largely hostile attention of the College of Physicians. For example, a widow, Mrs Ann Provost – not a mountebank of course, but a seller of medical nostrums – was informed on in 1627 by another irregular practitioner, Elizabeth Fennymore, a joiner's wife from Southwark. Four years later, Mrs Provost was questioned by the College and admitted only to having 'hunge out bills' in the past, although her accuser had alleged forty years of unlicensed medical practice (Pelling

[1] This advertisement is to be found in Oxford, Bodleian Library, Ashmole MS 1399.

2003: 94). A collection of such 'bills' survives from the late seventeenth century (Crawford 1984).

There was a close association between the selling of medicines and the selling of print products in early modern England (Isaac 1998). The chapmen who hawked almanacs, prognostications and ballads and chapbooks also distributed medicines available commercially. They were another form of easily portable goods to sell. In the second half of the seventeenth century, this association became closer still when pamphlets advertising the merits of proprietary brands of medicine began to be printed in considerable numbers. In her survey of popular medical books published between 1641 and 1740, Mary Fissell (2007: 116–17) found that of the 150–80 vernacular medical books published per decade 11 per cent could be classed as proprietary medicines. 'Daffy's Elixir' and 'Lockyer's Pills' were household names largely as the result of the successful advertisement of their merits in print. Almanacs too carried more and more advertising in the final decades of the seventeenth century, for medical services, appliances, books and medicines (Curth 2002).

A second scenario for understanding medical literacy in early modern England is the closet. The term is often found in the title of sixteenth- and seventeenth-century medical writings, usually in the context of the 'revealing' of the contents of the closet, which seems to be best understood as an inner private room in a dwelling, almost a roomier version of a medicine chest. Within the closet are books and private papers and the equipment to make up household remedies. We know that the closet was not just a literary conceit (though it makes frequent appearances in Shakespeare's plays, for example) but was a real location in households, referred to in private letters and diaries. The letters of Lady Dorothy Bacon and the diaries of Lady Grace Mildmay confirm that the closet existed as a place for making up remedies (Orlin 1998). In the sixteenth, and continuing on into the seventeenth century, the closet appears in the title and preliminary matter of books, first and foremost as a place for reading about as well as making remedies. But from the early seventeenth century onwards we also see the closet used in books in a more gendered way to describe the healing and nurturing activities of women, usually aristocratic women, who might be thought of as models for the behaviour of fine ladies. Some of these borrow the name and the prestige of the aristocratic lady to shed lustre on the remedies; others appeal more generally to a housewifely model, as with John Partridge's *The Treasurie of Commodious Conceits, & Hidden Secrets. And May Be Called, the Huswiues Closet, of Healthfull Prouision* (1573) and the anonymous *Closet for Ladies and Gentlewomen* (1608) filled with diverse syrups, medicines and salves. It is not clear that women were in fact taking over the medicinal closet, but certainly they were being used to good effect in the marketing of books with titles of this kind (L. Hunter 2002).

The most characteristic form of text to be found in the medicinal closet was the remedy or recipe book. This might include recipes for cooking, preserving or distilling, alongside more straightforward remedies. Such remedy books survive in large numbers in libraries and record offices today. They were owned by householders and were frequently added to in the hand of different generations of a family; thus, they were adaptable and readily passed from one person to another, but they were highly unstable as documents – added to, expunged or amended at will. Their fluidity as documents has often led to their being ignored or downplayed by historians as evidence for an important kind of medical literacy, although frequently alluded to as evidence for the practice of 'kitchen physick' in the home. In fact, they constitute our primary source for understanding the gathering, circulation and dissemination of medical information among laypeople in early modern England (Pennell 2004a; Leong and Pennell 2007). The sources of information for the remedies were often given in the text as a way of identifying and validating the recipe – they carry tags like 'given me by mistress' or 'Dr Butler's receipt' (Dr Butler was a famous Cambridge doctor who died in 1618, whose name lives on in many of these remedy books). Often the phrases 'proved by me' or '*probatum est*' were added to the recipe and witnessed to the successful use of the remedy in practice (C. Jones 1998). Some of the remedies evidently circulated in oral form before being written down and might be given as gifts or be bartered in exchange, thus constituting a kind of social capital; others were copied from contemporary printed books or from letters received.

Enterprising printers in the seventeenth century imitated the format and borrowed the contents of these manuscript remedy books, thus testifying to their importance. Gervase Markham's *Countrey Contentments or the English Huswife* (1615) is just such a remedy book in form, and it is noticeable how often these books claim that their recipes came from noble ladies. Thus, Markham credits one recipe he includes in his book to a manuscript he saw in the possession of a 'noble countesse'. As opposed to the manuscript versions, the main difference in these printed recipe books is their aspirational theme – hence Markham's encomium of the 'inward and outward vertues which ought to be in a compleate woman' (L. Hunter 2002: 517–19). The author or publisher (more often than not a man in fact) plays on the potential purchaser's desire not to be seen to be lacking in any of these virtues. They are in effect very similar to the lifestyle manuals of today. The ownership of such a printed remedy book provided ready-made access to a collection of recipes, though not of course the same sort of selective appropriation that a manuscript did: with a manuscript you tailored your collection to your interests, limited only by the sources of information you had to rely on. Nevertheless, you could still write any extra recipes that appealed to you in the margins and endpapers of a printed remedy book (Stine 1996; Glaisyer and Pennell 2003; Leong and Pennell 2007).

Our third scenario for medical literacy is the library or study (almost by definition a masculine space) as compared to the closet. The books to be found there were different in character to those in the closet. They were mainly printed and mostly contained Latin texts. The flood of printed medical literature in Latin that was imported to England, especially from 1550 onwards, overshadowed the development of vernacular medical books for scholars and gentlemen during the same period. This is easily forgotten or ignored by those who concentrate on the English language only or who base their research on the books noticed in the *English Short-Title Catalogue* (*ESTC*). For a more accurate idea of what medical books were to be found in English libraries at this period we need to look at the evidence that survives. We have valuable evidence for ownership of medical books in the probate inventories of possessions at the death of the owner. After 1550, Latin medical books were owned by medical doctors in much larger quantities than ever before, and the first large medical libraries were created by men such as Thomas Lorkyn, John Collins and William Paddy over the century before 1650 (P. M. Jones 2006). But, significantly, ownership of such Latin books was far from being restricted to medical men. The probate inventories show that university-educated men, gentry and merchants might own some medical books in both Latin and English. These were the books that could be studied in the library or study rooms of private houses, where large bookcases with reading desks built into them began to appear as staple items of furniture in a gentleman's house. The books in such libraries were not there to provide ready access to practical medical information, like those kept in the closet or in the still-room of such a house. Instead, they were emblematic of classical authority in medicine as a system of knowledge and of gentlemanly learning across a spectrum of natural philosophy and medicine (P. M. Jones 1996).

The English-language books in such a gentleman's library or study were far fewer in number than those in Latin, at least before the 1650s. This impression of English-language books being swamped is exaggerated still further when it comes to counting the numbers of both kinds of book in the probate inventories of libraries. Those who made the inventories may well have not bothered to record the titles of English books or dismissed them as 'a quantity of English books'. This was because their financial value was less than the larger Latin tomes imported from the Continent. Even allowing for this miscounting of English-language books of medicine, it is clear that they would have been a relatively small minority in the larger collections of medical books (P. M. Jones 2000: 119–20). As we shall see, the politics of medical literacy in this period assumed that authority in medical matters and Latinity went hand in hand, and, of course, the reading and writing of medical books in Latin connected England to the advanced medical centres of learning in Italy, France, Switzerland and the Netherlands. Many of the books published in England in the vernacular in the sixteenth century were translations of Latin works on medicine (see Chapter 2), although this was not always acknowledged in the prefatory matter of the books themselves. Their presence in the gentleman's library or study may have been puny by comparison with works in Latin, but essentially both English and Latin books spring from the same sources of authority. Paul Slack (1979: 258–61) has drawn attention to the misconception involved in treating English books of medicine as examples of 'popular medicine'; their pricing and their prefatory material suggest a readership for them of gentry, merchants and the 'middling sort', rather than of the lower orders of society.

These three scenarios of medical literacy – on the street, in the closet, in the library – do not of course exhaust the possibilities in describing the kinds of place and occasion in which different social groups gained access to medical texts in the sixteenth and seventeenth centuries. Each of the variously literate groups who made a living from medical practice or from care of the body, whether surgeons, apothecaries, midwives, barbers or others, might have owned medical books and used them in the course of learning or passing on appropriate knowledge, for reference or even for purposes of display and gaining prestige. The best documented of these groups is the surgeons, who were keen users of print, as both authors and readers, and maintained a library at the Barber-Surgeons' Hall after 1540 (Symons 2006). Patients too were readers of course. The seventeenth-century physician John Symcotts, who practised in Huntingdon in the 1620s and 1630s, corresponded with some of his patients about their illnesses. He found that he sometimes had to deal with patients who read medical texts and had their own ideas about diagnosis and treatment, which they defended by reference to books they had read. This was the case with one Richard Powers, a coal merchant living in Ramsey, and Symcotts had to write to Powers in 1633 explaining his own diagnosis and prescription for a decumbent gout, while disparaging 'your author Vaughan' and his 'prognostic vain and frivolous' (Poynter and Bishop 1951: 25–6). Powers' reading is most likely to have been William Vaughan's *Naturall and Artificial Directions for Health* in one of the many editions between 1600 and 1633 (*STC* 24612–8). Self-diagnosis with the help of medical texts addressed to the layman originated long before the Internet.

## 3.3 The politics of medical literacy

Who had access to medical information and how that information was used were matters of public concern in early modern England. On the one hand, it was possible to claim that the dissemination of medical knowledge benefited the commonwealth by giving poor people the means to help themselves to avoid illness or to obtain relief from it. The Christian virtue of charity found expression in the sharing of medical knowledge, and the prefaces to works translating medicine from Latin into English often spoke of these charitable motives and of the poor who would benefit (Getz 1990). On the other hand, there were dangers attaching to medical literacy too. Those same poor people might be seduced by fraudsters whose only aim was to profit at their expense. Street advertising was a particular threat. It allowed some practitioners to exploit medical literacy for their own selfish motives, at the expense of unwary readers. Who was to guarantee the safety of the medicines promoted in this way or protect the unwary from parting with their money to unscrupulous salesmen peddling worthless or even dangerous medicines? As early as 1485, Thomas Forestier, a French medical practitioner living in London, had warned of the dangers posed by notices 'placed upon gates and churche dores' by people he called 'false lechys' (Walton 1982: 72). The arrival of print made things worse by multiplying the numbers of posters, broadsheets and pamphlets put into circulation which so provoked the College of Physicians (as in the Fennymore case above). Uncontrolled medical reading was therefore potentially a threat to the commonwealth, and professions of benefit to the public on the part of those selling their services or remedies in print had to be treated with suspicion. The dangers that accompanied the exploitation of print for the purpose of advertising remedies and practitioners, and the circulation of remedies in recipe form, were emphasized by critics who themselves voiced their alarm in print. Thus, London barber-surgeons such as George Baker and William Clowes used print to conduct a campaign against unlicensed practitioners who were peddling chemical nostrums through their various publications, directing their fire at the apothecary and author John Hester as an exemplary target. They were seeking at the same time to promote the corporate identity of the Barber-Surgeons' Company and to protect themselves against the accusation of tolerating or even encouraging those who were ignorant of learned medicine (Harkness 2007: 88–96). According to these critics, the exploiters of medical literacy promoted their selfish interests at the expense of their unwary readers (and patients), and so print itself threatened the health of multitudes. These claims and counter-claims, expressed in a language framed in terms of the health of the commonwealth, constituted a politics of medical literacy. Of course, the economics of the 'medical marketplace' were very much implicated in this political language.

To counter the threat to the health of the commonwealth posed by the proliferation of medical print, and its accessibility to those with very limited degrees of medical literacy, the weapon of intervention by the state itself was of little use. Religious or political propaganda might tempt the state into action in an attempt to prevent the publication of some kinds of inflammatory views, but the only health threat sufficiently serious to concern the Privy Council was that posed by epidemic disease. The Tudor and Stuart state was not prepared to act to curb the proliferation of medical publications, or act as censor, nor even to delegate powers to the College of Physicians. Therefore, the policing of medical literacy largely fell to various corporations acting at the local level. The College of Physicians, the Barber-Surgeons' Company, the Bishop of London and the City aldermen all had jurisdictions in London which might include the supervision of medical practice. None of the other three, however, placed as much emphasis on the significance of medical literacy as did the College of Physicians. Rather than simply deploring it, the College prosecuted medical illiteracy when it was combined with medical practice. The jurisdiction of the College of Physicians of London extended only to a seven-mile radius in London, however, and in other parts of England we do not find evidence for similar attempts to police medical literacy. Within its jurisdiction, the College could and did mount prosecutions to try to ensure that all medical practitioners had a licence from the College. The success of the College in cracking down on unlicensed practitioners was nevertheless extremely limited, and its authority was contested throughout the sixteenth and seventeenth centuries. One of the chief preoccupations of the College in prosecuting empirics was their claims to knowledge of medicine based on printed sources (Pelling 2003).

The most notorious and instructive case brought by the College was that of the astrologer and medical practitioner Simon Forman, who practised in London from the 1580s to the early years of the seventeenth century. Forman's prosecution shows up the politics of medical literacy at the individual level. He owned and annotated a medical book that he had acquired in Oxford in 1574 and continued to use until after 1600. It survives today at King's College, Cambridge, as MS 16. The two principal Latin medical texts in the manuscript were written by professional scribes in England in the fifteenth century, and Forman proceeded to interleave the manuscript with blank paper leaves which he then used to write a kind of extended commentary on one of the texts, the *Tabula medicine*, which is ordered alphabetically by disease and is essentially a compilation of medical remedies. Forman's commentary, written by hand in English, was a summary of medical learning that he found useful, including a figure of a bloodletting man, additional remedies that he had gathered from different sources, cases he had treated himself and extracts from a printed text, *The Breuiary of Helthe* of Andrew Boorde, first printed in London in 1547. Effectively, Forman created a medical book for himself that was a conflation of multiple sources, oral, manuscript and print, a hybrid of both Latin and English languages, and could serve multiple functions: a summary of learning, a justification of his own practice and an information resource for future treatments. No wonder he cited it in his defence when he came up before the College of Physicians in the 1590s for what the doctors termed illicit and unlearned practice without a licence. Despite the fact that the *Tabula medicine* was a learned Latin text, the doctors condemned Forman's book as obscure and his practice as ignorant. The confrontation between Forman and his accusers centred on the mongrel book he owned and the suspicions it generated of him as a reader whose reading could inform his practice and thus pose a threat to the health of the public (P. M. Jones 1995; Traister 2000; Kassell 2005).

Concern about the exploitation of medical literacy by printers in search of private profit, who thereby made medical knowledge available to readers and unlicensed practitioners of all kinds, was not confined to the late sixteenth century. Things only got worse, as the advance of 'selfish' private interests and quackery came to be thought of as unstoppable. The translator of Georg Wedel's *An Introduction to the Whole Practice of Physick* (1685) despaired of finding a solution for these problems other than by government intervention (quoted in Stine 1996: 201):

Some will say, Why should you translate so Excellent a Book, and make it common to the Silly and Unlearned Quacks? My Answer is, That 'tis come to pass now, that their Numbers can hardly be increased by translating of Books, or any other means, and seeing this Nation is so unhappy, as to swarm with thos Miscreants after such a rate, and no hopes of diminishing their Numbers, but by a new Act of Parliament.

The same translator's motive for his own writing, he confessed, was to get a little money, which he could not do otherwise in the medical profession because of the proliferation of the 'quacks' among the practitioners of his day.

There were, however, other ways of controlling reading than coercion or ridicule. There were good readers to be encouraged as well as bad readers to be condemned (Sharpe 2000: 40–61; Brayman Hackel 2005). Bad readers were those unable through their invincible ignorance and prejudice to see through the claims of the fraudulent. Good readers were those who read medical texts in order the better to fulfil their duties as householders, good neighbours and dispensers of charity. These are the readers addressed so often in the epistles that preface vernacular medical texts printed in the sixteenth and seventeenth centuries. These epistles to readers and the other paratextual elements that inhered in the contemporary printed book could be used to invoke and address such good readers and to justify the production of the text proper in English. Authors and publishers of Latin medical texts would not have needed to address their readers in this way, but in any case there were so few Latin works on medicine printed in England as hardly to count, by comparison with the steadily rising tide of vernacular medical printing (Genette 1997).

The reader who is addressed in these paratexts may be designated by the author (or his/her friends or the publisher) as belonging to one of two groups. Either the reader is represented as him- or herself a practitioner of medicine, most usually a surgeon or midwife, or as a householder who dispenses treatment to that household, to neighbours or to charity cases. The first kind of reader is the one addressed by the surgeons George Baker and William Clowes (see above), for example; the second kind of reader is the one addressed in the great majority of English books of medicine. He or she – for increasingly the desirability of women fulfilling their domestic role in dispensing medical help with the help of what they read is emphasized in these addresses – is envisaged in the paratext as the reader who can be trusted to employ their medical literacy for the good of the commonwealth. This reader is not going to seek profit from the use of what he or she reads but to store up that reading as a practical resource. It is assumed usually that the reader does not have ready access to professional medical assistance, that such assistance is too costly or at too great a distance to call on for all one's medical needs. For such a reader, Latin texts are assumed to be out of reach, and often the English work is presented as attempting to translate the substance of Latin medicine into a vernacular that is accessible to this reader.

Paratexts, as is well known for Early Modern English books in general, were designed to both seduce and control the reader. Medical books in English, except the most primitive almanacs, came accompanied almost invariably by introductory dedications, verses praising the author, epistles to a patron or esteemed colleague, to the readers themselves and sometimes by printed marginal notations that guided reading of the text, to say nothing of indices, tables of contents and other reader aids. These paratextual elements must have been expected by the readers, who would have been disappointed by a book without them. Nevertheless, the paratextual elements themselves could become a subject of dispute. After 1649, they could seem to some critics as both old-fashioned and characteristic of a relation to the reader that relied on patronage and condescension. An example of this criticism is that of the York doctor William Simpson, launching an assault in 1669 on his rival Robert Wittie, the author of books praising the Spa at Scarborough. Simpson has little time for such paratextual elements in comparing his own *Hydrologia Chymica* with Wittie's *Scarbrough spaw*:

> No flattering Encomiasticks shall usher in this work nor pedantick Rapsodists attend these lines; nor need we Casta Napsaearum to adorn our Water-Nymphs; nor let the Reader expect our Contemplation upon our Waterworks; nor yet any Chronogram or Anagram to sound abroad our fame; nor shall we court great Patronages to cast a favourable aspect upon it … For if the substance of the Discourse, and what the piece itself offers, give not matter of Entertainment for the reader, whose genius bends that way without such previous antick-Stage-Playes: or if it sound not harmoniously in the Readers ear, without such pratling School-Boy Preludes, let it be thrown by and for ever buried in Oblivion. (Poynter 1953: 75, quoting Simpson 1669: sig. A10)

Nevertheless, we should note that this assault on the elaboration of antique paratexts does occur within the text of Simpson's own address 'To the Reader' that prefaces his work. Even if you took the position that the use of dedications and prefaces to flatter patrons or to beg favour was a betrayal of one's duty to a book's potential readership, or the commonwealth at large, you still had to use the paratextual means available to assert and maintain that position in print.

This chapter has attempted to sketch some of the different kinds of medical literacy that flourished from 1500 to 1700 and the political discourse surrounding medical literacy that is found in vernacular medical books. I have stressed variance, in the different senses of, first, distinctive levels of medical literacy and, second, in the adversarial positions adopted by authors taking political sides over the issue of medical literacy. Yet this is not to claim that there was a variety of medical cultures flourishing in early modern England. As Andrew Wear takes care to remind us throughout his magisterial survey of English-language medicine, *Knowledge and Practice in English Medicine, 1550–1680*, the violent disputes that took place in print between orthodox Galenists and Paracelsians or Helmontians, between proponents of writing in Latin and authors of vernacular works on medicine, between physicians, barber-surgeons, apothecaries and empirics, should not blind us to the fact that there was a single and unified medical culture in early modern England (Wear 2000: 6, 103, 154, 318). Wear maps the development of this culture as the result of a spreading of the influence of learned medicine from the Middle Ages onwards. Whatever the differences, sometimes violently expressed, between those involved in medical controversies in print, they shared a great deal of common ground about diagnosis and practice. Nor was this just a matter of the obstinate persistence of certain ideas and practices codified by the medieval scholastics right through into the age of the Royal Society. We can see this shared culture as also taking the form of willingness to use the medium of print to give expression to views on the politics of medical literacy, to seek ways of controlling or persuading readers to pursue the health of the commonwealth, or body politic, and to resist the blandishments of those who would exploit the ability to read to their own selfish ends. Opponents addressed each other in print across the various ideological divides in medicine using a shared politically charged language of duty and obligation to the public whose health was at stake.

# 4 Verbs of knowing: discursive practices in early modern vernacular medicine

TURO HILTUNEN AND JUKKA TYRKKÖ

## 4.1 Introduction

The concept of *knowing* is fundamental to the way we conceptualize the world around us – and to the way we discuss it. Being aware of what we know and do not know shapes our social and cultural landscape, situates us in relation to our neighbours, and, to paraphrase Francis Bacon's famous aphorism, either gives us power or deprives us of it.[1] Unsurprisingly, the nature and properties of knowledge and knowing have been a commonplace throughout much of Western philosophy, playing a key role in both philosophy and theology since antiquity. In the sciences, the pursuit of new knowledge has been a central feature since the early modern period.

In medicine, perhaps more than in any other field, the traditional understanding of knowledge has consisted of two complementary properties: *episteme*, theoretical knowledge, and *techne*, knowledge associated with skill and practical ability.[2] Medical practitioners have always acknowledged the need for both, but the understanding of how the two best relate to one another has been a point of great contention. During the Middle Ages and early Renaissance, the divide between theory and practice formed one basis for defining the relative roles of medical practitioners (see, for example, Siraisi 1990; Getz 1998; and French 2003). In this framework, university-trained physicians represented the epistemic side of medical knowledge, drawing on Aristotelian natural philosophy to understand the complicated theories of humoral balance that explained most ailments. By contrast, surgeons, apothecaries and other less formally trained healers often possessed practical skills that theoretically oriented physicians did not (see Wear 2000: 213–18). On the other hand, their practices were less strictly based on theory, and

[1] Bacon's oft-quoted phrase, 'scientia potentia est', first appeared in *Meditationes Sacrae* (1597).

[2] On *episteme* and *techne*, see Parry (2007). A similar taxonomy, used primarily in medieval learned epistemology, uses the term *scientia* for exclusively theoretical works, *scientia operativa* for theoretical works oriented somewhat more towards practical application and *ars scientifica* for knowledge gained by experience and practice in addition to theory. See, e.g., Selosse (2005) and Taavitsainen (2004: 39).

only the top end of surgeons and apothecaries were able to relate to complex Latinate concepts.[3]

Although the juxtaposition between branches of medicine persisted well into – and, in some respects, throughout – the Renaissance, it is safe to say that in the course of the early modern period the prevailing attitude to knowledge came to be characterized by the discovery not only of new knowledge but also of new definitions of knowledge itself (Spiller 2004: 1; see also Harrison 2001). The early modern medico was in many ways witness to, and a participant in, a profound shift in the overall attitude to both the sources and dissemination of knowledge. Scholastic didacticism, characterized by a logocentric and gnostic view of knowledge (see Pahta 2001: 212–13), slowly began to give way to a new kind of scientific writing which replaced medieval *disputationes* with raging controversies conducted on the pages of pamphlets and printed books (see Ratia and Suhr, this volume, Chapter 10).[4] As part of this process, the centuries-old infallible truths contained in the words of the ancients were cast into doubt, and the concept of knowing itself became an object of an entirely new kind of attention (see Taavitsainen 2009c). The practice of medicine became more professional and organized, with increasing commercial as well as scientific motives. The regulation of medical practice under royal charter, started under the Tudor era, afforded those with recognized knowledge a position of authority in society.[5] The persona of a 'rational and learned physician', as defined by French (2003), was not merely a reflection of elevated scholarly ideals but a guise necessary for financial profit and social standing. From this perspective, knowledge references had a third function in addition to the scientific and social: as calculated turns taken in the discourse of the contemporary medical marketplace.[6]

This chapter approaches knowledge in medical writing by means of a detailed syntactic and discursive analysis of *knowing-verbs* (see also Hiltunen and Tyrkkö 2009). Our intention is not so much to discuss how knowledge was produced or how it was conceptualized but rather to investigate when and why the act of knowing was overtly mentioned in written medical discourses. The argument will be made that overt references to knowledge, in

[3] Notably, the elite surgeons and apothecaries were Latinate, and some travelled to Europe for education. Nevertheless, discussions of the philosophical basis of medicine were restricted to university-trained physicians. See French (2003: 95–9) and Wear (2000: 220–2).

[4] The *gnostic* approach to knowledge, characterized by its focus on the knower, can be juxtaposed with the *epistemic*, which affords primary interest in the process by which something is known. See Bates (1995a: 3–5).

[5] The College of Physicians was founded in 1518, the Worshipful Company of Barber-Surgeons in 1540 and the Society of Apothecaries in 1617. See, e.g., Porter (1989a: 21–30).

[6] Increasing attention has been paid recently to the role commercial interests played in shaping medicine in the Middle Ages and the Renaissance (see Wear 2000: 28–9; French 2003). Early physicians and healers were not only driven by benevolent and scholarly motives but rather competed for customers in a complex and largely ungoverned marketplace of medical services.

this instance propositions that openly refer to the act of knowing by means of a verb, served a particularly salient role in communicating attitudes about, and the understanding of, knowledge within the professional community as well as outside of it. Consequently, by analysing such propositions in detail, we are able to identify developmental trends in the underlying styles of thought.

The results of the analysis will show that the use of knowing-verbs fell into three primary discursive *topoi*. In classical rhetoric, *topos* refers to general argumentative patterns which find their instantiation in concrete arguments (see Rapp 2002). Modern rhetoricians, such as Perelman and Olbrechts-Tyteca (1971) and Fahnestock and Secor (1988, 1991), have successfully used this concept in the analysis of specialized texts, treating it as a commonly held warrant operating in both the construction and interpretation of arguments. The concept is useful in the analysis of specialized discourse because, as pointed out by Perelman and Olbrechts-Tyteca (1971: 99), particular audiences are characterized by the kinds of agreements they adhere to, which are not necessarily held by society at large. Despite its internal diversity, the medical discourse community of the early modern period can be seen as forming this kind of specialist audience which shares certain values and perceptions (see, for example, Swales 1990: 24–7). When addressing this audience, then, a writer may appeal to these values in order to ground the discourse in familiar terms and to make it persuasive.

The evidence presented here indicates that the didactic orientation of scholasticism declined steadily over the early modern period and was replaced by a new assertive style primarily concerned with arguing a case rather than with disseminating knowledge held to be canonical. Observations concerning specific syntactic features, such as the polarity of knowing references and the use of modal auxiliaries, give additional credence to the conclusion that the discursive practices of knowing-verbs reflect the underlying thought-styles not only of medical discourse on the whole but also of particular parts of it, and that with detailed analysis changes in the scientific world view can be traced by the linguistic and discursive features of a small set of conceptually central lexical items.

## 4.2 Medical knowledge in the early modern period

In early modern England, medicine was practised by a colourful spectrum of professions ranging from university-trained physicians who rarely examined patients in person to barber-surgeons and apothecaries with rudimentary Latin skills and learning based on apprenticeship, to midwives and bone-setters who practised their art with little, if any, book-learning (see Wear 2000: 21–8).[7] This complex arrangement of healing services naturally raised

[7] See, further, Pelling and Webster (1979).

questions about the veracity of knowledge: whose knowledge was sound, and how could one tell the quacks and charlatans from those who truly understood medical matters? Traditionally, learned physicians, trained at Oxford and Cambridge (and, to a lesser degree, abroad), occupied the most privileged position. Their knowledge, based on age-old scholastic natural philosophy, was primarily concerned with the underlying principles of balance and harmony of the four humours (see French 2003: 88–127). The theoretically oriented knowledge of the 'ancients' had the highest currency (see Taavitsainen 2009c). For example, Edward Jorden, a royal physician and chemist, wrote:

But Hyppocrates, Galen, Auicen, and most of the best Authors in our profession do affirme that very often there happeneth an alienation of the minde in this disease, whereby sometimes they will waxe furious and raging depriued of their right iudgement and of rest. (*EMEMT*; Jorden 1603: 13v)

Although Aristotelian and Galenic knowledge retained authority, new medical theories such as Paracelsianism and chemical medicine (*iatrophysick*) began to gain ground, particularly in the seventeenth century (Wear 2000: 360–8; see also Debus 1987). Their growing popularity was at least partly connected to the increasing role of printing, some of it taking place abroad (see Furdell 2002: xi). New theories shunned by the conservative College of Physicians could be disseminated more efficiently than before, and medical practitioners' access to a wider range of titles allowed them to compare and consider different theories.

Surgeons and apothecaries occupied the second rung of the professional ladder.[8] They were generally in a subservient position to physicians, ironically in part because of the greater emphasis they placed on practical skill and knowledge gained by personal experience and observation, an approach to knowledge university-trained physicians considered trivial next to the Aristotelian natural philosophy of the Latin tradition (see French 2003 and Furdell 2002). Nevertheless, the upper echelons of both surgeons and apothecaries were organized and Latinate and shared the same underlying theoretical beliefs with the physicians (Wear 1995a: 293). Perhaps none emphasized the importance of formal knowledge more than prominent surgeons keen on promoting the profession: 'But if any reply, that there be many which doe the workes of Chirurgery, without any knowledge of such like things, who notwithstanding have cured desperate diseases with happy successe; let them take this for an answer, that such things happen rather by chance, than by the industry of the Art' (*EMEMT*; Paré 1634: 92).

[8] Wear (2000: 28) identifies physicians, surgeons and apothecaries as the three groups of medical practitioners with institutional identities. In this sense, the three were clearly at the top of the professions in comparison to the myriad of lay practitioners who were far greater in number.

Surgical books were first and foremost practical guidebooks. The complex discussions of natural philosophy included in Latin texts of the highest strata were often left out, although the surgical reformers of the sixteenth century made an effort to improve the standing of the profession by adopting Latinate terminology and aligning surgical theory more closely with university physic (see Wear 2000: 221). New discoveries by anatomists such as Andreas Vesalius and William Harvey demonstrated the value of first-hand experience and the fallacy of blind faith in ancient authorities.[9]

On the third rung were the midwives, bone-setters and other assorted healers. Few written records produced by such practitioners themselves are extant, most having been illiterate, particularly in the early centuries. Among these groups, knowledge was mainly circulated in manuscript form (see Jones, this volume, Chapter 3). Practically oriented skills were passed on through apprenticeship and experience, with only passing reference to contemporary medical knowledge. Over the early modern period, apothecaries and midwives organized into clearly defined professions.

The reality of a multitude of different kinds of practitioners operating at the same time naturally had a profound effect on the early modern medical marketplace. With effective licensing of medical practice still in its infancy, various descriptions of medicos vied vigorously both for patients and, perhaps more importantly, for recognition in society. The sheer scarcity of university-trained physicians, as well as the cost of their services, meant that most turned to surgeons, apothecaries and other available healers for treatment.

In medical writing, as in other learned domains, both epistemic and practical questions concerning the nature of knowledge itself were often discussed in prefatory material, where authors sought to define their own position in relation to both ancient and emerging contemporary authorities (see Taavitsainen 2002; Taavitsainen and Pahta 1998). These discussions were routinely also informed by concern over the transmission of professional knowledge to laymen, or beyond the perceived confines of a particular community of healers. Even most of the well-known proponents of the vernacular dissemination of medical knowledge such as Thomas Gale and Nicholas Culpeper only sought to do so within the medical community (Furdell 2002: 82–4). From the end of the sixteenth century onwards, health guides and regimens were produced for the wider audience in ever-increasing numbers, and the emerging literate middling class read medical treatises with interest (see Chapters 2 and 3). Written assertions of knowledge

[9] The importance of Andreas Vesalius' *De humani corporis fabrica* (1543) was not restricted to marking a new era in terms of medical illustration. Vesalius also vigorously criticized the very basis of Galenic knowledge, even suggesting that Galen had never dissected a human body (see French 2003: 141–4). William Harvey's discoveries concerning the circulation of blood in *Exercitatio anatomica* (1628) likewise undermined the veracity of ancient medical wisdom.

now took on an even greater commercial significance, because the reader of a medical book was also a potential patient (see French 2003; Furdell 2002). The contrast between these two approaches to medical knowledge is seen in the following quotation by Philip Moore, an early proponent of the dissemination of medical knowledge to the poor: 'And therefore, this litle perswadeth them that any arte maye preserue a man lo~g in health: to whom I answere that there is greate difference betwene those that study Phisicke only to get a liuing thereby, and them that searche out the knowlege therof to guide their liues accordyng to the doctrine of it' (*EMEMT*; Moore 1565: 3).

Medical books were furiously marketed on the strength of the unique knowledge they professed to disclose, with commonplaces such as 'the queen's closet' appearing in the title of many a treatise. Shades of the scholastic logocentric paradigm continued into the seventeenth century and beyond, with the name of a highly regarded physician serving as proof of the veracity of the knowledge in the book.

Against this background, the analysis of discursive practices involving knowing-verbs can be seen as a window into the different rhetorical strands at work in medical writing. Underlying the examination that follows is the premise that consequent to the importance of knowledge at both the communal and societal levels, assertions concerning knowing had a particular discursive significance. To assert knowledge was to claim power, and to acknowledge it was to share it with a colleague, a faction or a community or peers. As will be shown, knowing-verbs have a relatively well-defined set of distinct discursive uses in early modern medical writing. Furthermore, proportional differences and diachronic changes in the frequency of these different discourse topoi can be used as a reasonable representation of changing scientific, social and commercial thought-styles over the timeline.

## 4.3 Knowing-verbs and their properties

This chapter is concerned with verbs of knowing, defined here exclusively in reference to the core sense of the word, rather than to related fields such as teaching, learning and belief.[10] The hierarchical modelling of cognitive processes is an onerous task (see, for example, Kay 1994), certainly beyond the scope of this study. The argument behind the approach taken here is that references to knowing, that is, to the immediate possession of knowledge, can be analysed separately from references to its dissemination. Importantly, we are not suggesting that overt expressions of knowing would not at times be discursively utilized for related purposes such as knowledge

[10] Relevant sections of the *Historical Thesaurus of English* were consulted in the process of defining the field. For discussion, see Hiltunen and Tyrkkö (2009).

dissemination – and indeed we shall argue that this is one of their main functions – only that there is a distinction to be observed between the two. While verbs that denote knowing are necessarily arguments concerning a state of abstract possession, those in adjacent semantic fields are more varied and often perform their knowledge-related functions via implication; for example, when the verb 'to read' is used as a knowledge-acquisition verb.

Although the semantic field of knowing comprises several nouns, adjectives and adverbs, the number of verbs belonging to it is very restricted (see Hiltunen and Tyrkkö 2009). In Early Modern English medical writing, only three verbs are relevant: 'know', 'understand' and 'wit'. The last of these, 'wit', is very scarce and completes a semantic shift away from knowledge during the sixteenth century.[11] Notably, the reduction in the repertoire of available knowledge verbs was a relatively recent phenomenon, as lexical items such as 'can' and 'do' still had clear knowledge-related senses in the Middle English period. This study focuses exclusively on the three primary knowing-verbs.

Taking into account all grammatical forms and their variant spellings, there are 1,932 occurrences of knowing-verbs in the *Early Modern English Medical Texts* (*EMEMT*) corpus: 1,631 of the lemma 'know', 285 of 'understand' and sixteen of 'wit'.[12] The overall number translates to a frequency of 1.02/1,000 words, which is more or less the same across the Early Modern English period (Figure 4.1).[13]

Differences between the categories are slight.[14] The aberrantly high variance seen in the category 'General Treatises' is explained by the composition of the corpus, which in turn reflects contemporary textual reality; complete medical treatises were scarce in the seventeenth century, and thus inordinate weight is given to the few individual extracts (see Chapter 2). A modest decrease is noted in 'Regimens' and 'Surgical Treatises', while the other

[11] The knowledge-related sense of 'wit' persisted longest in formulaic expressions such as 'wit thou' and 'it is to wit(en)' (see Taavitsainen and Pahta 1997b). Such formulaic phrases were primarily found in translation from Latin, and they mostly disappeared by the end of the Middle English period (Rissanen 2006: 234; see also Rissanen and Koivisto-Alanko 2002).

[12] The following variants are found in *EMEMT*: **know**: 'knew', 'knewe', 'kniw', 'know', 'knowe', 'knowen', 'knowest', 'knoweth', 'knowing', 'known', 'knowne', 'knows', 'knowyng', 'knowynge'; **understand**: 'understand', 'understandeth', 'understanding', 'understands', 'vnderstand', 'vnderstande', 'vnderstanded', 'vnderstanden', 'vnderstandeth', 'vnderstanding', 'vnderstandyng', 'vnderstond', 'vnderstonde', 'vnderstondes'; **wit**: 'wit', 'witteth', 'wyt', 'wyte', 'wytteth'.

[13] In Hiltunen and Tyrkkö (2009), the frequency of knowing-verbs was found to follow a steeply decreasing cline from the Middle English period to the nineteenth century, after which usage appears to level off and remain consistent until the present day.

[14] Kruskal–Wallis non-parametric ANOVA $p = 0.0459$. No category comparison is significant on a Dunn's multiple comparison post-test. The study was conducted with a pre-release version of the *EMEMT* corpus. Its composition and size is close to the final release version.

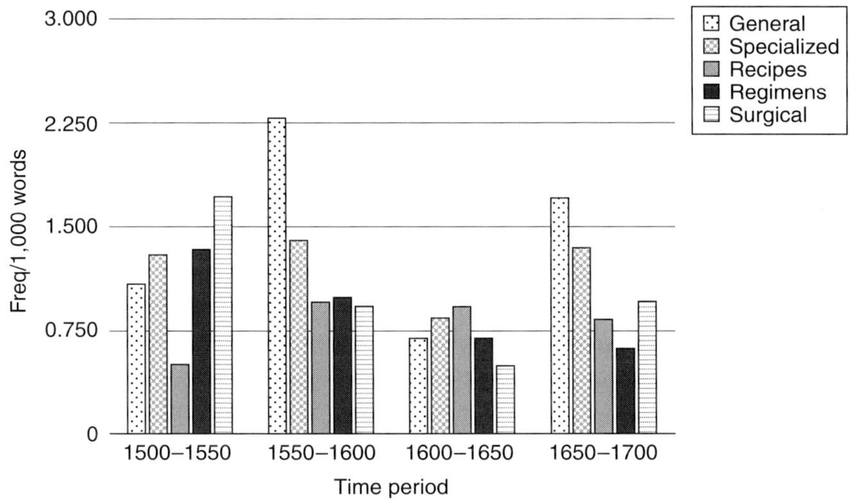


Figure 4.1 Frequency of knowing-verbs by corpus category.

categories show a moderate increase. The *Philosophical Transactions* (*PT*) category, not shown on the chart, appears at a frequency of 0.82, thus fitting in with the other texts of the final fifty-year period.[15]

However, when it comes to individual texts within and across categories, a considerably more divergent picture emerges. Texts from all categories and all time periods are represented in equal measure at both ends of the spectrum. It is clear that the linguistic choices of individual authors and translators, as well as the topics of texts, play a more significant role in determining how frequently knowing-verbs are used in a given text than the category to which the text belongs. The frequency of knowing-verbs in extracts longer than 2,000 words (Figure 4.2) ranges from a low of 0.08/1,000 words in John Hall's *Select Observations* (1679) to a high of 3.86/1,000 in Leonardo Fioravanti's *Treatise of Chirurgery* (1652b) – an almost fifty-fold difference. The first text is a collection of case histories, detailing the ailments of dozens of patients; the latter is a translated surgical textbook by a prominent sixteenth-century Bolognese surgeon.

The nature of knowing-verbs in the lexico-grammatical continuum is naturally a major contributing factor to their use in discourse. While clearly content words in the sense that they can carry topical relevance, knowing-verbs also have other pragmatic uses without particular reference to knowledge or knowing as concepts (see, for example, Van Bogaert 2009). Thus,

[15] In a small corpus such as *EMEMT*, diachronic division into relatively short sections is inherently precarious, as sometimes the difference of a single year could mean that the number of text samples may shift significantly (see Studer 2008: 33–5).

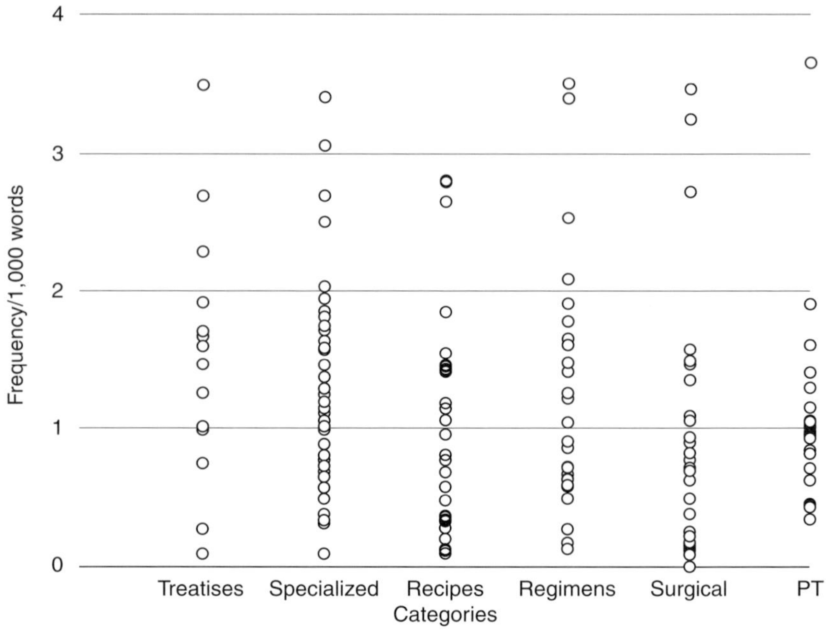


Figure 4.2 Frequency of knowing-verbs in extracts longer than 2,000 words.

a comparison of frequencies of occurrence without taking into account additional syntactic or discursive parameters holds little interest and may even be misleading.

We shall therefore begin by looking at a number of syntactic features of the three knowing-verbs that potentially indicate the perspectives on knowledge taken by medical writers. The analysis of grammatical subjects along with the semantic classification of their referents relates to the possessor of knowledge, polarity to its rhetorical expression and the use of modal verbs to issues such as certainty or importance.

All concordance lines containing either finite or non-finite forms of knowing-verbs are included in the analysis, but they are treated somewhat differently. Both finite and non-finite forms are analysed for the presence of modal verbs (either deontic, epistemic or none) and polarity (either positive or negative). Each concordance line containing either a finite verb form or a non-finite form preceded by a modal verb is analysed for voice (active or passive). The grammatical subject is identified for active knowing-verbs; second-person singular and plural pronouns are collapsed. Finally, for each instance of knowing-verbs, we identify the 'knower', that is, the party whose knowledge is referred to in the sentence. With finite verb forms in the active voice, this amounts to simply identifying and classifying the subject of the verb, but for concordance lines that do not indicate the agent of the verb (non-finite forms and agentless passives), it has to be inferred from the context. 'Knowers' are classed according to the model introduced in Hiltunen and Tyrkkö (2009).

For the syntactic and discursive analysis, the concordance lines were analysed without regard to the corpus category or publication date of the text in question. This was done to ensure objectivity at the next stage of analysis concerning the development of scientific thought-styles. Given that the data set of 1,932 items includes all instances of 'know', 'understand' and 'wit' in the *EMEMT* corpus, the findings constitute a comprehensive profile of the way these three verbs were used in the corpus and thus, by extension, in the domain of medical writing in the early modern period. To this end, it is of interest to begin by discussing their syntactic behaviour first and then to move to the discursive practices to which they are party.

### *4.3.1 Modal auxiliaries*

The meaning of modals depends on the context in which they are used. Modal auxiliaries used with knowing-verbs in the corpus can be roughly identified as falling into two groups. The forms 'may', 'might' and 'can' tend to have epistemic meanings, whereas 'must', 'ought', 'should' and 'shall' nearly always express deontic modality (though 'shall' is more often used epistemically than the others in the latter group) (see, for example, Palmer 2001 and Biber 2004b). Overall, 385 instances of modal auxiliaries and/or modal structures were observed, a figure that comes to 20 per cent of all instances of knowing-verbs. Comparing the proportions of deontic and epistemic modals to non-modal constructions, we observe that the usage is fairly even with recipe collections and the '*PT*' showing a significantly lower frequency (Figure 4.3).[16]

Deontic modals are more frequent in the categories where didactic discourse features prominently (see Section 4.4.2 below). On the other hand, 'Specialized Treatises' and '*PT*' exhibit a proportionately higher incidence of epistemic modals concerned with evaluating both the veracity of knowledge and, less frequently, the possibility of knowing something at all. In addition to formally epistemic contexts, epistemic modals such as 'can' and 'may' are also used in discourses of practical knowledge to convey the means or grounds by which something is known, as exemplified in (1).

[16] $\chi^2 = 64.89$, df = 10, $p < 0.001$.

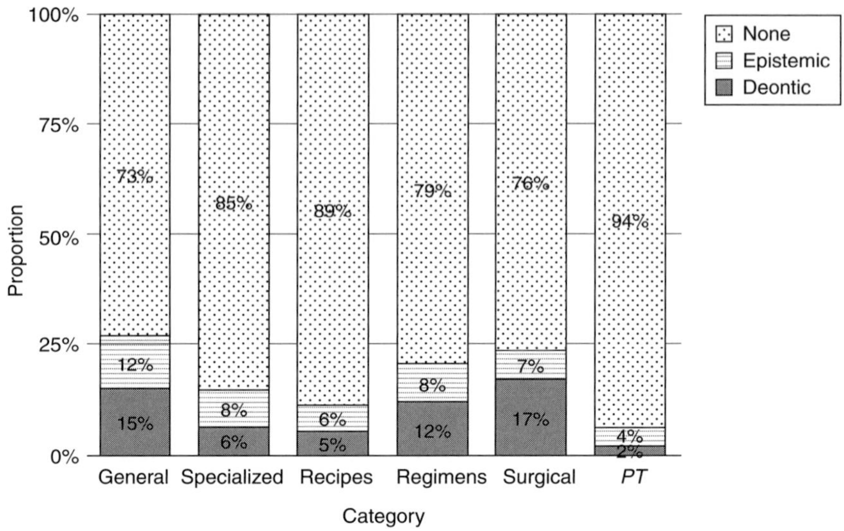


Figure 4.3 Modal auxiliaries and their type by category.

(1) and boyle them moderately vnto the wasting, not onely of the wine, but also of all the watery substance of the hearbes, which you may **know** by the ceasing of the reake or steeme Note that you ought to be carefull during the whole time of boyling, (*EMEMT*; Bonham 1630: 14)

When it comes to the use of modal auxiliaries, a diachronic development can also be observed (Figure 4.4).[17]

The decline in the proportional use of deontic modals, from slightly over 30 per cent in 1500–50 to around 10 per cent in both 1600–50 and 1650–1700, reflects a shift away from a didactic style of instruction.

### *4.3.2 Grammatical subjects and polarity*

The grammatical subjects of knowing-verbs are overwhelmingly realized as pronouns: 86 per cent of all subjects are pronouns and 14 per cent nouns. Pronominal subjects generally refer to the author, the reader or a person already mentioned in the text, while nominal subjects naturally tend towards new referents (see also Section 4.3.4).

Interesting parallels emerge between the categories 'General Treatises', 'Regimens' and 'Surgical Treatises', on the one hand, and between 'Specialized Treatises', 'Recipe Collections' and '*PT*', on the other (Figure 4.5), when the distribution profiles of personal pronouns in the grammatical subject position

[17] $\chi^2 = 63.22$, df = 6, $p < 0.0001$.

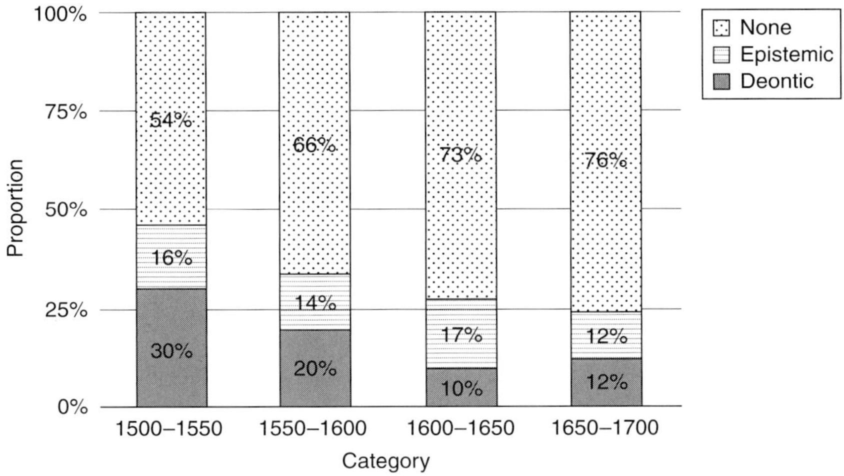


Figure 4.4 Modal auxiliaries and their type on the timeline.

of active verbs of knowing are compared. Figure 4.5 also gives the proportion of positive and negative polarity in relation to grammatical subject.

The high proportion of second-person singular verbs in 'General Treatises', 'Regimens' and 'Surgical Treatises' can be interpreted as suggesting an orientation towards the reader. In broad terms, the three categories comprise texts mainly written as textbooks and guides for students and lay audiences. The use of the second-person singular, overwhelmingly in the positive, thus refers to the reader's knowledge.

By comparison, 'Specialized Treatises', 'Recipe Collections' and '*PT*' appear more author-driven, as indicated by the frequent use of the first-person singular.[18] All three categories represent text types characterized by an intra-disciplinary focus, and it is clear that the authors themselves are positioned as the central figures. A diachronic shift can also be observed when it comes to the pronominal referent. In the sixteenth century, first-person accounts of Galen and other ancients continue to be published (see Taavitsainen 2009c), while in the seventeenth century personal observations, made in a characteristically author-oriented style, particularly in the '*PT*', raise the figure (Atkinson 1999).

The occurrence of negative polarity in the first-person singular often denotes a self-reflective stance, with the author discussing his own lack of knowledge, as in Example 2:

[18] Palander-Collin (2009: 111–12) notes an increase in the use of the self-referential first-person singular in personal letters from the sixteenth to the eighteenth century and argues that the development is indicative of a shift towards a more involved style of written discourse.

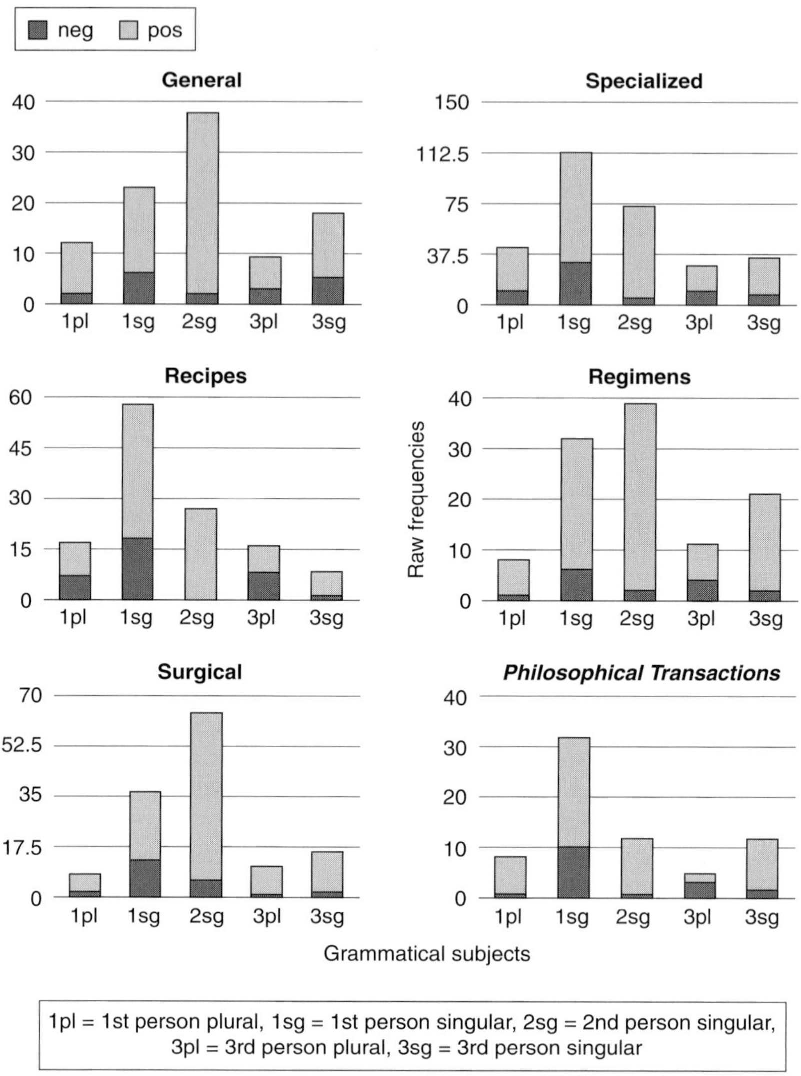


Figure 4.5 Trends in the use of pronominal subjects in the categories. *Note*: the charts feature raw frequencies. Note the difference in scale between the charts.

(2) And many others have written upon this subject, which knew nothing but what they had collected out of books, to what end, I **know** not, unless it were to draw other learned men unto them, thinking to gain some knowledge by their conference. (*EMEMT*; Hartlib 1655: 61)

Notably, the pragmatic function of what appears to be negative polarity may in fact be the opposite. In the following example from an early treatise on mental illnesses, negation is used to emphasize the breadth of the author's understanding (Example 3):

(3) Which producing I **vnderstand** not a discouerie only, as by withdrawing availe, to shew that which lay behind it, but a generation and coupling of matter with the forme: which forme it bringeth not with it, but receaueth it as it were an impression from the part. So then, as euerie thing is not made of anye thing (*EMEMT*; Bright 1586: 12)

Across the categories, the proportional distribution of polarity is relatively level. The only notable, and statistically significant, difference is observed in the category 'Regimens', where a lower proportion (8 per cent) of negative polarity can be observed (Figure 4.6).[19] This is not surprising, as the category is comprised of texts produced for the education of the emerging middling classes rather than professional medicos. Negative statements about knowing generally occur in the discursive context of discussions concerning the lack of knowledge exhibited by a particular faction of contemporary medical practitioners.

When polarity is observed in relation to the timeline, an increasing use of negative references is observed (Figure 4.7).[20] This development can be interpreted as a reflection of the numerous controversies raging between schools of medicine, and of the growing interest in the exploration of new phenomena for which no explanation was readily apparent.[21] A change is also observed in the underlying style of thought; while the scholastic style of the sixteenth century predicated an assertive and self-assured attitude to the knowledge of established authorities, the seventeenth-century medico was more apt to admit to his own lack of knowledge.

### 4.3.3 *Classifying the knowers*

By classifying types of 'knowers' more precisely we can begin to uncover the socio-historical context and suggest answers to questions such as whose knowledge was considered worth discussing and how the knowing of different groups was evaluated by writers. The classifying was carried out along a six-tier model introduced in Hiltunen and Tyrkkö (2009), reproduced here as Table 4.1.[22] The model pertains only to the class of knower as identified in context and not to the nature or veracity of a particular act of knowing.

19 $\chi^2 = 29.6$, df = 5, $p < 0.001$.
20 $\chi^2 = 31.77$, df = 3, $p < 0.001$.
21 Negative attribution of knowing figures prominently here. Forty per cent of such instances refer to laymen, 34 per cent to members of the medical community. On the discourse of medical controversies, see Ratia and Suhr (Chapter 10, this volume) and Ratia (2005).
22 For a similar classification of person references on the basis of sociocultural parameters, see Marttila (Chapter 8, this volume).

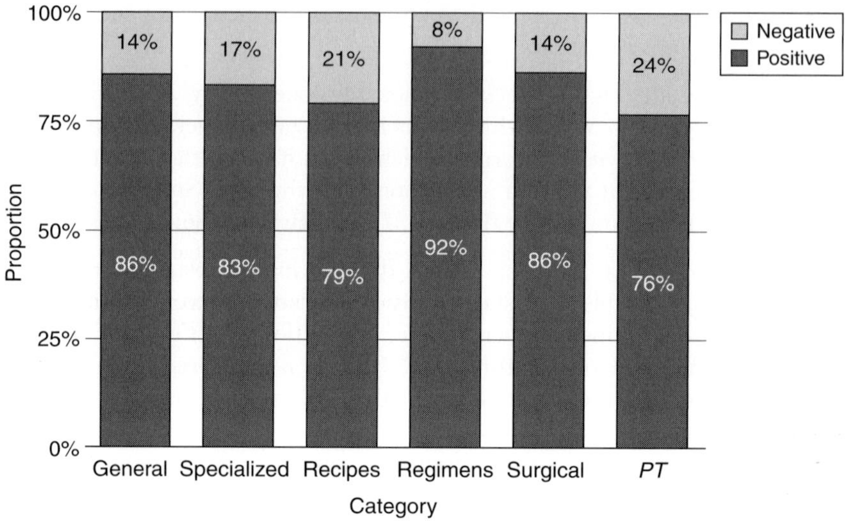


Figure 4.6 Polarity in relation to category.

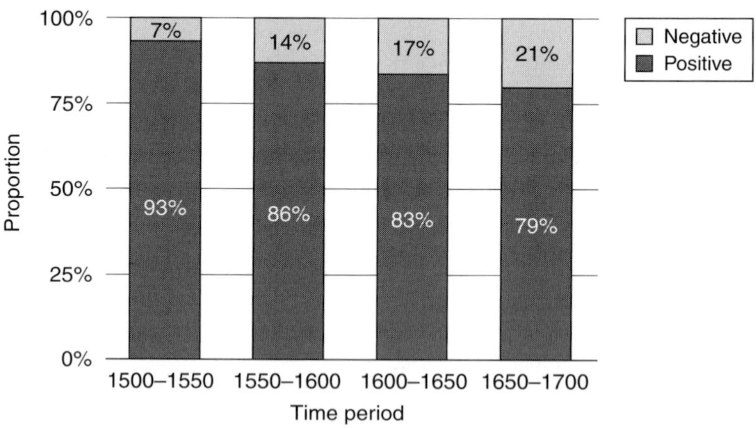


Figure 4.7 Polarity in relation to timeline.

Ten instances of knowing-verbs had a semantic subject that did not comfortably fall into one of the six classes. These included types of animals, witches and conceptual entities ('every Age of Antiquity knew it self better'), none of which can be reasonably ascribed as knowers in the same sense as human subjects (*PT*, 18, 1694: 274).

The frequency distribution of knower classes shows a statistically significant development over the 200-year time span (Figure 4.8).[23] The increase

[23] $\chi^2 = 159.00$, df = 15, $p < 0.001$. The figure includes both active and passive voice, the latter having been determined from the agent.

Table 4.1 *Classification of knowers.*

| Knower class | Description |
|---|---|
| Divine | God or the Devil; access to omniscient knowledge that transcends to the absolute and infallible. |
| Authority | A recognized medical or philosophical authority; primarily ancient (Galen, Aristotle); later on may include well-known contemporaries (Harvey). |
| Author | The author of the text. Texts attributed to an ancient authority but clearly written by a later author are assigned to this class as well. |
| Medical community | The medical community at large or a specific faction thereof: physicians, surgeons, apothecaries, etc. The reference may be to the author's own community or to a rival one. |
| Reader | The reader or addressee of the text. Often positioned as a student of medicine. Manifest in the text lexically or through the second-person pronoun. |
| All/lay | Knowers without medical training or not practising medicine. The category includes members of other professional groupings as well as laypeople, often represented by 'shepherds', 'boys' and 'women'. |

in the frequency of self-references by the author, from a mere 3 per cent in the first half of the sixteenth century to more than six times as much 100 years later, reflects a profound shift in scientific thought. As new theories began to replace the old, a new breed of medical authority began to appear: more self-assured, ready to claim centre stage. As part of the shift to a more author-centred style, the proportional frequency of references to the reader decreased by nearly half. Interestingly, references to the knowing of authorities, members of the medical community and laypeople remain more or less stable.

Although proportional number of references to the class 'All/lay' remains more or less unchanged, it does not mean that the nature of such references would have remained unchanged across the timeline. Whereas earlier references frequently remark on the knowing of non-medical people as an example of general knowledge, seventeenth-century texts show increasing interest in the notion of popular education (see Example 4):

(4) I will therefore give you some instructions by which <u>every one may</u> **know** whether shee bee with child or not. The signes of conception shall bee taken from the woman, from the urine, from the infant, and from experiment. (*EMEMT*; Sadler 1636: 143–4)

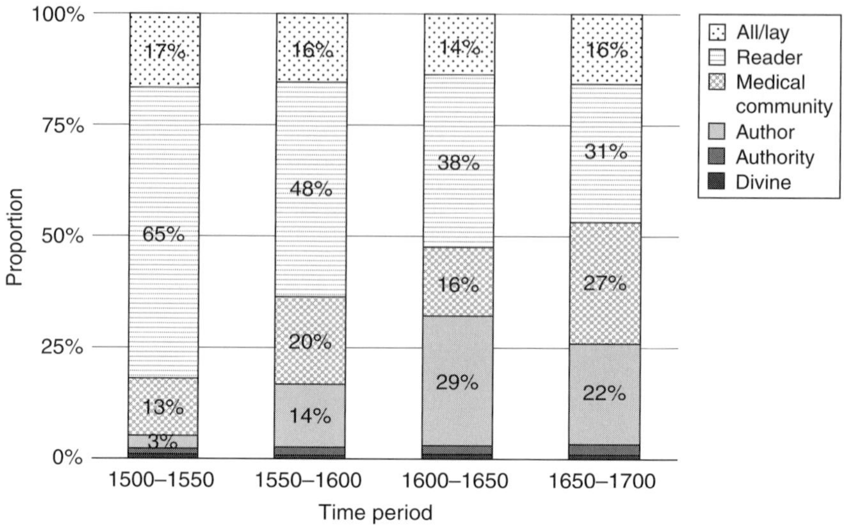


Figure 4.8 Changes in the knower class on the timeline.

The trends observed here follow a longer diachronic development, as Hiltunen and Tyrkkö (2009: 79) have shown that the didactic use of the second-person singular subject was even greater in the Middle English period, accounting for nearly 79 per cent of all occurrences of knowing-verbs there. By the same token, references to the author accounted for only 3 per cent in the Middle English period, thus rising nearly tenfold between the fifteenth and the seventeenth centuries. The other categories remain essentially level, with references to the things the medical community knows or should know regaining ground after a slight dip in the early seventeenth century.

The low frequency of knowing-verbs associated with medical authorities deserves a note, particularly because references to medical authorities are otherwise not infrequent in this period. As discussed by Taavitsainen (2001b: 45–6), the scholastic strategy was to allude to the knowledge of established medical authorities by means of reporting verbs, and the strategy continues well into the early modern period.

### 4.3.4 *Relations between grammatical and semantic subjects*

As noted, the vast majority (86 per cent) of the grammatical subjects of knowing-verbs in the corpus are pronouns. The only significant difference can be observed with the knower class 'All/lay', where the ratio of pronominal and nominal subjects is 1:1, as opposed to the 9:1 ratio in the other classes. This can be explained by the fact that references to the knowledge of

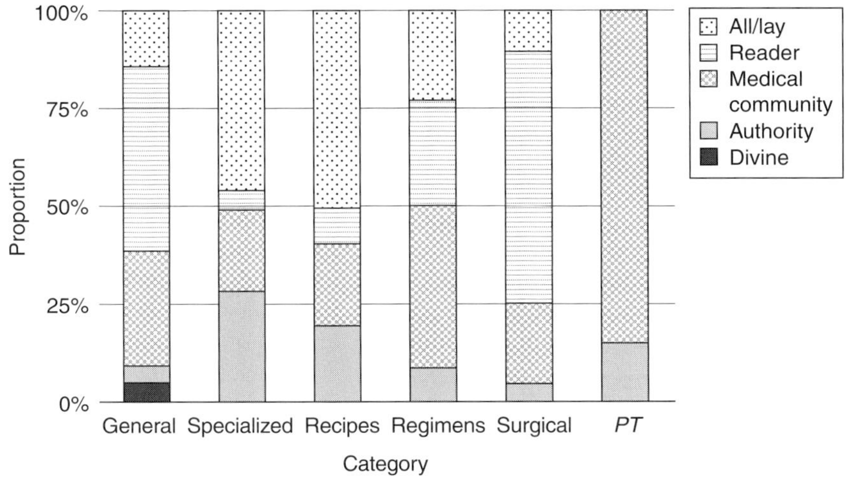


Figure 4.9 Knower classes of third-person singular subjects in relation to category.

members of the 'All/lay' class – e.g., shepherds, boys, women – are generally given as examples and are therefore restricted to a single instance, while the knowledge of medical professionals is more likely to feature as a continuing topic of discussion, which in turn allows the use of pronouns as subjects once the referent has been identified with a noun.

The use of most pronouns is relatively straightforward. The first-person singular almost invariably denotes the authors themselves, and second-person singular is used to refer to readers. The third-person plural is more or less invariably used in reference to the medical community at large, usually by reference to a particular group (surgeons, apothecaries, etc.). Altogether, these three pronouns account for 74 per cent of all pronouns. More referential variance is seen in the remaining pronouns, namely the third-person singular and plural.

In the third-person singular, considerable differences can be observed between the categories (Figure 4.9).[24]

Perhaps surprisingly, 'Specialized Treatises' and 'Recipe Collections' appear to consider the knowledge of laypeople more often than the other categories, as shown in Example 5:

(5) First therefore I wyl shew the causes of the disease: & secondly preseruatiues whereby a man may be kepte from the sicknesse: thirdly, the tokens, whereby he that is diseased maye gather, and **vnderstande**,

[24] $\chi^2 = 66.4$, df = 20, $p < 0.001$.

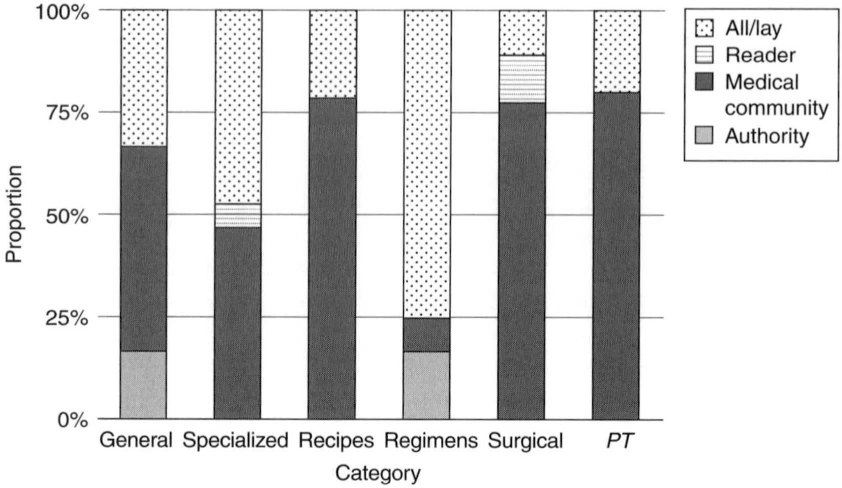


Figure 4.10 Knower classes of third-person plural subjects in relation to category.

whether he be infected wyth the plague or no: (*EMEMT*; Brasbridge 1578: A4r)

The emerging professional orientation of the *PT* is strikingly reflected (Figure 4.9). All knowledge references in the articles pertain to either medical authorities or to the medical community at large.

The third-person plural denotes a reference to someone other than the author or the addressee. A wide variety of referents can be identified, and some category-specific differences become apparent (Figure 4.10).[25]

While references to the members of the medical community predominate in all other categories, 'Regimens' are predictably more concerned with the knowledge of the target audience of ordinary, non-professional readers.

## 4.4 The topoi of knowing in medical discourse

Having examined the syntactic and semantic behaviour of knowing-verbs in detail, we now move to their use in medical rhetoric. First, we must briefly return to the premise that the act of knowing is fundamental both to the practice of science and to the scientific community. When it comes to the practice of medicine, it is imperative to communicate correct information and to identify things worth knowing from those that are not. References to

[25] $\chi^2 = 26.96$, $df = 15$, $p = 0.029$.

knowing need to be carried out following fairly well-defined discursive practices to avoid lack of clarity. On the other hand, for members of the medical community, overt references to knowing are invested with the performative force to attribute the quality of knowing to an individual or a school of thought. As political and communal discursive turns, they are always made deliberately and with much care (see Butchvarov 1970: 58).

The rhetorical function of knowing-verbs can be identified by analysing their phraseologies. For example, there are 260 instances of knowing-verbs following a first-person singular pronoun, and 41 instances of a knowing-verb following a second-person pronoun and the modal 'may'. Both these groups also seem rather uniform in terms of their function in the text. However, it would be problematic to assume that all instances of knowing-verbs that are used in the same grammatical context would be used rhetorically in exactly the same way. Phraseologies may imply different things depending on where they occur in the discourse, and, conversely, a given rhetorical function may obviously have several syntactic realizations. To illustrate this point, consider the following two examples which both have the auxiliary 'shall'. The first, demonstrating deontic use, clearly imposes a requirement on the reader, while the second, an epistemic example, has a wording suggesting a more polite tone. Similar situations are common in the data set, which shows that rhetorical analysis cannot rely on phraseology alone (Examples 6 and 7).

(6) How thou shall **knowe** yf the brayne panne be broken. (*EMEMT*; *Treasure of Pore Men* 1526: 11r)

(7) First you shall **understand**, that the Gout of what kind soever it be, either hot or cold, or of any other temperature, they all come of one onely cause, although they work divers Effects, which Effects come through the complexions of them that have that infirmitie: (*EMEMT*; Fioravanti 1652a: 28)

That said, phraseology is often indicative of the rhetorical function that the knowing-verb has in the text. For this reason, we make use of syntactic information in analysing the rhetorical function of knowing-verbs, but additionally the discourse function of each item in the data set is considered. Combining these two strands enables a detailed description of the rhetorical function of each knowing-verb, which is at the same time sensitive to individual discourse contexts. To describe the rhetorical function of knowing-verbs, we use the concept *topos*.

In our analysis, the use of knowing-verbs falls under three primary topoi of knowledge: *assertive*, *practical* and *epistemic*. In addition, we consider it useful to identify six sub-topoi, which, although clearly falling under one of the primary topoi, merit individual attention by having a distinct rhetorical or discursive purpose. Table 4.2 summarizes the three topoi and their main subtypes.

Table 4.2 *Topoi of knowledge.*

| | |
|---|---|
| Assertive knowledge | assertion |
| | negative attribution |
| | declaration |
| Practical knowlege | practical knowledge |
| | didactic knowledge |
| Epistemic knowledge | epistemic |

It is inevitable that circumstances would arise where more than one topos appears to be invoked with a single instance of a knowing-verb. In classifying such instances, a decision is made on which of the invoked topoi is primary. In this sense, the topos categories are treated as mutually exclusive, although it is acknowledged that some instances are more prototypical members of their category than others.

### *4.4.1 Assertive knowledge*

The first primary topos concerns the discourse representation of assertions about knowing. This topos encompasses a variety of assertions. The prototypical assertion has a knowing-verb in the active voice, preceded by the first-person plural pronoun 'we' as the subject (Example 8).

(8) Finally upon sure grounds we **know** that we have no Anatomicall kindred with the Archevs of vegetables, whether we respect the whole or the parts: For the endowments of simples are from the Creation, and not from the usurpation of possession. (*EMEMT*; Biggs 1651: 34–5)

Similar assertions are also frequently made in the passive voice. Although the passive clause in Example 9 does not indicate the agent of the verb, we can assume that, as in the previous example, the writer refers to what could be loosely described as the community of medical professionals, and therefore it can be analysed as having a discourse function similar to that of Example 8.

(9) The water of this bath is **knowen** to be salte and alumish / and haue some part of brimston as may by sight be well perceyued som deale of ashes. (*EMEMT*; Turner 1562: 7v)

It is possible to distinguish a major type of assertion, the declaration made by the writer emphatically in the first person (Example 10).

(10) But this I **know** and can testifie that there is but one Way, and but onely one Regimen, no more Colours than ours, and what we say or write otherwise, is but to deceive the unwary, for if every thing in the

world ought to have its proper causes, there cannot be any one end, which is produced from two waies of working on distinct principles. (*EMEMT*; Starkey 1655: 41)

Within an assertion, the act of knowing may also be attributed to someone other than the writer. The entire sentence quoted below (Example 11) shows an assertion that contains an attribution: knowledge about the four vessels of the heart is attributed to anatomists.

(11) In a birth there are four vessells of the heart the vena cava, the vena arteriosa, arteria venalis, and the aorta, or arteria magna, and are otherwise united then in one come to age, which all Anatomists **know** well enough. (*EMEMT*; W. Harvey 1653: 28–9)

Here Harvey attributes knowledge to members of his own medical community, but there are also many other kinds of attributions. Knowledge may be presented as being possessed by an infallible knower such as God (Example 12) or an ancient medical authority such as Galen or, alternatively, by someone who is not a member of the medical profession (Example 13).[26]

(12) This matter I do remyt to y=e= iudgeme~te of the reders, for god **knoweth** that I do nat wryte halfe as it is or was, but that I do wryte is but to trewe, the more pitie, as god knoweth. (*EMEMT*; Boorde 1547: 6v)

(13) As a confirmation of the Truth of the two last Experiments, every body knows, that Mint, and such like Plants, being set in a Bottle of Water, flourish as much, or more than those planted in the Earth. (*EMEMT*; Colbatch 1698: 22)

A particular kind of assertion contains an attribution with negative polarity, exemplified in (14). The discourse function of these assertions differs from an attribution with positive polarity in that the writer's knowing something is contrasted with someone else's ignorance of the same thing.

(14) And that which causeth me to beleeve it is, that I have alwayes seen the most part of Chirurgians, when they should have any case in Chirurgery, they **knew** not what Unguent would help the sore, but many times they prove this, and that, and so continue untill they have found one that is convenient for the sore, whereunto it is applyed, and therefore this is a certain signe, that they know not by Science their Medicine to help the sore, but with experience they search it. (*EMEMT*; Fioravanti 1652b: 6)

[26] Religious references are considerably more frequent in early modern prefatory material than in medical texts proper (see Koecher 1950: 10), mostly because medical authors felt obliged to make references to religious motifs even though the understanding was well established that medical problems have natural rather than supernatural causes.

A knowing-verb may also be the main verb of a relative clause.[27] Such assertions have the function of specifying to whom the assertion of the main clause applies (Example 15).

(15) The first whereof is Physiology, no one can cure aright, that does not well **know** the constitution of the body he has in hand; which is properly natural Philosophy it self, translated to a medicinal use: for ubi desinit physicus, ibi incipit medicus; but the Natural Philosopher ends not but in Physiology and Pathology; so the study of Medicine is to begin with the Semeiotica or Therapeia. (*EMEMT*; Prat 1689: A6r)

### 4.4.2 *Practical knowledge*

The topos of practical knowledge corresponds most closely to the Aristotelian concept of *techne*. In medical writing, this involves knowledge about medicines and *materia medica*, the identification of diseases and their progression, treatments, surgical techniques and the like.

A typical instance of a knowing-verb that invokes the topos of practical knowledge tells the reader how some item of knowledge is acquired.[28] The subject of the knowing-verb is the second-person pronoun 'you', and the main verb is often preceded by an epistemic modal verb 'may', as in Example 16, or 'can'. Example 17 shows that the same purpose can be achieved by using the passive voice.

(16) You may **know** the Bone is well set, if it answer the figure of the sound part, if no inequality be felt, and the vehement pain be eased or gone, When what's bofore is done, put on Splints fixed, and well-arm'd with Linnen or Tow, tying them on with taps. (*EMEMT*; Cooke 1693: 6)

(17) For an hote euyl co~plexio~ of the vlcered place, is **knowen** by the rednes, infla~mation, and outward heate of the place, and of the partes there about, and by the runnyng out of thyn quytture, hauinge a redde, yelowe, or grene coloure. (*EMEMT*; de Vigo 1543: 120r)

Under the primary topos of practical knowledge, we distinguish the topos of didactic knowledge. By invoking this topos, the writer imposes an obligation on the reader of the text to acquire some relevant knowledge. Indicators of the topos of didactic knowledge include deontic modal verbs, such as 'must' and 'should', imperative forms and adjectives and adverbs indicating obligation and necessity (Example 18). The subject of the knowing-verb

[27] There are 362 instances of relative clauses, which comes to 18 per cent of all knowing-verbs.

[28] When employed for the purpose of providing information about the identifying features of a disease or other ailment, knowing-verbs take on functional characteristics close to those of defining and naming. See also McConchie and Curzan (Chapter 5, this volume).

is either the second-person pronoun 'you' or a noun such as 'physician' or 'surgeon', which in the context of the text in question refers to the reader.[29]

(18) Now ye must **vnderstande**, that all the flowers, herbes, and other thinges rehersed, are not fou~d together in one time and season: wherefore the said licour can not be made at one tyme, but beginnyng the firste or seconde weeke of Maie, it shall be at the least, the ende of September or October, before ye can make an ende. (*EMEMT*; Ruscelli, 1562: A4)

### 4.4.3 *Epistemic knowledge*

The third primary topos is less frequent than the other two but is conceptually as important. The topos of epistemic knowledge can be defined as a discursive element that invokes the issues of how something may be known and the limits of what can be known. The grammatical features most strongly associated with this topos are adjectives (and adverbs) commenting on the ease or possibility of knowing. In Examples 19 and 20 illustrating this topos, the adjectives 'impossible' and 'hard' control *to*-infinitive clauses containing the verb 'know'.

(19) And therefore saith he, it is impossible to **know** that which the Astronomers say, that there are some fortunate, and some vnfortunate starres, but this only may be knowne, that whereas all of them are good, that some of them are better then other some. (*EMEMT*; Lodge 1603: C1v)

(20) Paulus AEgineta saith, that the Gout by reason of so manifold causes whereof it may come, and are hard to be **known**, doth bring with it a very heavy conceit, to wit, that it can no way be cured by the Art of Physick. (*EMEMT*; Holland 1633: 24)

Explicit discussions concerning the limits of human knowledge are rare in the main body of early modern medical texts. If at all, such issues are raised in prefatory material (see Taavitsainen, this volume, Chapter 6). Note that references to the inadequate knowledge of a particular medical group or an individual rival (as in medical controversies) are analysed here as assertions (see Section 4.4.1).

## 4.5 Discursive topoi of knowledge as indicators of scientific thought-style

Having defined the topoi in terms of their discursive and syntactical properties, we can use them to examine the differences in thought-style across the

[29] As noted in Section 4.3.4, nouns as grammatical subjects are most closely associated with the semantic subject class 'All/lay'.

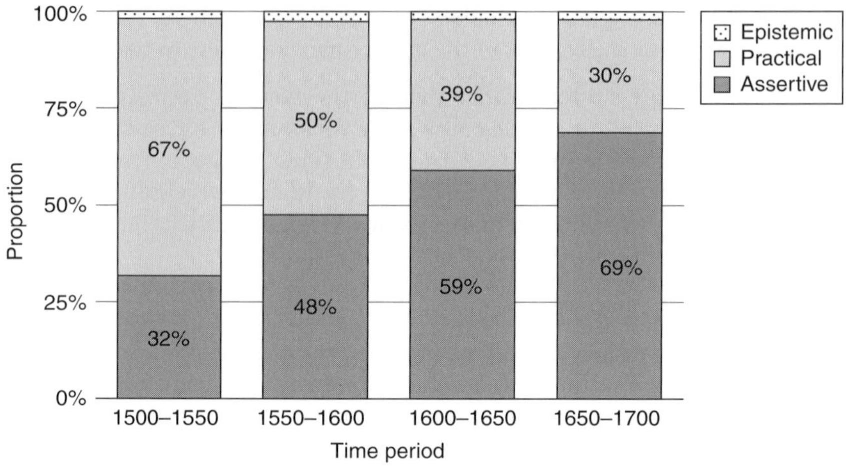


Figure 4.11 Topoi in relation to timeline.

timeline and between the various types of medical writing. The bulk of the observations will by necessity focus on assertive and practical knowledge, as the proportional frequency of the epistemic topos is both relatively stable and very scant.

Across the timeline, a clear trend towards a more assertive style is in evidence (Figure 4.11).[30]

Within the increase of assertive knowledge, the proportional role of the declarative sub-topos increases from the sixteenth century to the seventeenth at the expense of the assertive (Figure 4.12).[31]

As discussed in Section 4.1, the declarative sub-topos denotes direct claims of knowing made by the author of the text. The increase is thus a reflection of the growing role of the author himself rather than of assertions about the knowledge either of the medical community on the whole or of non-medicos. In the empiricist vein, authorial claims of knowing frequently take the form of reporting experiences or observations as the grounds of knowledge. Thus, the astro-physician Joseph Blagrave reinforces established knowledge with his own observations (Example 21):

[30] $\chi^2 = 136.08$, df = 6, $p < 0.001$. Figure 4.11 includes the category *PT*, which is nearly entirely assertive in terms of knowledge references (see below), but even if the last section were to be recounted without this category the cline would continue with the percentages for the assertive and practical topos at 64 per cent and 34 per cent, respectively.

[31] $\chi^2 = 23.47$, df = 2, $p < 0.001$.

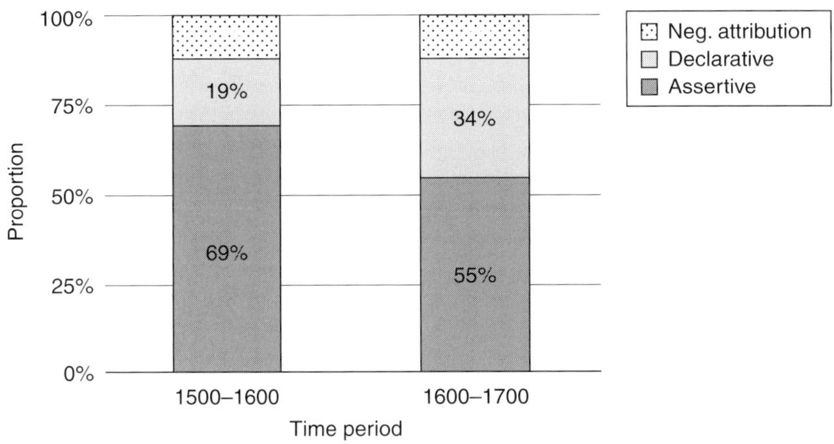


Figure 4.12 Sub-topoi of assertive knowledge.

(21) although what is already written, I have **known** <u>by good experience</u> to hold true by many examples it being for the most part the method of my daily practice; (*EMEMT*; Blagrave 1671: 28)

By contrast, use of the topos of negative attribution remains stable. Despite this, however, a shift can be observed in the referent of the sub-topos. While in the beginning of the timeline the sub-topos is typically invoked in reference to laypeople (Example 22), towards the end it is predominantly used in reference to members of competing medical groups (Example 23):

(22) there be <u>many men and women</u> thynkes them selfe wyse and knowes and lernes many thyngis but that that they be bounde to lerne & knowe that <u>they</u> **knowe** <u>not</u> as fyrste the x. commaundementis of god and the v. com~aundementis of the churche that euery creature that purpos to be saued shulde lerne and knowe and have them as perfetly as there pater noster. (*EMEMT*; Kalendar of shepherdes 1506: 7)

(23) and I know not one <u>Alchymist</u> this day, nor ever did, to whom, if I should have given him the true dissolvent in one hand, which is a ponderous bright water, and the dissolvend in the other hand, which is a powder, or filings of mettal: ye <u>he</u> **knew** <u>not</u> how to dissolve it. (*EMEMT*; Hartlib 1655: 56)

The sub-topoi of practical knowledge undergo similar developments. The role of didactic knowing – that is, obligations concerning the acquisition of a particular piece of knowledge – decreases, and the discursive focus shifts

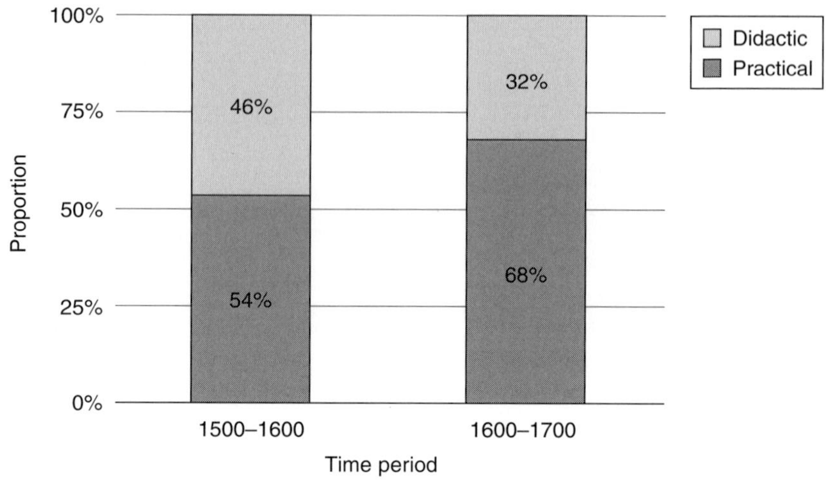


Figure 4.13 Sub-topoi of practical knowledge.

towards knowledge of specific, concrete pieces of information (see Figure 4.13).[32] Although much of the discussion still focuses on the reader's knowledge (78 per cent of all occurrences of practical knowledge), the syntactic realization does not include a deontic modal.

The proportional distribution of the topoi depends on the category in the corpus. Generally speaking, assertive and practical topoi can be conceptualized as forming two distinct groups. In the categories 'Specialized Treatises' and '*PT*', assertive claims concerning knowledge predominate, while the discourse of the other categories is more geared towards instruction or the dissemination of medical knowledge (see Figure 4.14).

The continuity of thought-styles can also be accessed through the use of discursive topoi. The didactic sub-topos, the predominant style of scholasticism, is strongly associated with the continuity of the Galenic tradition. Thus, in the latter part of the sixteenth century, the highly influential barber-surgeon Thomas Vicary assumes a didactic tone reflecting the scholastic mood when reiterating Galenic anatomical theory (Example 24):

(24) And you shal **vnderstande**, that the necke is all that is conteyned betweene the head and the shoulders, and betweene the chinne and the brest. It is compounde and made of foure thinges, that is to say, of Spondillus, of Seruicibus, of Gula, and of Gutture, the which shal be declared more playnely hereafter; (*EMEMT*; Vicary 1577: 45)

[32] Fisher's exact test, $p < 0.001$.

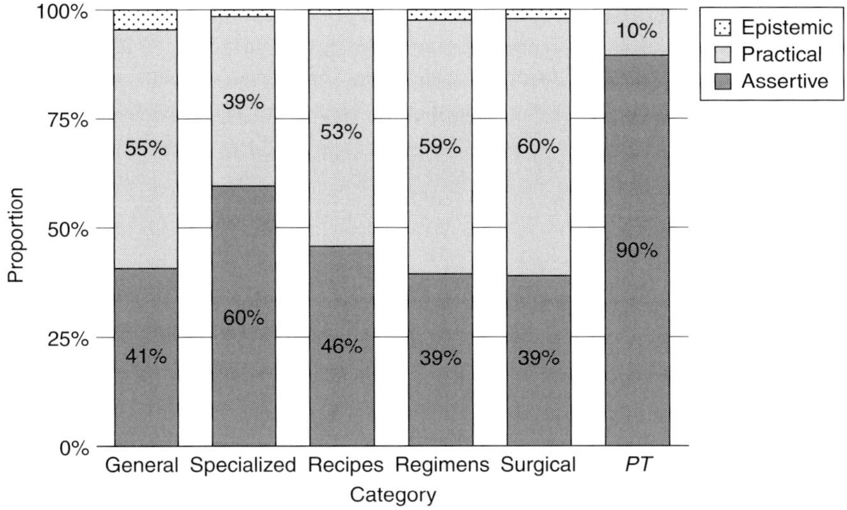


Figure 4.14 Topoi of knowledge in relation to category.

A hundred years later, the physician Gideon Harvey, a staunch critic of contemporary empiricists such as Thomas Sydenham (see Cunningham 1989), assumes a very similar style (Example 25):

(25) 3. The Physica Specialis depends upon the application of a forementioned, to every Subgenus, Species, and individual Body, and by that you are to **know**, what any particular Body is, of what it doth consist, and how each is differenced from the other. 4. What sound this modern Science of Bodies makes upon an Anvil, the following recital will inform you. (*EMEMT*; G. Harvey 1700: 8)

By invoking the didactic sub-topos, Harvey not only tells the reader how one piece of information is to be derived from another but also significantly draws on an established scholastic discursive pattern in an effort to reinforce the message – and to mark the distinction from the declarative style often favoured by contemporary empiricists.

In addition to diachronic developments in the use of topoi, we may also comment on the associations of specific categories of the *EMEMT* corpus with certain topoi (Figure 4.14).

Significantly, the two categories most strongly associated with the assertive topos also represent the highest end of medical writing.[33] The *PT*, in

[33] $\chi^2 = 153.09$, df = 10, $p < 0.001$. No significant difference exists between treatises, health guides and surgical texts ($\chi^2 = 3.96$, df = 4, p = 0.42). Although the categories of the *EMEMT* corpus are not explicitly defined by educational level, it may be said that the majority of texts in the 'Specialized Treatises' and '*PT*' categories were, relatively speaking, written by the members of the top-end of the profession.

particular, differs dramatically from all the other categories, being almost entirely assertive when it comes to the use of knowing-verbs. While there is nothing particularly revolutionary about this discovery – recent scholarship has repeatedly described the *PT* as having been the first step towards modern scientific writing (see Gotti, this volume, Chapter 11) – it is nonetheless striking that the difference is as sharp as it is.

## 4.6 Conclusions

This chapter has applied a rigorous and detailed method of analysis to knowing-verbs. The findings may be considered interesting from at least two perspectives. First, the study has produced a comprehensive profile of the syntactical usage of knowing-verbs within the domain of medical writing in the early modern period. Second, the results show that the uses of knowing-verbs vary between different categories of early medical writing and thus provide evidence for the argument that historical corpora benefit from the kind of detailed stratification used in *EMEMT.*

The analysis of the frequency of knowing-verbs demonstrated that while the overall differences between the categories of medical writing are relatively small, there is considerable variation between individual texts. Notable differences can also be found in the use of syntactic features linked to knowing-verbs, which can be explained by variation in the discourse contexts in which these verbs are used. These syntactic features can also act as indicators of changes in the pragmatic function of texts; for instance, diachronic changes in the relative prominence of different 'knowers' are clearly linked with the partial decline of the scholastic medicine and the emergence of new learning. The analysis of discursive topoi revealed that historically attested changes in medical thinking over the two centuries are evident in the way overt references to the act of knowing were realized. The increase in assertive and declarative references to knowing and the concurrent decrease in practical and didactic references serve to indicate that the general attitude to knowing shifted from a gnostic to a more epistemic style of thinking. More specifically, the decline of authority-driven scholasticism can be seen in the increase of references to the author's own, sometimes incomplete, knowing, as well as in the greater emphasis given in expository texts to instruction rather than to the use of directives. On the other hand, references to the shared knowledge of the medical discourse community decreased markedly. The robustness of the analytical method was further attested by the topoic profile of the '*PT*' category, which was found to be almost entirely assertive in nature, as was to be expected.

As for conclusions specific to early modern medical writing, the chapter has revealed significant differences in the use of knowing-verbs across the socioculturally defined categories. When addressing different readerships, authors would want to position themselves appropriately to the concept of knowledge, sometimes emphasizing scientific styles of thought, at other times focusing on self-promotion or on practical applications. Overall, a shift is seen from a predominantly practical discursive orientation to an assertive one, culminating in *PT*. The growing use of the declarative sub-topos and the simultaneous decline in the use of didactic sub-topos were motivated by the need both to dissociate oneself from ancient doctrines (see Wear 1995b: 156–61) and to promote one's knowledge for social and commercial objectives (see French 2003: 118–22).

In broader terms, the research supports the argument that linguistic analysis has a place in the analysis of historical discourse far beyond the investigation of lexis. The fact that the close analysis of a small set of mid-frequency lexical verbs can produce results that corroborate – and perhaps supplement – our historical understanding of how the prevailing thought-styles of a domain of learning developed suggests that a more broad-ranging analysis of such linguistic phenomena would hold promise for a comprehensive modelling of the history of written records of ideational thought.

# 5 Defining in Early Modern English medical texts

ROD McCONCHIE AND ANNE CURZAN

## 5.1 Aims

In *An Essay Concerning Human Understanding* (1690), John Locke describes an encounter with a group of physicians immersed in learned debate about liquor in the nerves, a debate which captures the importance of definitions in medicine:

the Debate having been managed … by variety of Arguments on both sides, I (who had been used to suspect, that the greatest part of Disputes were more about the signification of Words than a real difference in the Conception of Things) desired … they would first examine … what the Word Liquor signified … upon Examination found, that the signification of that Word was not so settled and certain, as they had all imagined; but that each of them made it a sign of a different complex *Idea*. This made them perceive, that the Main of their Dispute was about the signification of that Term; and that they differed very little in their Opinions, concerning some fluid and subtile Matter, passing through the Conduits of the Nerves; though it was not so easie to agree, whether it was to be called *Liquor* (Locke 1997 III, ix, 16)

The 'examination' of the meaning of 'liquor' by these seventeenth-century physicians probably involved further discussion, rather than reference to dictionaries, which were available, but far from ubiquitous – and many would not have been helpful with a word as common as 'liquor'. Physicians in the early modern period often had to rely on their own resources – each other or published medical texts – to define key terms. They could not reliably turn to dictionaries. Indeed, it is arguable whether English lexicographers even led the way in developing what we now see as their stock-in-trade, their early productions relying largely on glosses and synonymy as definitions.

In the late seventeenth century, when Locke was writing, English lexicography was still in its infancy. The appearance of English monolingual dictionaries has traditionally been dated back to 1604 with the publication of Robert Cawdrey's *A Table Alphabetical*, but several scholars have highlighted Edmund Coote's formative lexicographic work with his table in *The Englishe Scholemaister* (1590). Seventeenth-century English dictionaries, far from today's comprehensive dictionaries, typically focused on a few thousand 'hard, usual words' (Cawdrey 1604, title page) with brief definitions and no etymological information, pronunciation guides, usage notes or other familiar features of modern dictionaries. Take Cawdrey's simple definition of *medicine*, for example: '*medicine*, remedie, or cure.'

Sixteenth-century Latin dictionaries had included medical terminology (McConchie 1997: 99–104), and the early English hard-word dictionaries contained some scientific vocabulary. The first specialized English medical dictionary, *A Physical Dictionary*, appeared in 1657 (see Tyrkkö 2009).

Long before the first medical dictionary, however, the authors of English medical texts were already defining in the vernacular. Central to their scholarly task, often, was the explanation of medical terminology, as part of explaining medicine itself; and during the Late Middle and Early Modern English periods, it often involved navigation among multiple languages – Latin, and to some extent Greek and Arabic. In the early modern period, English was emerging as a language rich and eloquent enough to be used for scientific purposes, which resulted in a proliferation of vernacular texts, such as those included in the *Early Modern English Medical Texts* (*EMEMT*) corpus. Although English was sometimes found wanting, Renaissance language scholars recognized that the act of writing works like these medical texts in English would further enhance the language, whether by borrowing terminology into English or by creating new vernacular terms. As the writers of medical texts incorporated these new terms in the service of medicine, they simultaneously put into circulation models for defining in the vernacular.

This essay explores definition in Early Modern English medical texts. We examine the strategies employed for defining medical terms, contextualizing these practices within the history of English lexicography. What can we learn from defining practices in medical texts that might inform our understanding of early English lexicography? Scientific vocabulary has been and remains a substantial part of the English vocabulary (see Landau 2001: 34). Yet definitional practices in early medical texts are not often considered an influence on early English lexicography.[1] For example, Read (2003: 187–8) outlines six sources of the character of English lexicography:

1. the dictionary as the 'schoolmaster's help';
2. the models provided by dictionaries of classical languages;
3. the tradition of glossing and interlingual dictionaries;
4. the emergence of the scientific study of language;
5. antiquarian and etymological dictionaries;
6. specialists' dictionaries.

[1] McConchie (2002) has already argued that medical practitioners were often involved in compiling dictionaries.

As we will demonstrate in this essay, Early Modern English medical texts also offered models. We propose that to understand the developing practice of defining scientific terminology, both in general and specialized dictionaries, it is useful to examine the medical texts also devoted to explaining the terminology.

To take an example that provides a striking contrast to Cawdrey's definition of medicine, consider Langton's claim to define *physicke* (medicine):

(1) I think it very necessarye and expedient to open and declare … what physicke is, whiche in Latine is called Medicina, & in Englysshe woorde for woorde, Medicine. Hyppocrates … affirmeth that Medicine or Physicke, is nothyng, but the adiection of that that lacketh, or the subtraction, or takynge awaye, of that whyche is superfluous, & redoundeth: the whych declaratio or definition, Gallen alloweth in manye places, & trulie not w~out a cause: For ther is no parte of phisike but it is co~prehended in thys finition. Auerroes … dothe define phisicke … in these wordes … Medic[^i^]na [^orig. Medic na^] est ars factiuarum vna, ratione, et experimento inuenta, que tu sanitatem tuetur, tum morbum depellit. whiche is as muche to say in englysh, as Phisike is one of those artes whyche dothe make thinges inuented, or found out by reason and experience, and the whyche partly defendeth health, and partly beteth away disease, and siknes. Herophilus woulde haue defined it … Medicina est scientia salubrium, insalubrium, et neutrorum. Whyche in englyshe is as foloweth. Physike is a science of thynges holsome, & vnholsome, and of neyther of bothe: Gallen vseth thys finition … where he sayeth that this worde scientia, must be taken accordynge to hys common significatyon, and not as it signifyeth properlye: wherefore phisike is an arte, and no science … (*EMEMT*; Langton 1547: Ai$^{v}$–Aii$^{v}$)

Christopher Langton (1521–78), a university-trained physician, proves particularly interesting for the frequent and explicit attention he gives to the practice of definition. In this passage, he offers definitions of medicine by renowned authorities. Reliance on the definitions of others has long characterized English lexicography, but it is typically a silent practice (hence the frequent use of the term 'plagiarism' to describe it); here Langton uses others' definitions more the way later English dictionaries would use citations: as evidence for how readers should think about meanings. He also employs glosses of the Latin as well as the classical practice of situating a term in relation to a broader category – in this case 'a science' or 'an art'.[2]

[2] This distinction is roughly that between knowledge, especially systematic knowledge of a discipline (science), and the skill required to apply such knowledge (art). Taavitsainen (2004: 40) provides a more fine-grained account of this distinction. For a closely related discussion, see Hiltunen and Tyrkkö (Chapter 4, in this volume).

Similar definitional practices surface in a range of medical texts from the period, although not always with as much explicit discussion as Langton provides. The next two sections address two central methodological challenges for this study. We then turn to the definitional strategies in these early medical texts, which should be recognized as part of the historical, scholarly context for the beginnings of English lexicography.

## 5.2 Defining definition

Definition has been an issue in philosophy at least since Aristotle, who calls a definition 'a phrase signifying a thing's essence' (*Topics*, I, 5). Philosophers generally concentrate on such questions as the truth-value of definitions and whether they are tautological (Robinson 1954: Chapter 2) rather than the more practical issues applying in either lexicography or medicine.[3] For lexicographers, as Sidney Landau points out, defining is 'not a theoretical exercise to increase the sum of human knowledge but practical work to put together text that people can understand' (2001: 121).

The naming of things dominated English lexicographical practice through the seventeenth century and into the eighteenth, since one-to-one correspondence, first between words and realia and then between words in the lexicons of two or more languages, required no lexical definition. Words were the names of things, and definition pointed at the real world not at other words (see Lancashire 2002). During the early modern period, glossing, the rationale for which is synonymic naming, was slowly giving way to a more modern conception. The appearance of more elaborated monolingual dictionaries meant a gradual shift to the 'lexical definition', which described the headword primarily as a linguistic phenomenon. Since the dictionary of Charles Richardson (*A New Dictionary of the English Language*, 1836–7), English lexicographers have increasingly assumed that citations define the headword and that the definition merely crystallizes its senses into a conveniently stylized verbal form.

To examine the definitional work in Early Modern English medical texts, we define the word 'definition' broadly, to encompass a wide range of means for helping readers to understand and to use a term. This seems particularly appropriate to the Middle and Early Modern English periods. The Middle English *diffinicioun* was not necessarily clearly distinguished from related terms. The *Middle English Dictionary* (*MED*) provides a citation in which 'definition' is linked appositively with both 'description' and 'describe':

(2) Bi þe diffinyciou[n] or discripciou[n] or þe descryuyng bifore sett of prudence, prude[n]ce is a ku[n]nyng, dressyng, reulyng and techyng vs in oure gouernau[n]cis of doyng and suffryng. (Pecock, c. 1454)

[3] Robinson (1954), which remains a definitive account of the subject, provides a rare full-length philosophical treatment of definition.

This use of 'definition' does not seem to imply a form of words that captures the essence of the thing described and ignores features which are either non-essential or are shared by other entities, as we might expect from what Aristotle writes. It does, however, define in another Aristotelean sense, by providing the *genus* (*kunnyng*) and *differentia* Aristotle's *Metaphysics* delineates as the classical form of definition, whose first element is the broad classification (*genus*) and the second the characteristic or characteristics that uniquely differentiate the definiendum (*differentiae*). The minimum requirement is not to provide a full account of the characteristics of the definiendum but to obviate its being confused with other members of that *genus*.

The broader definition proves particularly useful for Early Modern English medical texts for, while sometimes relying on the familiar *genus–differentia* formula, they often provide much fuller descriptions – not surprising given their practical nature. Though glossing is also an important practice, the medical texts demonstrate that knowing what a disease is often involves inferring its nature from its symptoms or apparent signs, which requires definition far beyond a 'dictionary definition' as currently understood. To know that a person suffering from the falling sickness may fall and have a fit is not necessarily to know what the falling sickness is, which is often seen as knowing its cause. Our broader definition of 'definition' allows many ways of understanding a disease – that is, of using conceptual characteristics to make sense of the outward symptoms – to be part of the act of 'defining' it. And defining in the texts examined here often means a listing not merely of selected symptoms but also of all the known symptoms of a complaint.

The wide-ranging methods of defining terms in these medical texts escape any easy categorization, but patterns in the definitional strategies do emerge. We will focus on three major forms of explicit definition:

1. synonyms, which can include glossing in another language;
2. categorization, which may involve *genus/differentia* definition;
3. relation, typically to symptoms or causes of an ailment, or, with definitions of body parts, to other body parts.[4]

These definitional strategies will look familiar to users of a modern dictionary, although their manifestations in the medical texts often bend and exceed current lexicographical practice. Perhaps equally familiar is the inclusion in these medical texts of etymological information about technical medical terms. While not always a defining strategy per se, the etymological information is often presented as informative about the word's meaning – an assumption that still underlies modern lexicographical practice. It also provides

[4] Robinson (1954) usefully distinguishes between the purpose and method of a definition. In terms of purpose, we will focus on nominal definitions. In terms of method, these three categories are adapted from three of the seven categories proposed by Robinson.

writers with a kind of definitional authority, which was clearly a concern for some of these authors and which we discuss in the final sections.

## 5.3 Data for the study

One of the challenges of this study was how best to exploit *EMEMT* to examine definitional practices. Searching the terms 'define' and 'definition' turns up only a fraction of the ways that authors explain unfamiliar terms in medical texts. Accepting the impossibility of locating every passage that might constitute a definition, we compiled a list of twenty-one lexeme groups and phrases that we thought might occur in passages with definitions. These were the following (base verb or noun only listed): 'betoken', 'call', 'clepe', 'declare', 'define', 'demonstrate', 'denominate', 'explain', 'expound', 'interpret', 'name', 'nominate', 'note', 'signify', 'specify', 'style', 'term', 'token', 'translate', 'turn' and 'that is to say/wit'.

Not all were productive, but they did uncover a range of definitional practices which we describe below. 'Betoken', for instance, yielded only data to do with the significance of symptoms, not with defining. We have not covered everything; the copula as a search term seemed too daunting given the time constraints, and we did not search for 'sayeth that' and its variants, a formula sometimes introducing ascriptive definition discussed briefly by Taavitsainen (2004: 60–1).

The analysis is entirely qualitative in its approach, attempting to categorize different practices and to determine their potential significance for the development of English medical texts and English lexicography. For our purposes, quantitative analysis did not seem fruitful. The corpora searched were *EMEMT* (for all of the above lexemes) and *Middle English Medical Texts* (*MEMT*) (when relevant for specific lexemes).

We first describe *EMEMT* material in which authors reflect on the act of defining, including their anxiety about the status of English as a language of medicine. We then turn to different methods of definition, including the deployment of synonyms, categorization and relation. Finally, we examine the use of etymological information and ascriptive definitions – including exploitation of the first person – as part of authors' defining practices and negotiation of the authority to define.[5]

## 5.4 Metacommentary on defining

Were the writers of these medical texts aware of their role in developing a set of practices for defining in the vernacular? The evidence is mixed, but at least some writers in the corpus provide metacommentary about the defining

[5] For an account of defining based on the *MEMT* corpus and related issues in medical texts, see Taavitsainen (2004), especially pp. 208–10.

that the texts require of them. And this metacommentary reveals their anxieties as well as their strategies for locating their own authority.

Christopher Langton proves unusual in the explicit interest he shows in finding the appropriate English gloss and defining the terms inherited from the Latin tradition. He also sounds strikingly defensive of English's ability to cope with the demands of developing a full repertoire of medical terminology as well as insistent on the benefit to English speakers of doing so. As he writes:

(3) The thyrde chambre is behynde in the laste parte of the heed, … in latyne it is called Cerebellum: in oure tungue we haue no propre name for it, whiche I can do no lesse then count the negligence of our Phisitions to be the cause of: for yf they had wrytten of theyr arte in theyr mother tunge, as they do in other places, why shulde we lacke englysh names, more then we lacke eyther Latyn names or Greke names? and yet to saye the truthe, it is better for vs English men to haue English names, then eyther Latyn or Greke. (*EMEMT*; Langton 1545: Dii$^{v}$–Diii$^{r}$ [fols. xxvi–xxvii])

Later in the text, Langton provides 'meate pype' as a synonym for 'wesaunt' and then parenthetically asks: 'for why shoulde we be ashamed of these names, seynge we haue no better' (Diiii$^{v}$–Dv$^{r}$).

Yet, elsewhere in the same text, Langton appears, at least initially, to dismiss the definitional problems of navigating among the terms in different languages; he writes: 'in dede so that we vnderstande the thynge, it shall make but lytle matter for names' (1550: Eiiii$^{v}$). Despite making light of the problem, however, he then immediately continues with an explanation of what Galen says about the terms in question (*Porta* and *Caua vena* – see Example 31 below [p. 90]).

Langton is exceptional in providing this kind of metacommentary on defining. However, many of these Early Modern English vernacular medical texts at various points are immersed in the practice of definition through a range of strategies, as detailed below, and some authors highlight the activity and its importance.[6] For example, John Jones (*fl.* 1562–79), author of several medical works, begins his discussion of an ague with the explicit recognition that defining the term will aid the discussion:

(4) WHEN … I entend to declare thoccasion of Agues … it behoueth fyrst to define what an ague is folowing Cicero, which saith that euery thing which we purpose to speake of must rise of his definitio~. an ague is nothing els but an vnnatural heate or caliditie, which taketh his beginninge at the harte, disperseth all ouer the body by the artiers and veines, and so

[6] A recognizable trend in explicit use of the terms 'define' and 'defining' across time emerges, with few references before the mid sixteenth century, a rapid increase thereafter and a continuing, although less innovative, trend through the seventeenth century.

hurteth the actions therof. Thys laste parte of the definition is necessarily adioined to the same. For although a ma~ be made hotter the~ he was before (as it often chaunceth to dauncers, ru~ners, laborers and leapers. &c. yet it can not be said to haue an ague. (*EMEMT*; Jones 1566: Cv$^{r-v}$)

Jones is aware that a definition ought to describe the essence of the phenomenon – in this case, that being heated does not entail having an ague. Another author who is concerned with the defining process itself is Timothy Bright (see Section 5.9).

Explicit discussion also sometimes takes the form of questioning others' definitions, which may serve several purposes. It may question an established authority, thus raising the questioner's status by implication; it can also serve as a rhetorical strategy for advancing the argument and the text structure.[7] In general, it probably advances the emergence of independently derived, rationalized, empirically based and ultimately lexical definitions. In all cases, it emphasizes the importance of definition to medical practice and the writing of medical texts. William Clowes provides a useful example when he asks whether the disease *lues venerea* is caused by the liver:

(5) sith in the liuer is made the separation of all the humors of mans body, as by the good temperature and disposition thereof good humors are bred: euen so by the euill disposition thereof, corrupt humors are ingendred, so that is not to be doubted (saith he) but that the corruption of the liuer is the roote of this disease.

And if it be obiected, that the disease is taken by externall meanes as aforesaid, by kissing, eating and drinking, clothes infected, milke of nurses, &c. and therefore the liuer is not the cause, and so the definition then can not be true: (*EMEMT*; Clowes 1596a: 153)

John Caius (1510–73), the author of an original vernacular text rather than a translation, *Against Sweatyng Sicknesse*, is interesting for adding linguistic comment. Caius points out that this disease is 'almost proper' to the English, having not been noted elsewhere, a fact he finds appropriate since:

(6) it followeth somoche English menne, to who~ it is almoste proper, & also began here ... Whiche thing I suppose may the better be done, because I se straunge and no english names both in Latine and Greke, by commune vsage taken for Englishe. As in Latin, Feure, Quotidia~, Tertian, Quartane, Aier, Infection, Pestilence, Uomite, Person, Reines, Ueines, Peines, Chamere, Numbre, &c. a litle altered by the commune pronunciacion. In Greke, Pleuresie, Ischiada, Hydrops, Apostema, Phlegma, and Chole: called by the vulgare pronunciatio~, Schiatica Dropsie, Impostume, Phleume, & Choler: Gyne also, and Boutyre,

[7] The defining process fits neatly into the traditional question–answer dialogue format often employed in medical texts; it can also lead to a methodical point-form exposition of a subject, for example of the form 'The word X has two significations. One is ...'

Sciourel, Mouse, Rophe, Phrase, Paraphrase, & cephe (*EMEMT*; Caius 1552: 9$^{v}$–10$^{r}$)

In defining stone, Edward Jorden (d. 1631) highlights the difficulty of agreeing on a definition by putting several authorities' definitions into conversation and pointing out problems in them:

(7) Stone is another Minerall substance … and our Minerall men confound themselues much in the definition of it. Wherefore Fallopius implores the helpe of Marcus Antonius Iunica about it, as one of the most difficult points in Philosophie: but … defines it by his want of dissolution … either by heate or moysture. And whereas it is manifest that some Stones will melt, he imputes it to the admixture of some mettall, among which he receiueth glasse. Others define it by his hardnesse, wherein commonly it goeth beyond other Minerals. But you shall haue some stones softer … and therefore the definition is not good. (*EMEMT*; Jorden 1631: 18)

Thomas Gale probes the definition of surgery at length (we quote only an excerpt below), challenging authorities, noting corrupt terminology and seemingly anticipating the physicians' conversation about liquor that Locke described:

(8) I pray you, what call you Chirurgirie?

Iohn Yates. Guido de Cauliaco … defineth it in this sorte. Chirurgirie is a parte of terapentike helinge men by insition, vstion, & articulation.

Iohn Feilde. Those wordes, are taken out of a booke ascribyd to Galen, … But he should not haue called it corruptly terapenticke, but therapeuticke. For Therapeuticon is that part of phisicke, which curyth. this part consisteth eyther in curyng by conuenient diet: eyther by medicyne: or els by outwarde vse of the ha~de. there Galen (or he that was author of the booke aboue said) affirmeth howe +y=t= which healith by the hande, is a portion of the curatiue parte. this helpeth men by incisions, vstions, and reducinge the bones into their naturall seate. (*EMEMT*; Gale 1563c: F2$^{v}$)

This kind of deliberation about definition does not go unchallenged, however. William Bullein urges physicians to keep their focus on practical concern for the patient:

(9) I praie you, so spende no more tyme any lenger in definisions, names, causes, and signes, of apostumacions, but rather I praie you, begin the maner of their proper cures, and helpes (*EMEMT*; Bullein 1562: xij$^{r}$)

Bullein's caution notwithstanding, key to the cure seems to be understanding the terms, from the labelling of body parts to the naming of diseases, all as part of mastering the practice of medicine. The metacommentary reveals some medical writers' awareness of the importance of definitional authority as part of that practice.

## 5.5 Synonymy

Glossing is perhaps the least surprising form of definition in these vernacular medical texts. English lagged far behind Latin and Greek, the traditional languages of science and medicine, in terms of prestige, perceived eloquence and acceptable naturalized vocabulary through at least the first part of the early modern period. Defining in vernacular medical texts, therefore, sometimes involves negotiating the relative prestige of the languages from which terminology comes and supplying English with the vocabulary needed to discuss medicine. Many glosses are introduced with the lexemes 'call' and 'name', and in most sixteenth-century texts, even the collocation of 'call' with 'may' is rare; these texts only infrequently express judgement about what is to be called what when glossing terminology. Most are simple introductions to glosses, usually in Greek, Latin or English, and occasionally in Arabic, a practice that parallels the glossarial convention in contemporaneous dictionaries. Most authors are not explicit about the hierarchical linguistic situation, simply introducing glosses between English and foreign languages without comment. For example, Andrew Boorde equates terms simply in *Breuiary of Helthe*:

(10) CAros is the greke word. In latyn it is named Crepula. In englyshe it is named a surfyt. (*EMEMT*; Boorde 1547: Book 2: 3$^{r}$)

*Prognosticacion* (1554) introduces fever this way:

(11) Pronosticacion of the Feuer or Ague, whiche is called in laten Febris offimera. (*EMEMT*; *Prognosticacion* 1554: Aii$^{r}$)

Occasionally, when English has no equivalent term, the authors offer an English description instead – and often with no apology for English lacking a clear synonym. Boorde provides an example:

(12) DEmoniacus or Demoniaci be the latin words, In Greke it is named Demonici, in Englishe it is named he or they the whiche be madde and possessed of the deuil or deuils, and their propertie is to hurt and kyl them selfe, or els to hurt and kyll any other thyng (*EMEMT*; Boorde 1547: Fiiii$^{v}$)

The texts also provide examples of synonymy that do not involve glossing. For instance, Walter Bailey (1529–92), in *Three Kindes of Peppers* (1588), turns not to foreign languages but to synonyms in English to explain stonecrop:

(13) Likewise the herbe which we call Stonecrop, is also named mouse pepper. And som do cal diptander, herbe pepper, and some sauery pepperwort. (*EMEMT*; Bailey 1588: A4$^{v}$)

The concision of this definitional strategy is reminiscent of the earliest English dictionaries, such as Cawdrey's *A Table Alphabetical*. Occasionally, synonymy is supplemented by additional information. For instance, in the following excerpt, Langton first defines an element as 'a beginning of any thing' and then supplies examples, creating a more elaborated form of definition (more so than many modern dictionaries):

(14) I wyl (by goddes grace) fyrst declare the signification of this worde Elementum, which we maye verye well call in our tonge a begynnynge of any thynge: and thereof it co~meth y=t= the Alphabete letters be called eleme~tes, bicause they are beginners of al maner of languages, & the principles also of euery arte be called Elementes, bycause they are begynners of the same. (*EMEMT*; Langton 1545: Biii$^{r–v}$)

The next two definitional methods also go beyond the content typical of contemporaneous dictionaries – as well as sometimes contemporary ones.

## 5.6 Categorization

In medical texts, as alluded to earlier, the practitioner and reader often depend on full rather than minimal descriptions of diseases in terms of their symptoms or 'accidents'. One result is that categorization by *genus* and *differentia* in these early modern medical texts can expand to encompass extended lists of symptoms of a condition – which could also be seen as defining by relation (see Section 5.7).[8]

Example 15 employs the expression 'that is to say' to introduce a fairly succinct definition relying on the *genus–differentia* model:

(15) but after these elementes be once mixte in the body they can no more be called elementes, that is to say pure, and simple bodyes, & that y~ is made of them, is a bodye mixt, and corruptible. (*EMEMT*; Langton 1547: B6$^{r}$)

Put differently, an *element* is a body which is pure and simple, or is one which is not mixed and hence corruptible; that is, it is not an instance of simple synonymy but of categorization.[9]

A second example from Langton (Example 16) shows that the integration of definition into medical prose can reverse the now traditional ordering of definition, with the lemma first, followed by the definition/explanation/equivalent. In this case, an 'if … then' puts the characteristics of the sickness (in this case, symptoms) to the left and a proposed nomenclature to the right.

[8] Given that the taxonomy of definitional strategies is our modern, artificial imposition onto the data, we simply note that the listing of symptoms can straddle these two categories – examples appear in this section and in the next. Earlier examples of definition by categorization in vernacular medical texts do occur, as in Arderne's treatise on the fistula p. 20; see *MEMT.*

[9] In philosophical terms, this would be considered an intensional definition.

(16) Yf the naturall egestions be holden to long, then the party hath a byndyng disease they saye: but yf they runne to muche, that they call an open disease: And yf a man be bothe bounde and lewse together, than they call that sycknes a combynation of bothe the fornamed euyls (*EMEMT*; Langton 1547: Av$^{v}$)

However, by the end of this passage, what we might consider definition has given way to description: the second 'call' also lacks the equivalent of a simple lemma, since the initial clause refers to 'being both bound and loose'. Logical structures, such as 'if … then', prove a useful device for identifying disease in these texts, often through a description of their outward signs.

Another manifestation of categorization differentiates the item explicitly in terms of the characteristics it does not possess (as seen to some extent with the definition of an element above) rather than those that it does. Robert Recorde describes urine as follows:

(17) It shall not nede here to reken exactly … the generation of vrine / but it shall suffyce … that of the meate & the drynke together concocted in the stomake, is made rude bloude (if I may so cal it) which rude bloud is wrought agayn and made more perfecter in the lyuer: and thyrdly yet more purifyed in the hollow vayne / where the vrine is separate fro~ it … but yet may not exactly be called vrine tyll it cum into the raynes (or kydnes) which draw it out of the hollow vayn by a certayne naturall power restyng in them / And then doth the raynes (or kydneys) alter it parfectely into vrine (*EMEMT*; Recorde 1547: 1$^{v}$)

This passage effectively describes what urine is not, focusing on the appropriate parts of the body and the appropriate process step by step. This example also usefully captures the blurry line between strategies of categorization and relation – in this case, relation to the bodily processes involved in producing urine.

## 5.7 Relation

Medical conditions are often described and defined in these texts in relation to their symptoms and body parts in relation to the body as a whole and to other body parts. We might call this symptomatological defining 'symptomography'.[10] John Banister explicitly links defining and symptomography, as in the ulcer

(18) whose species or kinde is Phagedaena, which is an ambulative Vlcer, which creeping here & there in y=e= skin and subject fleshe, doth

[10] The anonymous *Seynge of Uryns* (1525) and Robert Recorde's *Vrinal of Physick* (1547) prove to be rich sources of medical terms with long lists of symptoms and what they signify.

corrode and feede on the toppe or outward partes, but it neuer perseth inwardly (*EMEMT*; Banister 1575: 10[v])

as well as urging his preference for real definition over the words:

(19) EUerie vlcer hath his proper note or token, whereby he is discried and knowe~ from an other, and they are taken of the definitions of euery of them. Wherefore I suppose it to be worthy the labour here to recite ... the short definitio~s of the chiefe differences aboue me~cioned, wherein doing, wee woulde not haue the Reader to regarde so much the woordes as the thing it selfe. (*EMEMT*; Banister 1575: 10[r])

But, of course, the purpose of these medical texts is to provide the words that will help readers understand the thing itself. And pedagogical texts in medicine continue to rely on the listing of symptoms to understand disease, even if their glossaries and modern dictionaries opt to excise these lists for the sake of concision.

In defining specific parts of the body, early modern writers often understandably turned to maps of the body, as in the fugitive sheets, placing the referent of a term in relation to more familiar physiological terrain. In the following, Braunschweig provides a verbal map of the leg:

(20) THe fyrste that is namyd the thygh is a great mary bone and rounde at both the endys The vppermost roundnes is named Vertebrum and entreth in y=e= brode bonys of the hanches. The nether parte toward y=e= knee hathe .ii. roundnessys whiche co~me in .ii. holownessys of the fyrste shynne bone namyd Os focile and theron is a rou~d brode bone namyd the worle bone or knee shyue and so is the knee full made. Than foloweth the shynne bone and ther be .ii. bonis namyd focilia y=e= byggest in y=e= former syde makyd the gaderynge of the shynnes and co~meth downe from the knees vnto y=e= fote and maketh the anclewe on the inner syde. (*EMEMT*; Braunschweig 1525: Ci[v])

In Example 21, Braunschweig begins with definition by categorization, explaining the skin in relation to a broader category and its distinctive characteristics; as the passage continues, new terms are introduced and defined in relation to the skin:

(21) THe skynne is a couerynge of the hole vnyuersall body wouen out of the vaynes & senewes made for the defence of y=e= wyttes of man and y=t= same skynne is twayne indyffere~t. The one doth couer the vttermost membre & that is named the very skynne The other coureth the innermost parte of the membrys and it is named panniculus or pannycle & that is as a flece lyke as by the selles or chambres of the brayne and pyrocraneum is y=e= thyn flece aboue the braynpanne ... Here after foloweth the fatnesses som is within the skynne & that is

named grece som is within by y=e= bely aboute the kydneys and that is named tallow. (*EMEMT*; Braunschweig 1525: Aiv$^{v}$)

This kind of pedagogical defining practice still characterizes many academic texts, but it is not allowed by the structure of modern dictionaries.

## 5.8 Etymology

At present, a certain definitional authority seems to accompany etymology. It is expected of a comprehensive, authoritative dictionary and is assumed to illuminate the meaning of a word in some way, even if it has been borrowed across multiple languages and has undergone semantic shifts along the way. This study of early vernacular medical texts reveals that etymologies appear almost from the beginning as part of defining medical terms, particularly terms borrowed from other languages. For example, in *Seynge of Uryns* (1525), the author explains the origins of two terms, the first of which is more useful in understanding the definition of the term as used in English:

(22) Trifera sarasenica it is called Trifera bycause it maketh olde men to appere yonge men. And it is called Sarasenica bycause it was founde amonge the Sarasyns. (*EMEMT*; *Seynge of Uryns* 1525: Eiii$^{v}$)

*Prognosticacion* (1554) uses the etymology of *effimeron* as a way to explain the nature of the condition:

(23) THat feuer after Auicen is lyght to heale, and harde to knowe. He y=t= knoweth it can saye and afferme the same. For the feuer I Effirme of his kynde dureth not, but by space of one naturall daye. And therfore he is named … of Effimeron a worde of greke whiche is a name of a certayne fysshe in laten. For that fysshe dyeth y~ same daye that he is gendred. And so it is of this Feuer, for of his nature he endureth but .xxiiij. hours. (*EMEMT*; *Prognosticacion* 1554: Aii$^{r}$)

In *Quydos Questions*, the term 'anatomy' is broken down into its etymological parts:

(24) Anatomie is the right determination and diuision of euery particuler member of the bodye of mankinde. And is deriuate of Ana, that is to saye (n[sic]ight) that is to saye (diuision.) Thus Anatomie, is called n[sic]ight diuision of members, done for certaine knowledges (*EMEMT*; de Chauliac 1579: 5$^{v}$)

John Jones offers reasons in several examples for what things are called, as in:

(25) Diaria, in English an ague of one daye … is [so] called bicause it hathe but one accesse, and endeth by his owne nature in the space of one day (*EMEMT*; Jones 1566: Cvii$^{r}$)

Elsewhere he also comments that this fever is 'aptly' called a *diaria*, although not without interpolating a longer comment on his doubts about the propriety of this appellation:

(26) let none maruel that Galen and other old writers do cal this ague a Diaria feuer when as it is of y=e= substa~ce of a Diaria feuer for that it lasteth more then one daye, for although the name be repugna~t vnto it, yet bicause it hathe one nature wyth others, continuin[eth] his fit or peroxisme from the beginning to thend, co~tinually for the space of certain dayes, wherfore it is most aptly called a Diaria, especiallye wantinge a more proper or conuenyent name to terme it by. (*EMEMT*; Jones 1566: Dvi$^{r-v}$)

In these texts, etymological information can provide authors with the authority to explain terms and to judge the appropriateness of particular terminology. Medical writers appear to be incorporating etymology as part of defining in the vernacular significantly before this becomes a standard part of the English lexicographic tradition.

## 5.9 Ascription and authority

Authority can be appealed to much more straightforwardly in what we propose to call ascriptive definition, which accredits some authority with a definitive name or description for some medical phenomenon.[11] Ascription, which typifies our material throughout, may be subdivided into

- definite ascription, which is ascription to a specific author or source text and is the commonest form;
- indefinite ascription, which is ascription to an unspecified author or source text;
- auto-ascription, which is ascription to oneself.

The difference in implication is very considerable, since definite ascription is often used simply to appeal to authority, while indefinite ascription clearly invites questioning, discussion, disagreement and even controversy, as one might expect with ascription to 'some … others'; auto-ascription may announce a significant status for one's own claims.[12] There is also clearly a difference between the individual first-person singular and first-person plural, the latter claiming to represent a group or, very often, merely a language.

[11] We find this term more concise and less encumbered with connotations than Robinson's (1954) 'stipulative'.

[12] Compare the steady rise in negative polarity related to knowing-verbs noted by Hiltunen and Tyrkkö, which they ascribe to 'the growing interest in the exploration of new phenomena for which no explanation was readily apparent' (Chapter 4, in this volume).

The particular importance of this category for this study is the extent to which it reveals acceptance of and dependence on authority as against claiming that a definition is one's own or at least a conscious modification of the monopoly of a recognized authority.[13] As Pahta and Taavitsainen (2004: 2) point out, 'references to authorities are perhaps the most conspicuous feature of the logocentricity of medieval science', a characteristic which also runs through the early modern period, although with modifications. It has long been a truism of the history of science that this attitude severely constrained advances in scientific knowledge, even in the early modern period, given that appeal to and commentary on authority was 'appreciated above originality' (Taavitsainen 2004: 41).

In the period covered by this chapter, ascriptive definitions are often ascription of a name to a source, either the language or the authority in most cases, but sometimes to particular classes of people or practitioners.[14] These we have called 'ascriptive naming', and few would qualify as definitions in the Aristotelean sense. Ascriptive naming appears in some of the earlier *EMEMT*, for example, this use of 'some' in *Seynge of Uryns*:

(27) Uryne Citrinum or subcitrinu~ & thynne with a thycke substaunce in a womans water betokeneth the Syncopyne and that is faylynge of harte in moeuynge and some call it the Crampe of the harte. (*EMEMT*; *Seynge of Uryns* 1525: G2$^{v}$)

Surveys of authoritative views may be lengthy, as in the 1559 translation of Conrad Gesner on the nature of *aqua vitae*:

(28) Ray. Senior the philosopher saith this medicine is tourned and altered from coloure to coloure, and from taste to taste, and from nature to nature: and therfore the names therof are multiplied. Also Minois a philosopher, if a man aske (saieth he) why is it made rede before it receiued whyt: Answer, that it was twys made blacke, twys turnid into orrenge colour, and receiued twys red coloure. Seing nowe that it receiueth twys red coloure, as red wyne and mans bloud ... the old menne speakinge by similitudes called it red wyne, mans bloud, & dragons bloud, and suche lyke, &c. (*EMEMT*; Gesner 1559: 101)

Ascriptive definition occurs in Timothy Bright's *Sufficiencie of English Medicines* (1580), in arguing for his lengthy definitions of a remedy, a

[13] See Taavitsainen (2004) for a background discussion of the medieval disputation. See also Crisciani (1990) on the learned background to medieval medicine, as well as medicine as *scientia*.

[14] Ascriptive definitions also occur prior to 1500, as in de Chauliac's *Ulcers* f. 81a (*MEMT*), which roughly follows the *genus-differentiae* formula, while also dismissing a symptom considered definitive by another authority, Henry de Mondeville ('Henric').

medicine and a disease, which he pointedly does not ascribe to a conventional authority, using the first person instead. His definition of remedy is:

(29) a remedie … I cal the work of the Physician, wherby health may be repaired. Physicke is an art which taketh charge of y=e= health of man, preseruing & mainteining it present by the right vse of meate, drinke, and exercise, with other such helpes of nature: and restoring the same decayed, by diet, medicine, helpe of hand, or surgerie instrument seuerally vsed, or by ioynt force applyed. Which three are Physicke instruments, whereby the action of curing is performed, which action I call a remedie. (*EMEMT*; Bright 1580: 8)

Bright is also at pains to point out that commonly used nomenclature does not make medicines what they are, since the 'instruments' are not natural. What makes them medicines is the use to which they are put. It is not until the early eighteenth century that medical dictionaries provide an account of comparable length from the lexicographers.

Judgements, often expressed through conditionals, adjectives and adverbs, as well as direct comment, may also be regarded as integral to ascriptive definition, since both reporting the opinion of some authority and asserting the author's own authority should be seen as steps beyond simple synonymy. The following example feels pedagogical in nature, as Langton provides a definition and then seeks to clarify what he seems to anticipate as a point of confusion with another term:

(30) That which the action hath made & finished, is the worke: as bloud, fleshe, & bone, and as ye may call euery action a certayne worke of Nature, so ye can not call euery worke, an actio~: as flesh is a work of nature, & not an action. (*EMEMT*; Langton 1547: D6$^{v}$)

We have seen that Langton stands out among the early authors. In ascriptive definition, he is using techniques other than simple naming, as well as having something to suggest about defining itself. He also uses a range of qualifiers and forms of ascriptive definition, including uncertainties or even exasperation at having no authoritative ('proper') names in English:

(31) y=e= veyne which is called Porta, & also of y=t=, that is called Caua vena, we haue no names in our tungue whych be propre or peculier to them onely, but muste be fayne to call them master veynes, and in dede so that we vnderstande the thynge, it shall make but lytle matter for names: howbeit Gallen sayth, that the one is called Porta, bycause that the iuyce commeth through it, and the other I thynke is called Caua, bycause it is a great hollowe veyne, well what well what so euer it be called, it groweth of the liuer, and carieth blood from the liuer to the hert (*EMEMT*; Langton 1545: Eiiii$^{v}$)

First-person plural ascription ('we call') is fairly frequent throughout.

Auto-ascriptive naming seems relatively infrequent until the seventeenth century. The earliest instance found in this data is Recorde's

(32) of the meate & the drynke together concocted in the stomake, is made rude bloude (if I may so cal it) (*EMEMT*; Recorde 1547: 11$^{v}$)

but only a handful of pre-1600 examples have been found to date. It is also worth noting that the comparable search string 'I name' was not found at all in the data, perhaps because of the claim implied by the 'give a name to' sense of the word (see *OED*, sense I, 1a). Because ascriptive definition in its various forms is very frequent in the material and is a basic model implying deference to authority, changes in its application are vital to understanding how thought-styles in medical writing undergo change.

## 5.10 Conclusions

Corpus-based research opens up the exciting possibility of collecting data to begin to answer new questions. We had little idea of what to expect from these early vernacular medical texts and only slight theoretical or methodological guidance about how to pursue our questions. We believe our findings are just the beginning of an investigation in the definitional practices in early vernacular medical texts. We hope that others will refine the methodologies we have employed and build on our preliminary findings in order to pursue additional questions about definitional practices in play before the beginnings of English lexicography, as traditionally defined.

This study makes it apparent that defining techniques of university-trained scholars, in this case the physicians, although they were not perhaps all that one might expect given the pre-eminence of Aristotle and the medieval philosopher-theologians, were often in advance of the practices of the contemporaneous lexicographers. We hope this study will encourage other scholars to look beyond the sources of the character of English lexicography as described by Read (2003: 187–8) to the vernacular texts in the Early Modern English period and before which were immersed in the work of definition.

The various forms of ascription in questioning authority and provoking scientific discussion and controversy are clearly important for our understanding of the rise of the scientific method generally, although a study more specifically on particular authors and the chronology of the various ascriptive strategies is needed.

A point of particular interest is that surgeons do not figure as much in the present discussion as one might imagine. This is probably because defining and thinking about defining was part of a classical education and had little to do with the more practical training of the barber-surgeons. Despite leading the physicians in producing texts in the vernacular in the sixteenth century (McConchie 1997: 53–6), surgeons lagged in these more abstract conceptual matters.

Our approach has suddenly made visible authors one might not have expected, including the physicians John Jones, Robert Recorde and Christopher Langton, as well as the surgeons William Bullein and Thomas Gale. It broadens the scholarly lexicographic conversation, permitting a more encompassing history of English lexicography, particularly near its beginnings, and by uncovering the historical conversation about definition among physicians, as Locke so aptly described, and among physicians and early English lexicographers.

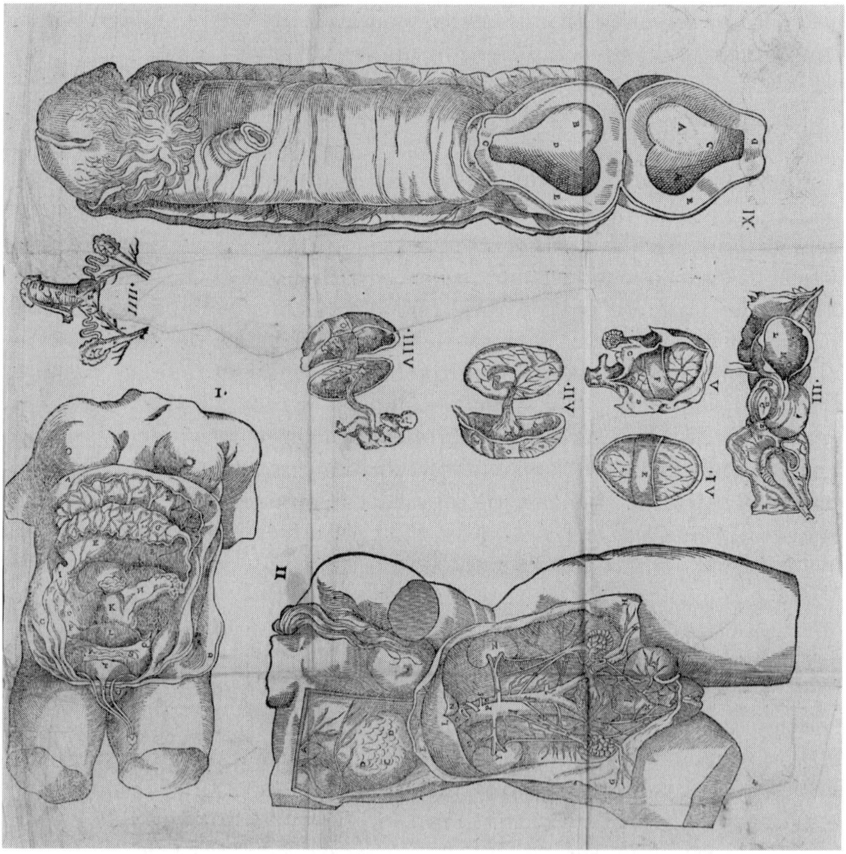

Plate 5 Anatomical diagrams of the female body from *The Birth of Mankynde* by Eucharius Rösslin, 1565

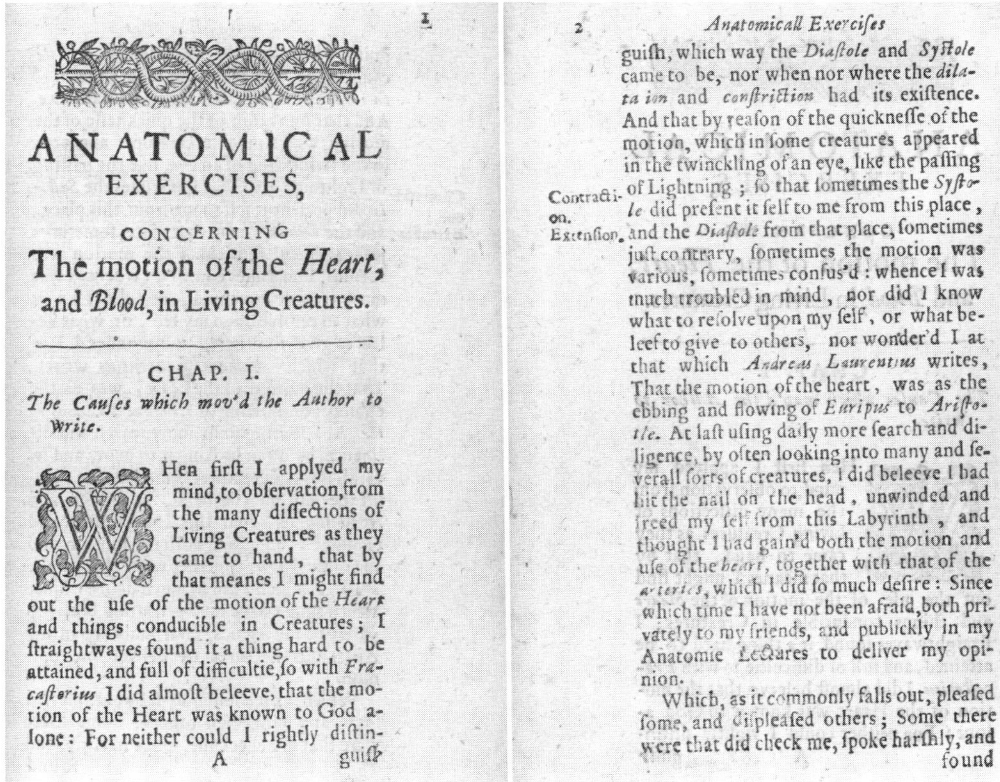

1

ANATOMICAL EXERCISES, CONCERNING The motion of the *Heart*, and *Blood*, in Living Creatures.

CHAP. I.

*The Causes which mov'd the Author to Write.*

WHen first I applyed my mind, to observation, from the many dissections of Living Creatures as they came to hand, that by that meanes I might find out the use of the motion of the *Heart* and things conducible in Creatures; I straightwayes found it a thing hard to be attained, and full of difficultie, so with *Fracastorius* I did almost beleeve, that the motion of the Heart was known to God alone: For neither could I rightly distin-

A guish

2 *Anatomicall Exercises*

guish, which way the *Diastole* and *Systole* came to be, nor when nor where the *dilata ion* and *constriction* had its existence. And that by reason of the quicknesse of the motion, which in some creatures appeared in the twinckling of an eye, like the passing of Lightning; so that sometimes the *Systole* did present it self to me from this place, and the *Diastole* from that place, sometimes just contrary, sometimes the motion was various, sometimes confus'd: whence I was much troubled in mind, nor did I know what to resolve upon my self, or what beleef to give to others, nor wonder'd I at that which *Andreas Laurentius* writes, That the motion of the heart, was as the ebbing and flowing of *Euripus* to *Aristotle*. At last using daily more search and diligence, by often looking into many and severall sorts of creatures, I did beleeve I had hit the nail on the head, unwinded and freed my self from this Labyrinth, and thought I had gain'd both the motion and use of the *heart*, together with that of the *arteries*, which I did so much desire: Since which time I have not been afraid, both privately to my friends, and publickly in my Anatomie Lectures to deliver my opinion.

Contracti-on. Extension.

Which, as it commonly falls out, pleased some, and displeased others; Some there were that did check me, spoke harshly, and found

Plate 6 Pages 1 and 2 of the beginning of William Harvey's discussion on the motion of the heart and the circulation of blood in *Anatomical Exercises*, 1653

# 6 Dissemination and appropriation of medical knowledge: humoral theory in Early Modern English medical writing and lay texts

IRMA TAAVITSAINEN

## 6.1 Introduction and aim of the chapter

The aim of this chapter is to demonstrate how the basic doctrine of humoral theory, with its applications, was disseminated and appropriated in early modern England. The early modern period provides a diversified picture of evolving practices of both professional and lay writing. The educational levels of authors and audiences varied, and we can expect multiple appropriations of basic cultural products like medical commonplaces that formed part of shared meanings, attitudes and values.[1] They found expression in symbolic forms, such as performances, artefacts and texts (Harris 1995: 1). Matters of health are of general interest, and knowledge of the basic doctrines must have penetrated all layers of society in some form. Humoral theory was derived from learned science and originated in academic settings, but in the fifteenth century it became modified for broader audiences: details became less specific; simplified applications were added for everyday use; and the underlying text type often changed from expository to instructive (Taavitsainen 2005).

Meanings and attitudes are encoded in texts, and an analysis of semantic and pragmatic features of language use provides a means to probe into them. My point of departure is the occurrence of the lexical item 'humour' in different contexts, as its occurrences should reveal how the humoral theory was disseminated and appropriated in the early modern period.[2] My hypothesis is that qualitative analyses of the linguistic realization of the relevant text passages reveal essential aspects of the dissemination and appropriation of the doctrine at a time when the world was widening to new continents and fundamental changes were taking place (see Taavitsainen 2009b). Context

[1] Commonplaces are shared cultural products. Before the development of strong vernacular and national intellectual traditions, scientific ideas spread through *loci communes* or commonplaces which circulated widely and belonged to the common stock of scientific ideas in late medieval and early modern England (Maclean 1980: 2).

[2] A preliminary study on semantic and pragmatic meanings of this word is given in Taavitsainen (2006).

provides the key to a multifaceted picture of several levels: semantic word meanings depend on accompanying words, the co-text; pragmatic utterance meanings may change according to context and situation; and larger units of discourse are negotiated at the genre level. Thus, context includes several layers from the immediate micro-level co-text to the macro-level of cultural, intellectual and historical contexts, but meanings and appropriations are elusive and difficult to capture. Language-external facts of the production process, time and situation and socio-historical parameters of authors and audiences are also needed if we want to interpret how people in the past negotiated meaning in these texts (Taavitsainen and Fitzmaurice 2007: 25–6).

In spite of the small number of learned physicians, the influence of the theories of learned medicine upon literate culture was remarkable, as educated laypeople took their knowledge from learned professional medicine; this knowledge often had a life of its own in a lay setting (Wear 2000: 116). The above statement is intriguing, but it needs further specification. Linguistic realizations are always based on choices made between various ways of communicating ideas to different audiences, and there is variation between genres of writing. I shall probe into this issue from the angle of professional versus lay appropriations and focus on cultural practices.

I shall begin my assessment with professional medical writing in the corpus of *Early Modern English Medical Texts* (*EMEMT*). Can linguistic patterns of different text types be detected and how much variation can we find within the corpus categories in the audience scale from learned to 'popular'? The high end of the scale constitutes university-trained physicians and the lower end illiterate people who achieved their knowledge by oral delivery, mostly from almanacs and pamphlets (Capp 1979; Fox 2000; Curth 2007; see also Marttila [Chapter 8] and Ratia and Suhr [Chapter 10] in this volume). After an assessment of medical texts, I shall move on to laypeople's writings and assess what they knew about humoral theory and how they used this knowledge in their correspondence, and to what extent and how fiction and drama refer to humoral theory.

## 6.2 The scale from learned to popular

It has been stated that in 1500 popular culture was everyone's culture and was not restricted to the 'unlearned' (Burke 1978: 207, 208, 270). But if the term 'popular' is understood as varied ways of using shared cultural products (Chartier 1988: 61), we can find evidence for a scale from learned to popular in the late medieval period. In my earlier study on the repertoire of genres in *Middle English Medical Texts* (*MEMT*), I established an inventory of distinguishing linguistic features in texts consumed by different audiences (Taavitsainen 2005). Learned texts give details that differentiate between various species and kinds, whereas more popular texts are satisfied with general statements. Specificity of reference indicates the level of writing in late medieval texts: learned texts state their sources with precision, whereas works for a general and heterogeneous readership often refer to unspecified 'philosophers' or 'wise men' (Taavitsainen and Pahta 1998). The vagueness of reference is in accordance with the idea that 'popular' in an early modern medical context indicates simplistic ideas, but the term 'popular' has also been defined as relatively cheap publications that would appeal to both professional and lay audiences (Curth 2007: 3–4).

My initial assumption was that early modern medical texts would continue the trends observed in late medieval texts, but the data proved more complicated than an issue of polarized 'high' and 'low' culture. Practices change in the seventeenth century, and a downward movement with stylistic shifts emerges: expressions that marked high scholasticism and learnedness in the fifteenth century found their way into more popular texts in the early modern period. In the seventeenth century, the earlier learned ideas and styles of argumentation occur in the most popular handbooks that reached the widest possible audience (Taavitsainen 2009c).

## 6.3 Commonplaces in early modern medical writing

Perhaps the most fundamental of all commonplaces, both from the medical point of view and from the common world view, is the theory of the microcosm of man and the macrocosm of the universe which was connected with humoral theory. This commonplace served to provide explanations for the world order as well as features of more private and individual concerns, such as illnesses or physiognomical features. In the Ptolemaic system, understanding of the natural world and conditions of human life were built on correspondences according to a system of physical and physiological fours: four bodily humours or fluids (blood, phlegm, choler and bile) were related to the four elements (fire, air, earth and water), the four qualities (hot, cold, moist and dry), the seasons of the year, the ages of man and the points of the compass; the twelve signs of the zodiac were treated in groups of four as well (Burrow 1986: 12–13; Siraisi 1990: 104–6; Wear 2000: 37–9). Health was understood as a balance between the humours and sickness as a disruption of this state, due to excess or lack of one of them; moral and religious reasons were also presented (see, for example, Getz 1998: 55–6). This doctrine was part of the cultural common ground in Western Europe and prevailed in all layers of medical and medico-astrological texts as a standard component of learning in the Middle Ages and beyond. Other commonplaces also included astrological elements; for example, the *homo signorum* doctrine of appropriate times and body parts for operating on, bleeding or taking medication was a standard component of medical texts. The Ptolemaic system was giving way to the Copernican: the position of man as the centrepiece of the universe was gradually changing, though the basic doctrine of Galenic medicine survived well into the seventeenth century (Grafton et al. 1992: 163). With the spread of the new Copernican world view, the old gradually became fossilized and lost its status; we can still find references to the old correspondences in the almanac literature of today.

## 6.4 The theory of appropriation and negotiation of meaning

According to the theory of appropriation, common cultural sets are understood and acted upon differently by different audiences. The term 'appropriation' means the process by which meaning is produced and the ways in which discourses affect the reader and lead to a new form of comprehension of oneself and the world (Chartier 1995: 89). In my earlier studies, I have argued for diverse and multiple appropriations according to the levels of audience, genres and text types of writing.[3] Dissemination can be studied by tracing the relevant passages of humoral theory in *EMEMT*, and these passages also reveal how the authors understood and chose to present the theory. But matters of health constitute a fundamental part of the common cultural ground and play an important role in society at large. Evidence of appropriation of medical theories can be found in letters and diaries and in contemporary fiction and drama, as well as in political and religious tracts (Wear 2000: 116).

How meanings are created is a central concern in both semantics and pragmatics, two closely connected and partly overlapping fields of study. The approaches can be used to complement one another, as this chapter demonstrates. Historical semantics traces semasiological and onomasiological changes of linguistic expressions, words and sentences and focuses on changes of meaning and restructuring of lexical fields. Recurring patterns show several unifying threads, and semantic change is closely connected with historical pragmatics, for example through speaker attitudes and politeness, and it is also connected with historical discourse analysis through changes in scope (Traugott and Dasher 2005).[4] Historical pragmatics takes the interlocutors into account and focuses on language in interaction between writer and reader, speaker and hearer, analysing utterances in context. Both sides of communication are considered: what speakers mean and how readers construct the meanings.

The beginning of the semasiological path of the word 'humour' (first attestations in the fourteenth century) shows negative polarity in collocations with technical adjectives mostly describing the unbalanced and disrupted states of the body in Middle English. In the course of time, the word develops into an abstract positive notion, collocated with pleasant ideas. All examples in *MEMT* pertain to the concrete, physiological meanings of the

[3] Genres are defined by external evidence according to their function, for instance, and text types defined by internal linguistic features (see Taavitsainen 2001a). This distinction provides a tool for more accurate descriptions and proved helpful in this context, too.

[4] Scope within the proposition > scope over the proposition > scope over discourse.

word. An assessment of the collocates of 'humour' in *MEMT* shows that 'hot', 'fiery', 'watery', 'moist', 'dry', 'black' and 'kind' are frequent; 'unkynd', 'corrupt', 'rawe' and 'malencolyous' occur as well. The semasiological pathway shows a change from constitutional physiological senses to temporary states of mind, a particular disposition or liking for some action without apparent ground or reason and a quality of action that excites amusement. Present-day 'humour' has come to mean the faculty of perceiving what is ludicrous or amusing, or it describes the mood. 'Humour' has completed the first step, from concrete to abstract, but the word has not developed markedly subjective meanings.[5]

## 6.5 Data and method

The data of my study is divided into two kinds: professional and lay writing. *EMEMT* was searched for medical texts (see Chapter 2 for a description). My method of assessment is qualitative, but the passages were located by the corpus-linguistic software WordSmith4. The word 'humour' was searched in *EMEMT* with the string *humo**, which catches the various spelling variants.[6] The KWIC (keyword in context) concordance option proved helpful as it indicated important discourse loci for the assessment of pragmatic meanings, and the narrow context of the concordance line showed attributes for the study of semantic meanings. The 'Main Sort on Left' (L1) function of the concordance viewing options sorts the entries according to the alphabetical order of the word immediately to the left of the search word, which makes it easy to assess the co-text of attributive adjectives. Collocations of words and word sequences group in interesting ways and have a tendency to occur in certain semantic environments (Sinclair 1991: 112; Hoey 2005: 22–3).

For lay appropriations of the term 'humour', a comprehensive database of correspondence, the *Parsed Corpus of Early English Correspondence* (*PCEEC*) was searched.[7] The word is not very frequent (0.14/1,000 words), as matters of health are not the main topic in correspondence, though they are an essential component in private communication. Yet some examples could be found, and they show how the term was used in both medical and metaphorical senses. For a better insight into laypeople's appropriation of the humoral theory, I made corpus searches with the same string *humo** in other contemporary corpora to locate relevant passages for qualitative analysis. I checked the *Corpus of English Dialogues* (*CED*) for the medical sense of 'humour', as fiction and drama have been mentioned as potential sources of

5 Its prototypical centres are 'mood' and 'amusement', but, unlike 'wit', it has not developed meanings associated with self-expression (see Koivisto-Alanko 2000: 240, 247).

6 The word list created with WordSmith4 of *EMEMT* was used to check the coverage.

7 *PCEEC* contains 4,970 letters in eighty-four letter collections, approximately 2.2 million words. For details, see http://www.helsinki.fi/varieng/CoRD/corpora/CEEC/pceec.html (accessed 27 August 2010).

information about how laypeople understood and appropriated medical doctrines.[8] This material shows that the meaning of this word was in transition, and references to the humoral theory were not frequent. Only a few illuminating passages could be found in contemporary handbooks and drama. They will be quoted as illustrations of the state of the semantic meaning. For the best example, i.e. a metatextual passage of the meaning of 'humour', I had to go beyond the corpus material.

## 6.6 Empirical study

The importance of the humoral doctrine in the medical corpus is manifested in the frequency of the word 'humour': it occurs more than 2,000 times in *EMEMT*.[9] Principles of humoral physiology formed part of the core of the academic training of sixteenth- and seventeenth-century university-educated physicians (Thomas 1980: 10). Society at large ultimately derived its knowledge of this theory from learned medicine. The point of departure in humoral theory is the definition of health as the balance of humours and sickness as a disrupted balance or corrupt humours generated within the body through some poison, as in plague. Curing procedures aimed at restoring the balance, and favoured therapies were bleeding, purging or vomiting in order to recreate a balanced humoral mix and to get rid of the plethora of excess humours (Wear 2000: 39). The frequencies of the search item in the categories of the medical corpus are given in Table 6.1.

### *6.6.1 General treatises or textbooks*

Out of the twenty texts in this category, sixteen contain the search item, with 282 hits in all. The highest frequency is found in Thomas Brugis' *Marrow of Physicke* (1648), with 6.24/1,000 words; next comes Leonardo Fioravanti's *Discourse of the Secrets* (1652a) with 4.77/1,000 words, and Petrus Pomarius' *Enchiridion medicum* (1609) with 4.65/1,000 words. I shall deal with this category in more detail than others, as the texts display different discourse forms and styles of writing and represent the scope of *EMEMT* as a whole, giving a good overview of the dissemination of humoral theory.

The discourse form of *Enchridion medicum* is dialogic. The doctor is examining a student, who answers according to scholastic conventions with absolute certainty and employs the enumerative text strategy. The dialogue

[8] *The Corpus of English Dialogues*, 1560–1760, contains 1.2 million words. It is divided into authentic dialogues (trial proceedings and witness depositions) and constructed dialogues (drama comedy, didactic works, miscellaneous works and prose fiction); see http://www.engelska.uu.se/Research/English_linguistics/A_Corpus_of_English_Dialogues (accessed 27 August 2010).

[9] An earlier version of *EMEMT* was used for the empirical part of this study. The corpus is compiled of text extracts, and only the more concise treatises are included in full; this means that passages of humoral theory may occur in parts not included in *EMEMT*.

Table 6.1 *Frequency of 'humour' in EMEMT.*

| Corpus category | Raw frequency | Frequency/1,000 words |
|---|---|---|
| 1. General treatises and textbooks | 282 | 2.15 |
| 2. Treatises on specific topics | 917 | 1.87 |
| 3. Recipe collections and *materia medica* | 169 | 0.59 |
| 4. Regimens and health guides | 468 | 1.79 |
| 5. Surgical and anatomical treatises | 378 | 1.22 |
| 6. *Philosophical Transactions* | 46 | 1.15 |

is built on short questions, often prefixed by an imperative 'Tel me what', or a somewhat longer and polite opening, and occasional feedback follows in phrases like 'That is very true' (see Taavitsainen 1999: 257–8; 2009a). The following example (1) also contains an extensive simile to make the discourse more vivid. In the examples, the main contents of the humoral passages are given in bold.

(1) **Doc**. I am also of your opinion, but I pray you go forwards, and declare vnto mee **the differences of humours**.

**Stud**. I will in no wise omit **the differences of humours**, which be in number **eight, foure naturall, and foure vnnaturall**: I haue alreadie shewed that the naturall is bloud, flegme, choler, and melancholy, the vnnatural is the same, turned by putrefaction, … **And euen as there perceiued in new wine, foure differences of humours**, viz. the flower or boyling of the wine, seco~ndly the watry substance of the wine, thirdly the feces or dregges thereof, and lastly the pure and sincere wine; (*EMEMT*; Pomarius 1609: 14–15)

After this, the discussion continues with direct questions: 'What is bloud/flegme/choler/melancholy, or black choler?' Each is discussed and defined briefly: 'Bloud is a temperate humour, hot and moist.' Authorities such as Galen are referred to occasionally. The dialogue form involves the reader with pronouns of the first and second person. The causes of diseases are also explained in terms of humoral theory:

(2) **All these foure humours**, as I haue said, being made vnnaturall, they turne to **the hurt of the body**, as when **melancholy** is burned, it beco~meth vitious, and causeth madnes: when it is mingled with too much **flegme**, it causeth a doltish disposition, and worketh cold diseases. When **blood** becommeth vnnatural, it is made wheyish and

watrish, and is very hurtfull, as in the hydropsie: when red **choler** is burned, it becommeth vitious and biting: when **flegme** is made vnnaturall through a weak digesture, it is made a watrish **humor**, and so hurtfull to the body. (*EMEMT*; Pomarius 1609: 16–17)

Dialogues are a common discourse form in textbooks of the early modern period. The target audience must have been students of the medical profession, as the text begins with the qualities of a good surgeon and proceeds to explain the basic conceptions and theories.

Leonardo Fioravanti's *Discourse of the Secrets* represents medical prose targeted at professionals. As in the previous examples, the writing is scholastic with an assured style and an enumerative text strategy, in accordance with the general trend of the textbook category (see Taavitsainen 2009c). Definitions are frequent:

(3) **SIcknesse** or Infirmitie **is** no other thing then **a distemperature of humours** in the bodies of creatures, as well reasonable as unreasonable, which are subject to sickness and to death (*EMEMT*; Fioravanti 1652a: 1)

The text discusses various diseases. Sicknesses are due to an imbalance of humours, and some, like the gout, receive a great deal of attention. Both aetiology and therapy are treated:

(4) **THe Gout** which cometh to men, **is a distemperature** and alteration, which is **caused of corrupt and undigested humours**, and also of feeding on meats that nourish much, and then to use no exercise (*EMEMT*; Fioravanti 1652a: 28)

(5) CHAP. XXXVIII. What order must be used in curing of the said Gout.

SEeing the Gout (as I said before) are grosse humours undigested coming of the aforesaid cause, **it were most necessary, if thou wilt cure them to do** three operations. **The first** of them is Phlebothomie, which **must be done** under the tongue, cutting overthwart one of those two veines: For that Phlebothomie evacuateth the stomocall humours that are cause of that corruption. **The second** operation **that is to be done**, is to assubtiliate the gross and rotten humours, and to evacuate them quite. **The third** operation **that is to be done**, is to preserve nature in good temperature, and to help the digestion, and thus doing, the said infirmity shall be extincted. (*EMEMT*; Fioravanti 1652a: 31)

The text which has the highest frequency count for the word 'humour' is *Marrow of Physicke* by Thomas Brugis, an English army surgeon who styles himself a 'Doctor of Physic'.[10] Although the title declares the text to be 'a learned discourse', it is more in accordance with late medieval compilations than professional treatises of the early modern period. The book contains a survey of the basic doctrines of humoral theory. Correspondences are given, and Avicenna and Galen are referred to. The section begins with a definition according to medieval naming practices (Taavitsainen 2002: 209):

(6) **AN humour is whatsoever is moist**, and liquid in substance, into which the nourishment is first converted in the body of living creatures endewed with bloud, **and is called an humour**, not because all of them have one, and the same force of moistning, but because all of them have a fluent substance. **For choler and melancholy** (according to Reolanus) **are drie humours**; humours because of their liquid consistence, and drie because they have the naturall force of drying. **The humours** are the first begotten matter, out of the mixture of the four elements; choler of fire; phlegme of water; melancholy of the earth; bloud of the aire; for it is hot and moist, as the aire (*EMEMT*; Brugis 1648: 21)

Reader involvement is created by references to the domestic environment and an inclusive use of 'we' ('the meate we eat'):

(7) **Blood in complexion is hot**, and moist, rather temperate, in colour Red, Rosie, or Crimson; in smell, not stinking, in taste savoury, of indifferent consistence, neither too thicke, nor too thinne, and is of **the nature of three signes** of the Aire, Gemini, Libra, Aquarius, and hath its originall in the very first minute of our creation, and is encreased by the meate we eat, ... **much like in consistence to almond butter**, and this is called the Chylus which is formed round, that it may be the better sucked out, for were it like a trough, that which was before concocted would be over much, (*EMEMT*; Brugis 1648: 21)

The vocabulary is somewhat simpler and less technical than in the two other works discussed above; for example, the description of death is straightforward and simplified:[11]

(8) **Blood** is the matter containing the spirits, of which the life, and every operation of the vegetative vertue consists ... for it **is the treasure**

[10] According to the *Oxford Dictionary of National Biography*, Brugis' medical qualifications are obscure. He practised for seven years as a surgeon during the Civil War and may have received his education in Paris.

[11] The blunt statement resembles that of *Sidrak and Bokkus*, the late medieval encyclopaedic work in rhyming couplets from the fifteenth century: 'And if a man of þise wantid oon / His body were deed anoon' (Burton 1998: 497).

**of life through the losse whereof followes death immediately.** (*EMEMT*; Brugis 1648: 24–5)

The text foregrounds astrological information, for example, the *homo signorum* commonplace of medieval medicine is repeated with planetary descriptions and symbols:

(9) **Cancer hath dominion** in the pappes, breast, ribs, the upper part of the belly, part of the stomacke, the spleen and lungs; **it ruleth over phlegmaticke humours, and denoteth** impediments in the eyes, darkenesse in the sight, spots and pustles in the face, the scab, leprosie, lithargy, galling of the skinne, and evill sickenesses of the body and face comming of phlegme.

... **Mars circleth** his sphere once in two yeares almost, he is a planet hot, and drie immoderately, governes the gall, veines, sinewes, and stones, **the humour cholericke, disdainefull, seditious, cruell, bold, and carelesse persons: the greatnesse of his body is once so bigge as the earth, and halfe so bigge, and an eight part, his character is thus.** (*EMEMT*; Brugis 1648: 14–15)

Similar texts circulated in the late medieval period, and passages like Examples 9 and 10 occur in multiple contexts from professional tracts to popular lore and almanac literature. Prognostications and physiological rules of recognition of various types of people achieve a prominent place in the following passage:

(10) **Those in whom this humour abounds are beautified** with a fresh and rosie colour, gentle and well natured, pleasant merry, and facetious; it is best generated in the **spring**, and accordingly in **youth**, that is to say, from the five and twentieth yeare to the thirtieth yeare of age. (*EMEMT*; Brugis 1648: 25)

In places, familiar non-medical items of information are brought in as illustrations of the physiological processes of the body. This device facilitates understanding as it presents concrete parallels from everyday life with abstract notions and is common in popular scientific writing even today.

(11) nature hath ordained these **phlegmaticke humours**, which as it were distilling out of the veines, doe water and moisten them; **not unlike the oyling the Axel-tree of a Coach, without which it would (as we see by daily experience) be burned into dust**; but **this office of this humour** is not profitable nor necessary for every one, for infantes, and weake impotent people, that can neither walke nor worke, but sit idle, doe not need this moisture; but those that labour hard, and go much, have extraordinary need of it. (*EMEMT*; Brugis 1648: 28)

The book was written to provide practical guidance and advice on how to deal with problems that people confronted in everyday life. The title page of the book explains that it 'shall be usefull and necessary in any private House, with little labour, small cost, and in short time'. Metadiscourse reveals the explicit purpose of the text: 'And these things thus understood, you may know what humour raigneth in the sicke, and at what time he shall be most grieved' (*EMEMT*; Brugis 1648: 35). The work is dedicated to a woman, Margaret Evre, confirming that the main target audience were women.[12] We have no records of the actual users of this book, but the 'Preface to the Reader' states that the book provides 'a plaine way to help the poorer sort' 'for the generall good' and is 'useful in a private house'; even the illiterate are mentioned as a potential audience: 'for if my booke come amongst the illiterate, let me make it the best waies that can be devised.' Women took care of the household and dealt with sicknesses and their cures but were not as well educated as men, and their degrees of literacy varied (see Jones, Chapter 3 in this volume). The contents of the book show what the learned author considered important and necessary for women to know, and it also explains how to act upon this knowledge.

### 6.6.2 *Treatises on specific topics*

The subcategories of treatises on specific topics show very different frequencies for the search item. Highest proportions are found in Categories 2a, 2b, and 2c, whereas Categories 2d and 2e are poorly represented.[13] Compared to the category of general treatises or textbooks, specialized texts form a fairly homogeneous group and discuss humoral theory in a professional way. The text often begins with definitions of humours or sicknesses (see McConchie and Curzan, Chapter 5 in this volume). For example, the text with the highest frequency of all in this category gives a definition of gout which is very similar to Example 4 from Category 1:

(12) **The Gout is a griefe of the feet, occasioned by some distemperature, or irregular humor**, which either is bred in the joynts of the feet, and toes, by some weaknesse thereof, or by deflux hath descended from some upper part thereunto. That the nature of the Gout may the better appeare, I will verbatim expound this definition (*EMEMT*; Holland 1633: 2)

The earliest text on melancholy, Timothy Bright's *Treatise of Melancholy*, defines the disease:

[12] Her name is not mentioned in the *Oxford Dictionary of National Biography*, which indicates that she did not belong to the highest ranks of society.

[13] The texts with the highest scores in the subcategories (see Chapter 2 for details): 2a: Philemon Holland, *Gutta podagrica* (1633) with 7.84/1,000 words; 2b: Simon Harward, *Phlebotomy* (1601) with 5.98/1,000 words; 2c: Thomas Russel, *Diacatholicon avrevm* (1602) with 6.77/1,000 words; 2d: Robert Pemell, *De morbis puerorum* (1653) with 2.69/1,000 words; 2e: Stephen Bradwell, *Physick for the plagve* (1636) with 2.25/1,000 words.

(13) **[M]elancholie ... signifieth** in all, either a certayne fearefull disposition of the mind altered from reason, or else **an humour of the body**, co~monly taken to be the only cause of reason by feare in such sort depraued. **This humour is of two sorts**: naturall, or vnnaturall: naturall is either the grosser part of the bloud ordained for nourishment, which either by abundance / or immoderate hotenesse, passing measure, surchargeth the bodie, and yeeldeth vp to the braine certaine vapors, whereby the vnderstanding is obscured; ... all organicall actions therof are mixed with melancholie madnesse; (*EMEMT*; Bright 1586: 1–2)

The most important forms of therapy are explained in various specialized tracts for professional practitioners of medicine. The main cures were all connected with humoral theory:

(14) **PHlebotomy is the letting out of bloud** by the opening of a vayne, for the preuenting or curing of some griefe or infirmitie. I take in this place bloud, not as it is simple and pure of it self, but as it is **mingled with other humours**, to wit, fleame, choler, melancholy, and the tenue serum, ... And although it still fall out that **other humours are also by Phlebotomy euacuated** out of the whole body, (*EMEMT*; Harward 1601: 1)

(15) A generall powder of Gold, **purging all offensiue humours** in mans BODIE: Good in generall for all diseases, where there needeth any Purgation:

As also for any sicknesse yearely incident, or which is feared to approach by the increase of **any euill humour**, distemperature of diet, or otherwise how so euer growing towards any disease, to preuent the same, and keepe the bodie in health. (*EMEMT*; Russel 1602: B1r)

(16) Of Vomits.

**IS the expulsion of bad humors** contained in the Stomach; upward it is accounted, if wisely administred, as to the mitigation of the violence rightly considered of, to be the wholesomest kinde of Physick, for those which are gross, or **full of humors**: (*EMEMT*; Culpeper 1659: 225)

### 6.6.3 *Recipe collections and* materia medica

This category contains texts that focus on the preparation of medicaments. It includes collections of recipes, herbals and instructions for preparation of substances.

Knowledge of humoral medicine forms the basis of treatment, but diagnostic skills are taken for granted, and humoral theory lies in the background.

An early text from 1528 continues the medieval tradition of lapidaries, which attribute magical virtues to stones. For example, it tells about the powers of a stone called 'the soryge':

(17) It is good also for the syckenesse of the stomake and **for the humours of a mans body** & agaynst all wode beest~ and the bytyng~ of other vermyns and venomous beestes if a man drinke of the water that this Soryge stone hath touched he shall be in no peryll nor daunger of all these thynges aforesayde. And also this sayd stone healeth a man in lykewyse of all maner of syckenesses of the stomake. **And also the body of euyll humours**: and he that shall haue and bere this sayd stone he ought to be honest and clene of his body. (*EMEMT*; *Lytell Boke of the .xxiiii. Stones*, 1528: B4v–5r)

All occurrences of the word 'humour' in remedy books reflect the underlying reliance on humoral theory; it provides the premise, and there is no need for further explanation.

(18) Headake vvhose cause is not knovven. Him also that hath headake and woteth not whereof it is mayest thou heale of thys wyse: Take a penyworth of pepper … let him kepe it thus in hys mouth a whyle and **it shall drawe the euell humors out of the head into the mouth**. Thys must be done fastinge and thre houres in the daye. (*EMEMT*; Braunschweig 1561: 5)

(19) For Warts, and Cornes. Warts are of divers formes, and very troublesome, by reason that for the most part, they are on the hands, which are continually used, **they proceede of a mellancholly humor**, and are cured according to their formes; (*EMEMT*; Hawes 1634: 29)

The following passage comes from the very end of the period. It is from William Salmon's *Phylaxa medicinae* and contains a similar discussion of remedies based on humoral theory:

(20) It is singular against the Plague, and **all other Diseases arising from sharpness and obstructions of the humours, or stagnation of the Blood**. It is an **excellent remedy in all cases of putrefaction of the Blood and Humours**; prevails against Rheumatisms and Gouts, … It is of singular use in easing Pains of the GOUT, **repelling of the Humors**, and resolving of the tartarous matter, by bathing the part affected therewith Morning and Evening, and applying Stuphes wet therein to the same. (*EMEMT*; Salmon 1700b: 11)

### 6.6.4 *Regimens and health guides*

The category comprises texts focusing on a good life and the preservation of health, providing advice on diet (food and drink) and various aspects of lifestyle, such as exercise, sleep, sexuality and the healthiness of environments. Philip Moore's *Hope of Health*, with 5.77/1,000 words, has the highest number of hits in this category. Correspondences are explained, and a definition of health is included:

(21) THere bee in the bodie of **all mankinde**, fower **sondrie humours**, that is, **bloode, fleume, choler and melancholie**: which humours are daielie nourished and engendred, of the iuise of meates and drinkes, receiued into the body, and there altered by naturall heat. **These humours, maie bee called the second elementes**, … **These .4. humours, as long as the bodie is in health, doe remaine in soche porcion, as nature ordained theim in at the firste generacion of the bodie**: (*EMEMT*; Moore 1565: 10v)

A discussion about healthy diet contains arguments from humoral theory. The text form is dialogic. It does not contain well-defined roles, like Example 1 above, but the author debates with an imagined audience:[14]

(22) But mee thinks I heare some, by reason of that which hath beene already said, aske mee a question, whether a draught of drinke in a morning fasting, be not, in the rules of wholesome diet, to be allowed of? Their colour to cleare this their custome, is this: a draught in a morning (say they) **washeth downe all ill humors, that lie in the stomack**, or places adjoining, and withall, is good against the stone. I answer, (*EMEMT*; Hart 1633: 112–13)

### 6.6.5 *Surgical and anatomical treatises*

Descriptions of human anatomy and books focusing on various aspects of surgery are placed in this category. In addition to the core material, these books contain advice on diet and exercise, remedies and recipes, so that there is an overlap with other categories. A surgical text from 1543 discusses phlebotomy in the following way:

(23) **FLebothomye (as the doctours testify) is a good euacuation of humours**, and surer, than a purgation receyued by the mouth, for it lyeth in the chirurgyens wyll, to emptye euyl blood, and kepe in the

[14] The text contains an innovative phrase (see below, Section 6.6.8) in a passage with a discussion according to humoral theory: 'Let Londoners, and others that frequent the city much, looke about them, and **moderate their insatiable wine-bibbing humor**, lest withall they drinke downe some of this stuffe, whereof Pliny here complaines. Sure I am our Vintners are as cunning' (*EMEMT*; Hart 1633: 122).

good, by closynge of the veyne. And it is a synguler remedye to heale diseases procedynge of **aboundaunce of bloode of euyll qualitie**, as Arnoldus de villa noua, declareth, gyuynge a good definition of the same, and sayinge: Flebothomye is the cuttynge of a veyne, **purgynge bloode and humours** rennynge therewithall. (*EMEMT*; de Vigo 1543: 221v)

A text from the middle of the seventeenth century, *Vade mecum* by Thomas Brugis, the author of *Marrow of Physicke* (Examples 6–11 above), also discusses humoral theory (5.54/1,000 words). His two texts are written for very different target groups, but both repeat the received wisdom of humoral theory and contain practical advice. In the example below, the readers are addressed using the imperative, and an application is appended at the end of the passage:

(24) **By Humor understand not**, with Philosophers, a quality opposite to driness, but a body, yet not any, for chyle, seed, milk, sweat, urine, &c. are not properly humors, but only the alimentary with their excrements: 'tis rashness to deny them, seeing they affect us in quantity, quality, &c. they're begot of the mixtion of aliments, four in general.

1. Natural, going under the name of **bloud**, whose **hot, cold, thick, thin** parts, are call'd **choler, phlegm, melancholy**; serum's their vehicle, expell'd by urine, sweat, tears, &c. **Pure bloud makes men blithe, florid, prudent, &c. but if it redound, foolish**, &c. (Brugis 1689: A5)

There was an overlap between physiognomy and practical medical texts from the late medieval period onwards, and a professional treatise such as *Vade mecum* shows both how fuzzy the borderlines are and also that practical applications such as physiognomical rules were appreciated by medical practitioners as well as by laypeople. This handbook became a best-seller and ran to seven editions, clear proof of the author's success in reaching his audience.

### *6.6.6* Philosophical Transactions

Texts in this category are extracted from *Philosophical Transactions* (*PT*), and they deal with physiology and anatomy or the nature of medical substances. They are accounts of medical experiments and discoveries or reviews of medical books. The passage below shows that a new phase in the treatment of humoral theory had begun in spearhead research. The old received truth is questioned, and reliance on empirical evidence enhanced.

(25) An Experiment of Signior Fracassati upon Bloud grown cold.

When any **bloud** is become cold in a dish, that part which is beneath the superficies appears much blacker, than that on the top;

and 'tis vulgarly said, that this black part of the bloud is **Melancholy bloud**, and men are wont to make use of this example to shew that the **Melancholy humor** as 'tis called, enters with the 3 others into the composition of the bloud. **But** Signior Fracassati maintains, that **this blackish colour comes from hence, that the bloud, which is underneath, is not expos'd to the Air, and not from a mixture of Melancholy**: to prove which he assures, that upon its being expos'd to the Air it changes colour, and becomes of a florid red. An Experiment as easie to try, as 'tis curious. (*EMEMT*; *PT*, 1667: 492)

Another experiment, from 1694, this time on worms, concludes with the following statement, which refers to 'humour' as a concrete substance:

(26) but why, I know not, they now all dyed the same day before I was got home, when as formerly I had kept them Fourteen or Fifteen days; they had fasted three days before I had them. I had the Curiosity to try whether I could find any Blood in them, but did not; **which makes me think they feed of the same Humour they are bred of**. (*EMEMT*; *PT*, 1694: 222–3)

### 6.6.7 *Lay texts*

#### 6.6.7.1 *Correspondence*

The word 'humour' does not occur very frequently in *PCEEC*, but the corpus provides a different array of examples from professional discourse in *EMEMT*. Royal letters by Queen Elizabeth I provide interesting examples. The author represents the highest level of education outside the professional circles, and these passages show familiarity with humoral theory and the appropriation of professional terms in new, more abstract and figurative ways:

(27) Elizabeth I to James VI of Scotland 1590
Eccept my howrely care for **your broken countrey**, to to muche **infected with the maladie of strangers humors**, and to receue **no medecin so wel compounded** as if the owner make **the mixture appropriatted to the qualetye of the siknes**. (*PCEEC*; Royal 1 1590: 57)

A similar use is also included in a letter by John Holles (Senior), to John Holles (Junior), from 1633, with reference to Queen Elizabeth:

(28) Mansfelds employments purged this realme of sum ill **humors**, yet like a fontanelle of good spirits allso: peradventure in regard of the party and the cause, many Voluntaries ar expected: but that **humor** dyed with Queen Elisabeth: (*PCEEC*; Holles 1633: III, 452)

The meaning of a temporary mood is also recorded in Elizabeth's letters:

(29) Elizabeth I to James VI of Scotland
I confes that diuers be the **affections** of many men, some to one, some to another, but my rule of trust shal neuer faile me whan it is **grounded, not on the sandes of euery mans humor, but on the stedy rock of approued fact** (*PCEEC*; Royal 1 1594: 103–4)

A reference to medical applications of the term is given in a letter between two aristocratic lady friends, the Countess of Bedford writing to Lady Cornwallis in 1626:

(30) I am very incredulous that itt can prevent my having more **fitts of the goute**; howsoever, when I am trobled with any, they are accompanied with such accidents of sicknes as shows **they proseed from such humors as phisicke uses to correct, against which I have too rebellious a spleene** I doubt to be brought into such obedience as not faster to power out the souernes therof into my stomache, and distill itt into other parts, then all the poticarie's drugs will be able to correct (*PCEEC*; Cornwallis 1626: 145–6)

The following example records the use of humoral commonplaces in a description that a patient gives about himself to his doctor. Sir Hamon L'Estrange writes to Sir Thomas Browne in 1653:

(31) **I am** aged neere yeares, **of sanguine humour, and a thinn cholerique frame of body**, and was taken with the Palsey 3 yeares since, though I prayse god I endure no great affliction or disability thereby: I doe not find but my cheife vitalls are well conditioned, onely some spleenatique obstructions, (*PCEEC*; Browne 1653: 286)

The above occurrences show a clear understanding of the medical doctrine among the upper classes of society. Humoral theory was part of the common cultural ground so that more abstract uses were possible. Elizabeth I was skilful in appropriating the theory in an extended metaphorical sense to describe the state of affairs in the realm. In another example, the meaning of temporal moods is foregrounded. Laypeople revert to humoral theory to describe their maladies, and human mental states are attributed to a bodily organ. A self-description relies on humoral theory and correspondences, appropriating the common ground that both the upper-class patient and the physician understood.

### *6.6.7.2 Handbooks*

In the *CED*, abstract meanings prevail, and only a few contexts refer to the original physiological sense. The clearest examples are found in handbooks. A text from 1625 contains a moralistic passage on the dangers of the lustful life engendering 'euill humours':

(32) Yea, I tell you the pure truth thereof: **for euery man that loseth the time after his lusts**, doth lose his courage: loseth his renowne: loseth

the force of his body: puts his bodie in many dangers: strayeth himselfe from the favours of God: tormenteth his conscience: **encurreth many excesses and scabs, excrements, cathaires and euill humours**. Moreouer, dulleth his noble memory (*CED*; Wodroephe, *The French Tongve*, 1625)

Another handbook contains the following passage referring to the medical theory of humours as the original cause of the states of mind, and it also refers to purging as the way to treat anxiety and to ensure peace of mind:

(33) [Ma.] Trust mee truly, hee comes ouer him with kindnesse; this hony was not fetched from the Bees hiue, but from the Aspes hole, more like to stir **choler** then to procure rest.

[Nick.] This tricke he learned in his passage of Charon the Ferriman; to looke towards peace with his face, and rowe towards discord with his pen. He sets out the Oliue branch for a signe, but his vessels are full of **gall** and wormewood within.

[Min.] If we may take his owne word in his owne worke, it is the gentle sound of a solid answere, **It is a purgatory sallet to purge his prophane humours**, made of fiue medicinable hearbs, (*CED*; *A Cvrry-Combe for a Coxe-Combe*, 1615: 9–10)

The above examples are in accordance with medical theory of the time and show that these cases were based on a firm and widespread general knowledge. Thus, humoral theory could be referred to in non-medical handbooks dealing with language teaching and moralistic didactic topics.

### *6.6.7.3 Drama*

In the lay material assessed for this study, the meaning of 'humour' as 'transient states of mind' prevails. In *CED*, the phrase 'your sonne Dowsecer hath made me melancholy with his humour' occurs in a comedy from 1599 (Chapman, *Humerous Dayes Myrth*) and refers to contemporary medical theory, but otherwise meanings implying transient states of mind are the rule. The meaning of transient states is so common that a whole genre of 'comedy of humours' developed round this notion (Sampson 1970: 251). The term occurs frequently in titles of plays, the most famous examples being Ben Jonson's (1573?–1637) *Everyman In His Humour* (acted 1598, printed 1601, revised 1616) and *Everyman Out of His Humour* (acted 1599, printed 1601). The term is discussed in the latter play, using physiological explanations, showing that the original physiological sense was common knowledge, but the transient moods and significations of outward features were already current as well:

(34) *Humor.* So in euery humane body
The choller, melancholy, flegme, and bloud,
By reason that they flow continually

In some one part, and are not continent,
Receiue the name of Humours. Now thus farre
It may by *Metaphore*, apply it selfe
Vnto the generall disposition:
As when some one peculiar qualitie
Doth so possesse a man, that it doth draw
All his affects, his spirits, and his powers
In their confluctions all to runne one way,
This may be truly said to be a Humour,
But that a rooke, in wearing a pyed feather,
The cable hatband, or the three-pild ruffe,
A yard of shooetye, or the *Switzers* knot
On his *French* garters, should affect a Humour!
O, 'tis more then most ridiculous. (Jonson [1601] 1954: lines 98–114)

Metatextual passages like the above are rare witnesses of how the concept 'humour' was misunderstood and appropriated in the early modern period.

### *6.6.8 Semantic collocations and meanings*

To probe deeper into the semantic development, I assessed the company the word 'humour' keeps in professional and lay texts, in both *EMEMT* and *PCEEC*. The main division is a positive and negative polarity, namely associations with pleasant and unpleasant qualities. Another difference can be located between technical and general terms. The difference proved striking: the collocations and phrases in professional writing clearly deviate from lay examples. Technical terminology prevails in medical texts, whereas adjectives are more varied and mostly occur only once. The scale from positive to negative is also more pronounced in lay texts.

#### *6.6.8.1 Medical (EMEMT, 151 attributive adjectives)*

**Technical collocations and phrases**: 'evil' (84 occurrences), 'melancholic' (71), 'raw' (59), 'corrupt' (48), 'gross' (48), 'cold' (47), 'superfluous' (43), 'ill' (42), 'vicious' (32), 'phlegmaticke' (24), 'bad' (22), 'choleric' (22), 'waterish' (21), 'hot' (18), 'putrid' (16), 'sharp' (14), 'christalline' (13), 'crude' (12), 'slymy' (11), 'rotten' (9), 'undigested' (8), 'tartarous' (4) and 'morbific' (3). In addition, several adjectives are found once, for example, 'acid', 'acrimonius', 'adust', 'albuginus', 'alimentary', 'aqueal', 'aqueous', 'ayere', 'bibbing', 'bilious', 'biting', 'black', 'burnt', 'catarrhous', 'clammy', 'clinging' and 'coagulated'. Positive adjectives, with the exception of 'good/better' (24), are rare: 'healthy', 'laudable', 'light', 'lucky', 'noble' and 'profitable' each occur once.

#### *6.6.8.2 Lay (PCEEC, thirty-three attributive adjectives)*

The repertoire of technical terms is narrow, and only 'ill' occurs more than once (seven occurrences). The following adjectives each occur once and are technical and/or negative: 'clouded', 'cold', 'complaining', 'current', 'dangerous', 'disorded', 'distrustfull', 'dull', 'frantike', 'giddy', 'goutish', 'jealous', 'lazy', 'melancholic', 'mutinous', 'sanguine', 'scorbutic', 'serious', 'sharp', 'strange', 'unpleasant', 'unquiet', 'wandring' and 'wanton'. In contrast to *EMEMT*, the list includes general adjectives connected with temporary states of mind and emotions. Positive notions are more common than in professional medical writing: 'good/better' (10); 'ambitious', 'cheerful', 'jolly', 'light', 'lucky', 'pretty' and 'quiet' occur once.

## 6.7 Discussion and conclusions

This study set out to provide empirical evidence for the dissemination and appropriation of the humoral theory by investigating how this central medical commonplace was reproduced in different contexts for different audiences and how the contents were understood and acted upon. It has been stated that there was no single coherent cultural entity called 'science' in the seventeenth century which underwent revolutionary change but a diverse array of cultural practices aimed at understanding and controlling the natural world, each with different characteristics and each experiencing different modes of change (Shapin 1996: 68). In this study, I combined semantic and pragmatic approaches and assessed the commonplace of humoral theory in medical literature and contemporary lay texts. Context provides clues to the ways people in the past understood scientific ideas and how they used them. The aim was to test whether there was a difference between the two sets of data and how large the possible overlap would be, as well as to find out what 'popular' means in this connection.

Semantic meanings are more salient, and the two kinds of writing, professional and lay, show different stages of semasiological development. In the medical corpus, concrete meanings relating to physiology prevail. In lay correspondence, the meanings are connected with mood, the willingness to do something or mental attitude, and more abstract uses with metaphoric expressions are also found. Negative polarity is evident in professional writing, whereas positive meanings are more common in lay texts, and concrete meanings have given way to more abstract and even figurative uses in lay-people's texts.

In contrast, pragmatic meanings are elusive and difficult to capture. According to my earlier observation on late medieval materials, learned writings deal with the doctrine in an expository way, providing definitions, whereas texts for more heterogeneous and more popular audiences are instructive, giving practical advice and applications. This tendency is evident in the treatment of humoral theory in the present material as well. The best example is found in a book mainly intended for women, *Marrow of Physicke*, where it is discussed in the context of other practical pieces of writing, miscellaneous recipes and cosmetic concoctions. The book was intended for domestic use as a 'self-help' guide. But the issue is not simple, as the same author employs similar applications in another text, this time aimed at a professional audience, which shows the wide appeal of practical applications. The distinctions are not clear, and there is a great deal of overlap. The term 'popular' requires further definition, and perhaps the notion of wide circulation in relatively cheap booklets, not only almanacs, applies to this material best; for example, Thomas Brugis' books belong to the category of widely spread treatises, some intended for a general audience, others for medical practitioners. A vast range of such medical books were printed in large quantities and distributed widely. They played an important role in disseminating medical knowledge and ideas about health and illness to laypeople in early modern England (Curth 2007: 27). It is likely that during this time it was thought that everyone could become well versed in making remedies, diagnosing illnesses and offering advice on regimen. A variety of English medical texts were written 'for a great number of people perish for want of meanes to procure the advice of a Physician; when perhaps with a little instruction, they might have cured themselves' (*EMEMT*; Brugis 1648: 1), and they give witness of 'a medical culture that was based on the transformation of learned medicine into a popularly accessible form, whilst still preserving the impression that there was a learned medicine, a higher level of expertise' (Wear 2000: 45). An assessment of the excerpts on humoral theory provided evidence for this statement, but it also showed how gradual the changes and how fuzzy the borders were where humoral theory was concerned.

# 7 Code-switching in Early Modern English medical writing

PÄIVI PAHTA

*The Queens Closet Opened.*
*Incomparable Secrets in Physick, Chyrurgery, Preserving and Candying, &c. Which were presented to the QUEEN: By the most experienced Persons of the Times, many whereof were had in Esteem when she pleased to descend to private Recreations. Corrected and Revived, with many new and large Additions: together with three exact Tables.*
*Vivit post Funera Virtus.*
*LONDON, Printed for Obadiah Blagrave, at the Sign of the Black Bear in St. Pauls Church-yard, 1679.*

## 7.1 Introduction

*The Queens Closet Opened*, one of the most popular seventeenth-century household handbooks first printed in 1655, is a collection of medical remedies, advice on preserves and culinary recipes claimed to be used in the royal household of Queen Henrietta Maria, the wife of King Charles I. On the title page, the anonymous author, W.M., describes the book in the usual persuasive market discourse of the period, promising the purchasers and readers access to the incomparable secrets of the aristocracy in diet and health. The target audience of the book was presumably the seventeenth-century general readership, particularly female readers in charge of similar concerns in their own households. What catches the eye of a researcher interested in multilingualism on this page is the lofty Latin sentence, *Vivit post Funera Virtus*, 'virtue outlives death'. Both in terms of language choice and actual meaning, this sentence seems out of place in a small and relatively cheap-looking practically oriented English-language quarto volume which in all likelihood is intended for a non-Latinate readership and directs the reader to better health and pleasures and luxuries of life rather than to concerns of moral values.

Why, then, has the author (or publisher) decided to insert this Latin sentence as a motto here? Where does it come from? According to Bensly (1904), this sentence, a common funeral phrase found on tombstones throughout the country, can be traced in England to 1557, when John Caius, a famous physician of his time, inscribed it in old St Paul's on the monument of Thomas

Linacre, another sixteenth-century giant of medical learning. The very same words, Bensly notes, were later inscribed on Caius' own monument in the chapel of his college in Cambridge. The same sentence is also part of a poem that Georg Sabinus, a sixteenth-century German humanist and poet, wrote in dedication of Cardinal Albert of Brandenburg, Archbishop of Mainz (d. 1545).[1] These associations with high culture and the learned traditions of medicine provide a key to understanding why the Latin sentence has found its way to the title page of a popular household handbook. Its function here is clearly emblematic: a phrase in the prestige language of medical learning, possibly familiar to some of the prospective readers from contexts connected with learned medical figures, is intended to lend an aura of credibility and prestige to the book by association. Thus, what we see on the title page of *The Queens Closet Opened* is in fact the author (or publisher) using his or her multilingual resources in a discursive practice that today is known as image creation. The ultimate purpose is probably to guarantee and boost the sales.

This example is one of the many instances of the co-occurrence and alternation of languages – a phenomenon known as code-switching – within printed English medical writings of the early modern period. In this chapter, I examine such multilingual practices in the material included in the corpus of *Early Modern English Medical Texts* (*EMEMT*; see Chapter 2). The carefully structured domain-specific corpus provides an ideal basis for studying code-switching practices in texts representing a wide range of medical writing of the period. My aim in this study is to provide a qualitative corpus-aided overview of code-switching in Early Modern English medical writing, analysing the forms and functions in which languages other than English occur in the data. The analysis combines an examination of the linguistic and textual structures observed in code-switching with an investigation of the communicative functions and contexts of discourse in which the code-switched segments are used in medical writings of the period. In order to trace the diachronic lines of development in domain-specific patterns, I will also compare the findings in early modern data with earlier findings in medieval medical materials. The study shows that the writers of Early Modern English medical texts make use of multilingual resources in a variety of ways, sometimes to create images and to build associations, as in the opening example, but more often to communicate a particular domain-specific meaning connected with the theory or practice of medicine as an area of special knowledge.

## 7.2 Multilingualism in early English medical writings

Multilingual practices in medical and scientific texts produced in medieval England have recently attracted considerable attention in philologically and

[1] Since 1720, the sentence is also part of Nottingham City coat of arms (Walker 1928).

linguistically oriented research, whereas in materials from the early modern period multilingualism has been largely overlooked. The research on pre-1500 writings has confirmed that medieval medical and scientific writing is in fact characterized by the presence of more than one language. In a social domain permeated by diglossia and inherent language contact on several levels, including the translation process in the production of vernacular medical texts, this is understandable (see Pahta 2004a). The scale of the phenomenon was revealed in Linda Ehrsam Voigts' study (1989b) of scientific and medical materials produced in England in the period 1375–1500, i.e. in the earliest phases of the vernacularization of science. Her quantitative and qualitative assessment of 178 manuscript units (entire manuscripts or leaflets) containing medical and scientific texts showed that almost 50 per cent had material in more than one language. The frequency of code-switching is also seen in Voigts' analysis of bilingualism in scientific and medical manuscripts (1996), in Hunt's studies on English–French–Latin multilingualism in medical texts from this period (2000, 2010; see also Hunt and Benskin 2001), and in my analyses on the uses of Latin in late medieval medical texts (Pahta 2003, 2004a, 2004b). The juxtaposition of languages is found on different levels: it is customary to find manuscript codices consisting of monolingual texts in different languages one after the other, but it is also common to find individual texts containing more than one language. The coexistence of English, Latin and French, and the various forms, functions and meanings of shifts from one language to another in codices and individual texts have been in focus in several studies (e.g., Voigts 1996; Hunt 2000, 2010; Pahta 2003, 2004a, 2004b). These studies have shown that it is possible to perceive some clear structural and functional tendencies as well as some textual and genre patterns in the use of multilingual resources in medical texts in the age of the manuscript (see Section 7.3).

The coexistence of Latin and English continued in medical and scientific writing after the manuscript era on many levels. The general macro-level lines of development in the domain are well known. Latin remained the language of institutional discourse and the international lingua franca in science and academic medicine well into the seventeenth century and, in some functions, even longer. At the same time, the vernacularization of medicine, instigated in many parts of Europe by the fourteenth century, gained momentum (see Chapter 2). Thus, in England, discrete texts in Latin and English continued to coexist in the domain as long as Latin was retained in use; many texts existed in both languages, often aimed at different target audiences. However, the general histories of science tend to present a somewhat simplified picture of the language situation, and our knowledge of the micro-level patterns of multilingualism in the domain is limited. For example, much remains to be discovered about situated, contextualized practices in the use of Latin and English texts in various communicative situations and discourse communities in the domain. Little attention has been given to the role of other European vernacular languages, although the period is characterized by an increasing number of translations into English made from, for example, German, Dutch and Italian. Similarly, multilingual practices within individual texts have been ignored, with the notable exception of research on medical terminology (e.g., McConchie 1997; Norri 2004).

Recent research has established that multilingual practices can be found in texts from all periods in the history of English medical and scientific writing, and pilot studies on small samples of Early Modern English medical and scientific writing suggest that new knowledge can be gained in this area. An overview of code-switching in the Helsinki Corpus of English Texts, a diachronic multi-genre corpus containing over 1.5 million words of running text from c. 700 to 1710, suggested that scientific and medical writings contain a higher number of foreign-language segments than most other types throughout the 1,000-year period examined, extending from Old English to Early Modern English (Pahta and Nurmi 2006).[2] Furthermore, a study of eight English medical texts written between 1552 and 1672 suggested that code-switching has important discipline-specific functions in early English printed medical texts (Pahta 2007). Finally, multilingual practices have also been recorded in the Late Modern English period in scientific texts on mathematics (Crespo and Moskowich 2006) and in scholarly writings in the humanities (Nurmi and Pahta 2010). In comparison with medieval medical materials, these studies also implied some interesting changes in the textual forms and communicative functions of switching that seem to be linked with language-external changes in the professional and disciplinary cultures and practices in medicine and in the society at large.

## 7.3 The object of enquiry: code-switching

Code-switching can be and has been defined in many ways. In this study, I use the term to refer to any identifiable alternation of languages in a communicative episode (Heller 1988: 1). This broad definition encompassing all language alternation phenomena, including those sometimes referred to as code-mixing or language-mixing, allows a data-driven approach, useful in charting the scope of multilingualism in the new material.[3]

Code-switching between different languages is a common and widely studied discourse strategy in bilingual communities, especially in spoken language, where it has been found to index various micro- or macro-social factors connected with speaker identity or interlocutor relationships or to mark changes in the speech situation (see Bullock and Toribio 2009). Switching also occurs in written language, but until recently there has been

[2] For information on the Helsinki Corpus, see, e.g., Rissanen et al. (1993), Kytö (1996), or the Corpus Resource Database at http://www.helsinki.fi/varieng/CoRD (accessed 27 August 2010).

[3] For a discussion of various definitions of the term, see, e.g., Bullock and Toribio (2009).

little research on the phenomenon in either historical or present-day writings (see Schendl 2002; Callahan 2004; Pahta 2004a; Bhatt 2008; Pahta and Nurmi 2009). In written language, too, code-switching practices are clearly conditioned by a variety of micro- and macro-social factors. The communicative situation is important, as writers, like speakers, vary their output according to the context of discourse, including the setting and scene, participants and their interpersonal relationships, the purpose or function of the communicative act and the social rules governing the event (see, for example, Hymes 1974 and Biber 1988). In writing, registers and genres are known to play a role in the quantity and quality of code-switching, as are the participants of the communicative situation. The writers' educational background bears on their code-switching practices, and the nature of the intended target readership has an effect on how the writers draw on the linguistic resources available to them (see Pahta and Nurmi 2006; Nurmi and Pahta 2010). Thus, the essential question is '*who* speaks [or writes] *what* language to *whom* and *when*' (Fishman 1979: 15).

The communicative episodes examined here consist of written texts, complete or extracts, representing a wide range of different genres, written by authors with varying social backgrounds and aimed at heterogeneous readerships (see Section 7.4). In texts written several hundred years ago, it is often difficult – virtually impossible – to define the communicative situation and its participants very precisely. In many cases, we do not know who the writer is and who actually read the text, and, thus, information on 'who speaks to whom and when' has to be gathered from external bibliographical facts, focusing on the production and reception histories of individual books and examining them as artefacts. The present study, aiming at a general charting of the phenomenon, will help to identify sites for more closely contextualized micro-level analyses of the interactional functions of code-switching in the material in later research (cf. Pahta and Nurmi 2009; Nurmi and Pahta 2010).

Various communicative functions of code-switching have been discerned in earlier research on scientific and medical writings. A corpus analysis of *Middle English Medical Texts* (*MEMT*), the medieval part of the Corpus of Early English Medical Writing, identified three distinct discourse functions where switches into Latin were frequent in late medieval medical texts (Pahta 2004a).[4] The most prominent function was related to professional discourse and included switched specialized terms and references to domain-specific sources of knowledge. Switches were common in religion-related discourse, such as embedded prayers and charms, connected with religious healing practices. Code-switching also occurred frequently in

[4] For information on the corpora, see, e.g., Taavitsainen and Pahta (1997a) and Taavitsainen et al. (2005, 2006), or the Corpus Resource Database at http://www.helsinki.fi/varieng/CoRD (accessed 27 August 2010).

various types of text- and discourse-organizing functions, for example, separating different voices in the texts or marking textual boundaries and different levels of text. Similar functions have been observed in other studies on historical scientific writings as well. In terms of their syntactic structure, the foreign-language segments also varied, ranging from individual words to longer stretches of unlimited scope. The segments commonly took the form of syntactic constituents, but not always. The most common code-switched grammatical structures were single nouns and noun phrases, although other constructions also occurred, including prepositional phrases, verbal constructions, clauses and sentences. Most switched segments tended to be short; for example, the average length of segments in the quantitative analysis of code-switched elements in scientific writings of the Old, Middle and Early Modern English periods in the Helsinki Corpus varied from 2.6 to 4.6 words (Pahta and Nurmi 2006; see also Pahta 2003).

## 7.4 Material and method

For this study, I analysed texts in a pre-final version of *EMEMT* in early 2008. All texts in the corpus at the time were included in the analysis, apart from the sub-category of '*Philosophical Transactions*' (*PT*), which will be discussed in a separate study, and the Appendix, containing texts on medicine in society (see Chapter 2). The data is thus derived from c. 250 medical texts or text extracts printed in the period 1500–1700, amounting to c. 1.7 million words representing a range of genres with various domain-specific communicative functions. The material includes extracts of comprehensive, book-length treatises of medical theory and practice, treatises on specific topics, recipes and *materia medica* texts, health guides and surgical and anatomical treatises. The target audiences vary, including medical professionals with varying social and educational backgrounds and lay audiences, general readers interested in matters of health – both men and women.

The actual code-switching data was extracted from the corpus texts using the Corpus Presenter software (Hickey 2003). The first step in the procedure was to generate lists of all lexical items in the text body of each corpus category using the word-list function of the corpus tool. From these category-specific word lists, all potential foreign-language elements were selected for scrutiny and analysed in their context by close reading of the text samples. This stage in the analysis involved a decision on which items should in fact be categorized as code-switches as opposed to, for example, lexical borrowings. In the extensive body of research on language alternation, this vexing theoretical question has been resolved in a number of different ways (for a discussion, see, for example, Schendl 2000 and Pahta 2004a). For the sake of comparison, I have used a broad definition here, as in my earlier research, and treated as code-switches all identifiable foreign-language items that do not show unambiguous morphological or orthographical accommodation into English and items that have been explicitly flagged as expressions in another language.

## 7.5 The languages and structures of code-switching

The most frequently occurring language in the *EMEMT* data in addition to English is Latin, the primary institutional language and lingua franca of science and medicine throughout the period of concern. As the examples provided in this study indicate, Latin is found in a variety of structural forms and functions across different types of texts in the corpus data. Example 1, illustrating its use, is from a mid-sixteenth-century surgical treatise.

(1) As touching the first, what venome or poyson shoulde be (which is called in Latine ***Venenu~***, and in Greeke ***Pharmacon***, it is no other thyng then ***res non naturalis***, a thyng not naturall (*EMEMT*; Gale 1563b: 1)

Example 1 also illustrates the use of Greek, the original language of Western science, which occurs in some texts with a considerable frequency. In Example 1, the Greek term is written in the Latin alphabet, but the material contains over 400 cases where the original Greek alphabet is retained, as in Example 2.[5]

(2) THere is also of the kinde of putrifying feuers, a feuer pestilential, of the Grekes called ἐπιδημιός, of y[e] Latines pestilens febris of vs properlye the pestilence, so called, bicause it spryngeth and groweth by inspiration and venemous ayre (*EMEMT*; Jones 1566: F3r)

There are a few embedded items representing Arabic, which had an important role as an interlanguage in the early transmission of scientific knowledge from Greek antiquity to the Latin Middle Ages through the Islamic world. Arabic segments are customarily transliterated using the Latin alphabet, as in Example 3, which shows a typical case of an Arabic noun embedded and flagged in the English text.

(3) ye marye of the backebone, whyche the Arabians call ***Nucha***, it is of the same nature, that the brayne is (*EMEMT*; Langton 1545: 21)

Instances of contemporary European languages also occur in the data, especially French and Italian, illustrated in Examples 4 and 5. However, these are relatively rare and do not play a significant role in the overall picture.

(4) Aetius founde ***Sulphure*** and Nitrum so farre from any venomous qualitie (*EMEMT*; Gale 1563b: 4)

[5] In the corpus data, the passages in the Greek alphabet have been left out and marked by a code '[^GREEK OMITTED^]'; thus, they can be easily retrieved from the original printed texts.

(5) This locust is a flie ... hauing ... an hedde like a horse, and therfore called in Italy ***Caualleto*** (*EMEMT*; Caius 1552: 14v)

The length and syntactic structure of the code-switched segments in the data ranges from single lexical items through phrase-level constituents to clauses and sentences and, in some cases, sequences of sentences. The majority of the switched segments are short, consisting of fewer than ten words; one- and two-word segments are by far the most common type. The syntactic types include intersentential switches, taking place at a boundary between two sentences or clauses and consisting of full sentences or clauses in another language, as in Example 6.

(6) the old Proverb is, and 'tis a good one, ***De mortuis nil nisi bonum***, speak nothing but good of them that are dead. (*EMEMT*; Culpeper 1652a: 17)

Most switched segments in the texts are intrasentential, consisting of words and phrases embedded within English sentence structure. The majority of embedded segments are nouns or noun phrases (see Examples 7 and 8), but other word classes and syntactic constructions also occur, for example, prepositional phrases (Example 9).

(7) They that were of the first sect, were called ***Empirici***: and they that were of the seconde secte, were called ***Methodici***: the last and best were called ***dogmatici***. (*EMEMT*; Langton 1545: 7)

(8) from the Guts there are the ***Venæ Lacteæ*** which have immediate communication with the mamillary Glands (*EMEMT*; *Letter Concerning Acid and Alkali* 1700: 30)

(9) you may apply fit remedies: as Pills ***de Tribus***, Rhubarb (*EMEMT*; Sennert 1662: 20)

Sometimes a switch coincides with a boundary in text structure so that the switched segment actually forms an embedded text component. This is illustrated in Example 10, where a passage providing information on the degrees of drought and heat, i.e. details of the prevailing humoral theory, is inserted in Latin within an early sixteenth-century English text that already circulated in medieval manuscripts.

(10) How thou shall knowe the pulse.

WHan thou towchest the pulse with thy foure fingers ... this betokeneth dethe.

**De gradibus siccitatis et caliditatis sciendum est.**

**PRimus gradus siccitatis & caliditatis est cum aliqua res habeat vna~ portionem frigiditatis et duas caliditatis / tunc res illa dicitur esse calida in primo gradu**

For the Dropsy be it hote or be it colde (*EMEMT*; *Seynge of Uryns* 1525: D3rv)

## 7.6 Code-switching as a communicative practice

Most foreign-language segments in the *EMEMT* material represent domain-specific language use, being connected with medicine as an area of special knowledge and practice. Three communicative contexts can be identified as particularly frequent sites for code-switching. They are all related to the specialized professional discourse of medicine but differ from each other in their scope and function. The first area of language use where foreign-language segments are frequent is special terminology, a key feature of any field of specialized knowledge. The second context of discourse is related to intertextuality and includes overt references to and quotations from earlier sources of knowledge. The third communicative site where foreign languages occur frequently is medical recipes. There is also a tendency towards a predictable form–function correlation in code-switching in the data so that particular structural switched segments are likely to occur in certain contexts of discourse.

The three contexts are not posited here as separate rigid categories, and some overlap between them is evident also in the extracts used to illustrate the practices in this study. For example, specialized terms are focal in some quotations and in all recipes, and recipes quoted from earlier sources at the same time exemplify intertextuality in medical writing. In addition to these domain-specific contexts of code-switching, foreign-language segments also occur in communicative functions connected more generally with the culture of knowledge and writing and literacy practices of the time. In some of them, as in the opening example of the chapter, the change of language seems more motivated by decorative or image-creating purposes than by a content-related communicative function. It is, however, important to bear in mind that the use of foreign-language segments that have a semantic connection to the actual subject matter also serve as indexicals by which writers consciously or unconsciously indicate their associations and aspirations and their ideas concerning their target audience (see Blommaert 2005). Hence, all code-switches in the data potentially index writer- and reader-identities and, as such, contribute to our knowledge about the communicative practices in different discourse communities of Early Modern English medical texts. Establishing detailed correlation patterns between types of multilingual practices and types of texts is beyond the scope of this qualitative study, but some tendencies in the co-occurrence patterns can be discerned and will be pointed out in the following sections.

### *7.6.1 Medical terminology*

Special terminology is a core component of the knowledge base of any discipline. Terms provide names for the disciplinary concepts and methods by which the professionals operate, and they are vital for the organization and systematization of domain-specific knowledge. They also have an important function as indexicals of group membership, forming an essential part of the in-group knowledge that the professionals within the field are expected to share. Thus, texts aimed strictly at medical professionals tend to show a high frequency of specialized terminology, setting them apart from texts targeted at a more general readership: hence the presence or absence of special terminology in the texts reflects their audience design.

The key role of the classical languages in medical terminology is a well-known fact. In the data examined here, consisting of different types of texts aimed at different types of audiences, the use of Latin and Greek technical terms varies a great deal from one text to another. In some texts, Latin and Greek are used almost exclusively to denote domain-specific concepts, whereas others favour native or anglicized lexicon in this function. The foreign-language terms primarily consist of single nouns or noun phrases and denote concepts connected with various fields of medical knowledge, illustrated in Examples 11–15. In Examples 11 and 12, the Latin terms denote medicinal substances, in Examples 13 and 14, Latin and Greek terms name sicknesses and body parts, and Example 15 refers to a particular technique for preparing a medicinal substance and names another.

(11) in Inflammations and Rhumes of the Eyes, I order a few drops of my ***Aqua Opthalmica***, to be dropt into the Eyes two or three times a day. (*EMEMT*; Packe 1693: 19)

(12) The best that I do know (that is to be had at the Shops) is that which is called ***Aqua Benedicta***; being an infusion of ***Crocus Metallorum*** of which (if the Crocus be good) one ounce (*EMEMT*; Lamport 1685: 20)

(13) Maister Doctour Cunyngham in my iudgement doeth of all other moste aptlye geue to name, ***Chameleontiasis*** (vulgarlye it is called ***morbus Gallicus***) as appeareth by hys booke written on the same. (*EMEMT*; Gale 1563b: 9)

(14) the Bloud being prest out into the ***Vena cava***, or rather hindred to flow in so fast by the Artery, may with more eagerness flow into the other side (*EMEMT*; Wiseman 1676: 343)

(15) Distillation ***per descensum***, yet it will still ferment with ***Aqua fortis*** (*EMEMT*; Tauvry 1700: 4)

The practices of integrating Latin or Greek terms into the texts vary. Sometimes they are preceded or followed by an English equivalent or explanation. This is seen in Example 16, where an English synonym is added as a doublet for one of the three Latin terms, and in Example 17, where a Greek term is explained by a longer phrase. In general, this explicatory practice seems less common in the early modern material than in medieval medical texts, where it is something of a rule (see Pahta 2004a). It is more common to explicitly flag the switched terms as Latin or Greek, as in Example 18.

(16) the Head inclining downwards towards the ***Cocyx*** or Rumpbone that joyns to the ***Os Sacrum***, which Bone, together with ***Os Pubis***, in the time of the Birth parts and is loosened (*EMEMT*; *Aristoteles Masterpiece* 1684: 22)

(17) the maner and space of the disease (by cause the same is no sweat only, as herafter I will declare, & in the spirites) make the name ***Ephemera***, which is to sai, a feuer of one natural dai. (*EMEMT*; Caius 1552: 10)

(18) Take of the best Bole of Armenia one ounce, or perfect Cinamom halfe an ounce, of the rootes of the hearbe called in Latin and Greeke ***Pentaphillon***, or else Tormentil, of each halfe an ounce (*EMEMT*; Lodge 1603: Chapter 6)

The study reveals great variation in the use of classical terminology across texts included in the *EMEMT* corpus, and no clear-cut differences between texts from different corpus categories can be discerned in a qualitative overview. As Marttila's detailed analysis of the use of classical terminology in nine recipe collections aimed at two types of audiences, professional and lay, shows (this volume, Chapter 8), the picture is complicated, with texts aimed at a general readership sometimes showing a greater tendency to use foreign-language special terminology than those aimed at medical professionals.

### *7.6.2 Expressions of intertextuality*

Intertextuality in texts consists of identifiable traces of other texts (see Mäkinen 2006). Its manifestations include overt reference to and quotation from other texts and various kinds of paraphrases based on earlier sources. Like special terminology, intertextuality is characteristic of organized disciplinary discourse, reflecting the transmission, accretion and dissemination of knowledge within the discipline. It also has important interpersonal functions, serving as a tool for the authors to position themselves in the theoretical frame of their discipline and allowing them to establish an expert identity (see Hyland 2000: 21 ff.). Thus, being essentially connected with the medical authors' sources of information, intertextuality is a sensitive index both of science as a social practice and of the epistemology of science: citation patterns indicate knowledge chains or circles and point out communities of practice, and changes in citation patterns, indexing changes in the sources of knowledge, can indicate shifts in scientific paradigms.

The great majority of texts in the material contain overt expressions of intertextuality. As in the case of special terminology, there is great variation between texts in the frequency of intertextual links and in the forms and rhetorical functions in which they occur.[6] This variation may reflect

[6] For a study of the rhetorical functions of citations in the *Philosophical Transactions*, see Valle (1999).

differences in the audience design of the texts, but a more systematic analysis of the texts in relation to their socio-historical background, beyond the scope of this study, is needed to verify the correlation.

The code-switched intertextual practices attested in the *EMEMT* data are in many respects similar to those witnessed in medieval medical texts (see Pahta 2004a; see also Taavitsainen and Pahta 1998). They include references citing authoritative texts by their Latin title, illustrated in Examples 19–24. These are found with varying frequency in the majority of texts. The titles are sometimes accompanied by a more specific reference to a particular section or chapter of the work, as in Examples 20 and 23.

(19) One other, a woorke of Erasmus ***de vera theologia***, the true and redy waye to reade the scripture (*EMEMT*; Caius 1552: 5)
(20) as the same Galen sheweth in the first page of his ninth booke ***de methodo medendi*** (*EMEMT*; Harward 1601: 15)
(21) Hippocrates ***de Offic. Medic. Vinculorum aliud per se*** (saith he) ***remedio est, aliud iis quae remedio sunt subservit***: Amongst ligatures, some of themselves are Remedies, others are servants to Remedies. (*EMEMT*; Wiseman 1676: 344)
(22) Gesner hath a Story, in his ***Observat. de Chirurgiae dignitate & praestantia***, of a Chirurgeon, who when he could by no means get forth an Arrow (*EMEMT*; Wiseman 1676: 341)
(23) you have sufficient examples in the ***Decoctum traumaticum*** of the ***Pharmacop. Lond.*** (*EMEMT*; Wiseman 1676: 347)
(24) And tho Dr. Sydenham in his last work, his ***Schedula monitoria***, only appoints purging in Fevers, and does not go the length of Vomiting. (*EMEMT*; Brown 1699: 8)

In Example 21, the reference is accompanied by a direct quotation from the work cited. As in medieval medical texts, quotations are also common in the early modern data.[7] Further examples from the present material are provided in Examples 25–31. Most quotations consist of a complete clause or sentence and thus represent intersentential switching. There are also cases where the quoted construction is a smaller unit, consisting of a phrase-level constituent, as in Examples 29–31.

(25) often according to the rule of Auicenna, **Melior est multiplicatio numeri quam quantitatis**. (*EMEMT*; Harward 1601: 4)
(26) But as 'tis not good to overact a Cure, so it is not safe to Dally and triffle away time, which is sometimes very Precious, ***Occasio præceps***,

[7] Switched quotations are one of the common functional types of code-switching in present-day spoken and written bilingual communication (see Gumperz 1982: 75 ff.; Callahan 2004).

Oportunity Slips and ***Medio Tutissimus ibis***, the midle way is the Safest. (*EMEMT*; Brown 1699: 12)

(27) And therefore that word of Hippocrates is not to be referred to the ioyning together of the vaynes one in an other, but to the rectitude of the whole parts of the body, ***quia dextra dextris & sinistra sinistris sunt*** ὁμόφυλα, because the right lims to the right, and the left to the left are as it were of one tribe or kinred, and therefore like good neighbours do one labour to help an other. ***Maior est vis in forti contentione obsessae partis quam in venarum situ***, There is a greater force in the strong contention and striuing of the side that is besieged or set vpon, then is in the situation of the vaines. (*EMEMT*; Harward 1601: 41)

(28) This liablenesse of ours vnto corruption the Philosopher speaks of, in that to him ***Omne sublunare est corruptibile***; all sublunarie things are perishable. ***Optima sanitatis tutela est non satiari cibis, & ad labores esse impigrum***; The best preservation of health is in avoyding of surfetting, and idlenesse (*EMEMT*; Ghesel 1631: f. A3v)

(29) And as for Campher, Galen knew it not. Avicen saith expressely of Campher, that although it bee ***odorata***, yet it is ***frigida***. (*EMEMT*; Jorden 1631: 27)

(30) Sennertus adds to his Definition, that it be done ***a re secante & acuta***. (*EMEMT*; Wiseman 1676: 339)

(31) This must be done (I say) first gently; ***sensim & sensim***, as Fallopius hath it, by little and little; not hastily at one pluck (*EMEMT*; Wiseman 1676: 342)

The code-switched quotations can simultaneously serve multiple rhetorical functions. The switched quotation can simply give credit to an earlier writer or recognize the original source of knowledge. They can be used to specify the topic of discussion or to bring in another, authoritative voice to support the writer's argument or recommendation. In some of the examples cited here, the Latin quotation is followed by an English translation or paraphrase, which indicates that the switched segment is not significant for its semantic content but rather it is the switch itself that is significant. In such cases, the indexical function of code-switching, constructing an author-identity of someone familiar with the prestigious Latin medical tradition, is important.

The range of writers cited as sources of knowledge in the texts is wide. It includes ancient and Muslim physicians and philosophers and medieval medical authors. The citation patterns change over time, as later texts clearly include more of both references to and quotations from contemporary authors and the author himself, as Examples 22–4 and 30–1 indicate (see Taavitsainen 2009c, and Marttila, Chapter 8 in this volume).

### *7.6.3 Recipes*

Embedded recipes provide an interesting site for observing multilingual practices from both formal and functional perspectives.[8] Sometimes the switched segment consists of an entire recipe. In cases like these, illustrated in Example 32, the switches to and from Latin coincide with the boundary between texts representing two different genres. The content of such recipes consists of the ingredients, their measurements and the instructions for preparing or applying the medicine. Most recipes are concise in form, making frequent use of various conventionalized abbreviations and contracted forms that at least the professional readers of the texts can be assumed to have shared.

(32) Aetius saith, when Struma beginneth in children, they must be molifyed and dispersed: And for mollifying in children is approoued this remedy following. ℞. ***Diachylon.*** ℥ ***iiii. Oesypi*** ℥ ***i. Radicum Ireos Pulueriset.*** ℥ ***iiii. Misce.***[9] (*EMEMT*; Clowes 1602: 22)

In some instances, a change of code occurs within the embedded recipe at a boundary between different recipe components. In such examples, the ingredients and measurement specifications are frequently given using Latin and Greek terminology and technical sigils, i.e. symbols belonging to a kind of language-free zone (see Voigts 1989a), while the instructions for preparing and applying the medicine are in English. Embedded recipes of this type are illustrated in Examples 33 and 34. In Example 33, the instructions follow the list of ingredients, whereas in Example 34 the instructions come first. Example 35 illustrates a more mixed style, where English instructions alternate with both Latin ingredients and Latin instructions. In some lists of ingredients, Latin nomenclature alternates with English or anglicized terms, illustrated in Example 36.

(33) Rec. Resinae abiectinae, v. vnce. Olei rosacei, ij. vnce. Sem. Hypericonis, v. dragmes. Sem. Momordicae, iij. dragmes. The seedes shall bee brosed, and put in a duble vessell with the oyles, and let them boyle halfe an houre. (*EMEMT*; Gale 1563b: 8)

(34) Wherfor it shal be wel done, if you take of this co~position folowyng euery mornyng the weight of ij. d. in vi. sponefulles of water or iuleppe of Sorel, & cast it vpon your meate as pepper. ℞ *sei~s citri. acetos. ros. rub. sa~dal. citrin. a~n.* ʒ *i, boli armeni orie~tal.* ʒ *i. s, terr. sigil.* ʒ *s, margarit.* ʒ *i, fol. auri puri. n°. iiij, misce. & f. pul. diuidatur ad po~d.* ʒ *s.* (*EMEMT*; Caius 1552: 23)

[8] For a discussion of embedded recipes in medieval medical texts, see Taavitsainen (2001c).
[9] Special characters in the recipes: ℞ = 'recipe', ℥ = 'ounce', ʒ = 'drachm'.

(35) A choyse and speciall mollyfying and resoluing plaister, and serueth well for the curing of this greeuance: As my selfe haue many times approoued.

℞. ***Serapini.*** ℥ ***iiii. Ammoniaci.*** ℥ ***iii. Bdellij.*** ℥ ***i. Galbani.*** ℥ ***i. Euphorbij.*** ℥ ***ii.*** Let these be dissolued in good Malmesey, and then adde thereunto. ***Ol. Lilior. Ol. Amigdalar. An.*** ℥ ***i. Propoleos.*** ℥ ***iiii.*** ʒ***s. Mise, fiat Implastrum.*** (*EMEMT*; Clowes 1602: 20)

(36) For Medicines, **Aromaticum Rosatum**, and **Aromaticum Caryophillatum**, **Confectio Alchermes**, Mithridate, &c. For Simples, Rue, **Angelica** Roots, Nutmeg, Cinnamon, Saffron, … and Flowers, **cum multis aliis quae nunc praescribere longum est**. (*EMEMT*; Culpeper 1652a: 35)

In addition to recipe ingredients and instructions for preparing medicines, some recipes also include Latin efficacy phrases (see Mäkinen, Chapter 9 in this volume).

As with other domain-specific code-switching practices, embedded recipes occur with varying frequency in the material. However, differences between different types of texts emerge more clearly than in the case of special terminology and expressions of intertextuality. Latin embedded recipes appear more frequently in texts connected with professional discourse communities, such as surgical texts and scholarly recipe books specifically aimed at medical professionals.

### *7.6.4 Textual organization and literacy practices*

Code-switching is common in text-organizing functions in various types of historical texts (see Nurmi and Pahta 2004, 2010; Pahta and Nurmi 2006, 2009). In such cases, a change of code occurs at a boundary between texts or text units. Within a text, a switch can separate, for example, an embedded text representing a different genre, as in texts containing embedded recipes (see Examples 32–6 above). Switches also frequently mark out direct quotations from the flow of discourse, distinguishing different voices in the text from each other (see Examples 25–31 above). In medieval medical texts, code-switches often separate the informationally distinct headings or subheadings from the body text or indicate beginnings or endings of texts or textual units (see Pahta 2003, 2004a). In the early modern data, code-switched headings and subheadings are rare, only occurring in the early part of the period (see Example 37). However, another conventionalized literacy practice carried over from the medieval period is the use of Latin to mark the end of a text, as in Examples 38–40.

(37) ***Subcitrina.***

Take powder of Plipedranis / Aloe epatyke and myngle them with Suger / and vse it in thy potage. (*EMEMT*; *Seynge of Uryns* 1525: H3v)

(38) Thus endeth the treatise of Gonneshotte, compiled and published, by Thomas Gale maister in Chirurgerie. ***FINIS***. (*EMEMT*; Gale 1563b: 19)

(39) Very true, and so is his time come that is hanged, although perhaps he might have lived much longer had not the Executioner's unlucky Knot prevented him. ***FINIS***. (*EMEMT*; Lamport 1685: 30)

(40) Haue care of your Health. ***Vale, te ipsum ne negligas***.
NIL VaLent DIVItIa VnIVersae, NIsI habeas In pretIo abstInentIaM. MDCXXXI (*EMEMT*; Ghesel 1631: f. B4v)

In comparison with medieval handwritten texts, a new literacy practice also drawing on multilingual resources emerges in the early modern data. This is the practice illustrated at the beginning of the chapter, i.e. the use of a foreign-language motto – 'a word, sentence, or phrase attached to an impresa or emblematical design to explain or emphasize its significance' (*OED s.v.* motto, *n.*) on the title page of a printed book. The custom, illustrated in Examples 41–3, is familiar from medieval literacy practices, which is also seen in the fact that it occurs already in the earliest manuscript-based texts in the material (Example 41), but it became more common in printed books.

(41) Here begynneth the seynge of Uryns / of all the colours that Uryns be of / with medycynes annexed to euery Uryne / & euery Uryne his Urynall / not Imprynted in englysshe before this tyme / moche profytable for euery man to knowe. ***Cu~ gratia et priuilegio a rege indulto***. (*EMEMT*; *Seynge of uryns* 1525: title page)

(42) Containing some Remarks, Pleasant and Profitable, concerning that Debate, And the Usefulness of VOMITING and PURGING in FEVERS. By AND. BROWN, M. D. ***Victrix causa Diis placuit, sed victa Catoni***. (*EMEMT*; Brown 1699: title page)

(43) A LETTER TO A PHYSICIAN CONCERNING Acid and Alkali. Being an Answer to a late Piece, Intituled, A Dialogue between ALKALI and ACID.
*Ìùμ ή όåôá ί τις μ ᾶ ëλον ἢ μιμήσεται ΔιοY*. ***Non soles respicere te, cum dicas injuste alteri? Plaut. in Pseud***. (*EMEMT*; *Letter Concerning Acid and Alkali* 1700: title page)

The corpus material only contains a few foreign-language mottoes – too few to allow any specific patterns to emerge. The mottoes that do occur, illustrated in the previous examples, serve to exemplify the multiple functions in which they can be used. Like an *ex libris*, a motto can identify ownership, dedication of the work to a specific person or a particular legacy to produce a work. It can also set the tone for the work or provide a guiding wisdom for the readers in the same manner as a proverb. As an indexical, a foreign-language motto is in many respects similar to the manifestations of domain-specific intertextuality discussed above, with important emblematic functions: a particular phrase or sentence connects the book with particular cultural or social spheres and acknowledges the author's bond with a specific tradition or ideology. In addition, the use of a language traditionally connected with the culture of science and knowledge in itself is a significant persuasive factor in the interaction between a book and its readers.

## 7.7 Conclusion

In this chapter, I have examined multilingual practices in sixteenth- and seventeenth-century medical writing, analysing material included in the corpus of *Early Modern English Medical Texts*, a sizeable domain-specific collection of writing in computer-readable form. The qualitative overview of the *EMEMT* data shows that authors and translators of vernacular medical texts in early modern England, like their medieval predecessors, indeed make use of multilingual resources in their writings. The most commonly occurring languages in addition to English in the material are Latin and Greek, but other languages also occur occasionally.

A contextual analysis of the multilingual passages in the data, concentrating on the most prominent formal and functional tendencies in the code-switching practices, suggests that foreign-language segments in medical texts of this period are particularly common in three partly overlapping domain-specific contexts: in specialized medical terminology, in overt manifestations of intertextuality and in embedded recipes. In addition, foreign-language segments are used in various more general literacy practices, including text-structuring functions and emblematic functions, associating the vernacular texts with the classical cultures and traditions of knowledge and learning.

In a diachronic perspective, a clear continuity in the use of multilingual resources can be observed from the medieval to the early modern period, as code-switches pertaining to the same three areas of domain-specific practices occur in texts from both periods. However, some changes are also in evidence. The most conspicuous differences concern switches connected with the domain of religion. In medieval medical texts, various types of code-switched prayers or blessings, Latin quotations from religious texts and religious set phrases are frequent, especially in recipe collections and other remedy texts. In the sample material from the early modern period examined in this study, such segments do not occur. This difference reflects the nature of the material on a more general level as well, as links with religion in general are not as frequent in the early modern data as they are in medieval medical texts. Some differences can also be observed in the use of code-switching as a text-organizing device. While medieval texts make frequent use of code-switched headings and subheadings to mark the beginnings or endings of texts or chapters, in early modern texts this convention has largely disappeared. The change in the writing conventions is parallel to the overall development of English as a fully fledged written language. At the same time, new Latinate literacy practices, like the use of foreign-language mottoes, were adopted.

Establishing the more nuanced patterns, including the possible correlation between different types of multilingual practices and texts with different types of audience design, is a task for further research. What this study has confirmed is that there is a wealth of data on multilingual practices to examine in medical texts from the early modern period. In view of continuity and change, the central concerns of this volume, the analysis of code-switching practices in Early Modern English medical texts in comparison with their medieval counterparts shows that despite some changes in the actual practices in using multilingual resources, multilingualism continues to be an essential characteristic of medical writing in Early Modern English.

A PRETIOUS

TREASURY:

OR A NEW

DISPENSATORY.

Contayning 70. approved Phyſicall rare Receits.

Moſt neceſſary and needfull for all ſorts of people to have in their Families.

Collected out of the moſt approved Authors, both in Phyſick and Chyrurgery: by *Salvator Winter*, and Signiour *Franciſco Dickinſon*, expert Operators.

*In two Bookes.*



London, Printed by *Tho. Harper* for *Richard Harper*, and are to be ſold at his ſhop in Smithfield, at the Bible and Harpe. *1649.*

Plate 7 Title page of *A Pretious Treasury: Or a New Dispensatory. Contayning 70. Approved Physicall Rare Receits* ... by Salvator Winter, 1649

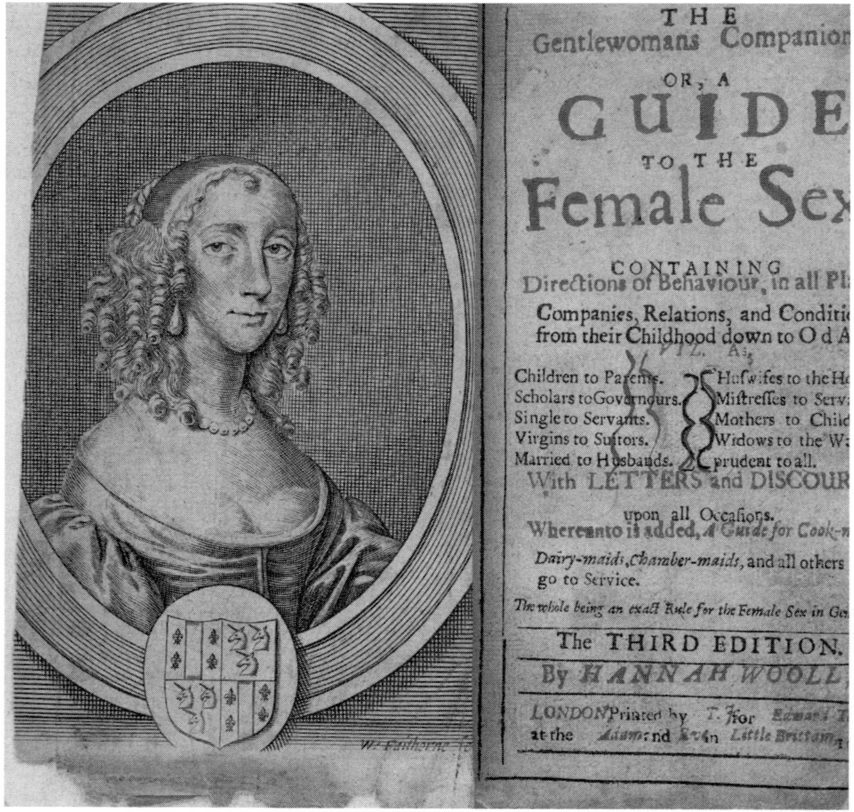


Plate 8 Frontispiece portrait and title page of *The Gentlewomans Companion or a Guide to the Female Sex* by Hannah Woolley, 1682

# 8 New arguments for new audiences: a corpus-based analysis of interpersonal strategies in Early Modern English medical recipes

VILLE MARTTILA

## 8.1 Introduction

It is commonly argued that in the early modern period remedy books formed the most popular end of 'a spectrum from popular to elite medicine', with theoretical textbooks at the most elite end (Wear 2000: 40). A more accurate description of the situation would be to say that remedy books spanned the whole spectrum from popular to elite medicine, as remedies were prepared by and for the rich and the poor alike and they constituted 'a shared material culture between lay people and medical practitioners' (Wear 2000: 103). Although the pragmatic and interpersonal aspects of medieval and early modern recipes and related genres have previously been examined by Taavitsainen and Pahta (1995), Taavitsainen (2001c), Mäkinen (2002) and Grund (2003) (see also Ratia and Suhr, Chapter 10 in this volume), their relationship to the intended audience as stated by the author has not been studied systematically.

This chapter examines the textual strategies that seventeenth-century writers of printed remedy books aimed at laypeople employed to make them more accessible to their stated target audience. The question is approached by comparing a selection of recipe collections, ostensibly aimed at common laypeople, to English translations of authoritative recipe collections meant for the use of the medical community. The interpersonal strategies employed by the authors of the nine recipe collections will be compared by looking at several indicators of interpersonal orientation, including overt reference to the reader in the text, the use of authority references to convince readers and the use of classical languages and terminology in the recipe collections.

The study takes a 'broadly function oriented' approach (Thompson and Thetela 1995: 104) to the interaction between readers and writers, concentrating on the ways in which the writers more or less overtly assume and assign roles for themselves and their readers and attempt to influence the readers' behaviour. It focuses on the interpersonal function of language, 'concerned with the social, expressive and conative functions of language, with expressing the speaker's "angle": his attitudes and judgements, his encoding of the role relationships in the situation, and his motive in saying anything at all' (Halliday and Hasan 1976: 26–7).

Within this interpersonal aspect of language, the focus here is on the 'interactional' function as defined by Thompson and Thetela (1995). It is approached from both 'information-oriented' and 'function-oriented' angles. The first of these focuses 'on the ways in which the writers take the (imagined) readers' expectations, knowledge and interests into account in constructing their text' (Thompson and Thetela 1995: 104). The second is concerned with the roles the writers project on their readers by overtly labelling them in the discourse, assigning them a role not only in the language event but also in the processes referred to by the language event (Thompson and Thetela 1995: 104–8).

The construction of roles in the early modern recipe texts is approached through the examination, both quantitative and qualitative, of overt interpersonal reference in the text: how frequently do the writers refer to their readers and how do they portray them in the text? The assumed expectations, knowledge and interests of readers are examined by looking at two separate but related features. First of all, the methods of authorizing the medical information are examined; i.e. what kinds of authorities do the authors use to assure their readers of the validity of their recipes and other medical information? Second, the amount and type of classical (i.e. Latin and Greek) terminology used in the text is examined in order to give an indication of the level of classical learning expected of the reader.

### *8.1.1 The remedy-book tradition*

The printed remedy book was a direct descendant of the medieval tradition of manuscript recipe collections, and there were close similarities between them. Both were practically oriented and contained little explanation of medical theory, focusing on listing practical remedies for various illnesses. Remedy books tended to be inherently conservative, and many sixteenth-century collections were based on remedies already circulating in earlier remedy books, their authors often being anonymous and not always professional physicians – only a third of sixteenth-century remedy books whose authors are known are by established doctors. Many were written by learned men who had studied some medicine but who also wrote on a variety of other subjects (Slack 1979: 252–3). The mid sixteenth century also saw the first printed medical works specifically intended for laypeople, such as the *Apoteck für den gemainen Man* by Hieronymus Braunschweig, translated into English in 1561 as *A Most Excellent and Perfecte Homish Apothecarye or Homely Physick Booke* by John Hollybush.

Although this genre of medical works intended for the layperson 'achieved instant success' (Slack 1979: 241) in the sixteenth century, it was in the 1650s that the printing of medical texts – especially cheaper and more popular ones, such as remedy books – really took off (see Chapter 2 in this volume). The increase in print volume brought prices down and placed the cheaper sort of remedy books well within the reach of the lower middle classes. At the same time, learned medicine was also being standardized and codified, first and foremost by the College of Physicians, founded in 1518 to grant licences to physicians qualified to practise medicine and to punish unqualified practitioners. To regulate the variety of practices in the production of medicines and to standardize medical compositions, the College of Physicians prepared the *Pharmacopœia Londinensis* in 1618. It defined standard versions of all common recipes, and its use by doctors and apothecaries was enforced by a royal decree. It was also translated into English – albeit without the approval of the College – by Nicholas Culpeper in 1649, bringing learned medicine within the reach of the non-Latinate lay population. While printing as a medium was increasing its influence throughout the early modern period, it should be kept in mind that the medieval traditions of oral and manuscript transmission of recipes continued alongside the printed tradition (see Chapters 2 and 3 in this volume).

### *8.1.2 The readership of vernacular medical texts*

In the seventeenth century, '[s]urprisingly few books are completely mute about their intended audiences' (Fissell 2007: 111). Since the title page and the possible preface had a crucial advertising function, they often described the intended audience in some detail. For example, the title page of Owen Wood's *An Alphabetical Book of Physicall Secrets* (1639) states that the book was 'Collected for the benefit, most especially of House-holders in the Country, who are either farre remote, or else not able to entertaine a learned Physician: as likewise for the help of such Ladies and Gentlewomen, who of charity labour to doe good' (*EMEMT*; Wood 1639: title page).

This is not surprising, since 'the primary arena for medical treatment in the premodern era was the household' (Leong and Pennell 2007: 134; see also Chapter 3 in this volume), and the employment of 'kitchen medicine' almost always preceded the intervention of an outside medical practitioner. According to Slack (1979: 260), remedy collections were used especially by women – both by the housewife among her own family and by women who visited and cared for their sick friends, neighbours and the poor who came to them for aid. Although Slack's estimate of the primary audience of remedy collections coincides with Wood's stated audience, he nevertheless concludes that such claims of popular utility were nothing more than 'pious hopes or calculated advertisements rather than statements of fact' (Slack 1979: 237). He goes on to claim that these works 'can scarcely have reached the illiterate poor, and the extent of their diffusion even among the literate may well be questioned' (Slack 1979: 237). The same sentiment is echoed by Fissell for the seventeenth century:

These descriptions of audience cannot be taken literally. Literacy was not so extensive that many agricultural day labourers or others 'of the meanest capacity' were likely to be reading them. Rather, such claims were rhetorical, perhaps signalling that not much knowledge nor deep literacy skills were required to use the book. (Fissell 2007: 111)

On the other hand, she does concur that 'early modern printers and publishers were highly effective at marketing their product, and we should take their designation of intended readership seriously' (Fissell 2007: 111).

With regard to the cost, Fissell has calculated that the median price of vernacular medical books in the seventeenth century was around 1 shilling 6 pence, which equates to about a twentieth of the weekly income of lower-middle-class people or a quarter of a labourer's weekly income. While this would rule out the very poorest as potential buyers, it means that especially cheaper medical books, which include many remedy books, would have been well within the reach of the lower middle classes. Furthermore, vernacular medical books seem to have circulated widely in the used book market of mid-seventeenth-century London, bringing second-hand recipe collections within the reach of even the lower classes (Fissell 2007: 112). This also meant that medical books were not ephemeral but could have a long life of over a century and 'were a common item of print for those who owned more than just an almanac and a religious work' (Fissell 2007: 114). Remedy books especially, being published and printed in large quantities, had a wide potential readership (Slack 1979: 258). Although printed books were more numerous in the capital and in other large cities, the potential readership of vernacular remedy books extended even to the countryside, where many householders collected private manuscript recipe collections and would thus be interested in printed collections as sources for new remedies.

The degree of literacy in early modern England – as well as the definition of literacy itself – has been a matter of debate among historians (see Chapter 3 of this volume). The differences between different social and occupational classes, between city, town and country and between early and late seventeenth century make it difficult to quantify the degree of literacy among the population. Qualitatively, however, it could reasonably be argued that the potential readership for medical recipe collections by the mid seventeeth century would probably have extended from the whole of medical and other educated professionals and clergy to most of the gentry and upper-class merchants, a fair part of yeomen and craftsmen and even some labourers and servants.[1]

The above is not intended to suggest that vernacular medical texts were intended only for medical laypeople. Not all early modern medical

[1] It is good to bear in mind that a single person with sufficient literacy in the household or community allowed the entire household to profit from a printed recipe collection.

professionals were necessarily fluent in Latin and they would have found vernacular texts very useful. In 1551, William Turner, in the preface to his new English herbal, referred to the dangerous consequences of apothecaries and surgeons not knowing Latin:

Then when as if the potecari for lack of knowledge of the latin tong, is ignorant in herbes: and putteth ether many a good mā by ignorance in ieopardy of his life, or marreth good medicines to the great dishonestie both of the Phisician and of Goddes worthy creatures, the herbes and the medicines: when as by hauyng an herball in English all these euelles myght be auoyded: ... The same reson myght also be made of surgeons, whether it were better y[t] they shuld kyll men for lack of knowledged of herbes or y[t] an herball shuld be set out vnto them in English, whiche for the most part vnderstand no latin at all, sauyng such as no latin eares can abyde. (Turner 1551: A3v)

As Wear (2000: 40–1) points out, '[d]istinctions between lay and medical readerships were blurred and both groups might read works which were ostensibly for the other'. Many of the more 'popular' medical works also seem to be 'intended in part for practitioners' (Slack 1979: 256), perhaps with the purpose both of educating popular practitioners or apothecaries and of raising the overall level of medical competence in the community (Slack 1979: 257). Vernacular works could also have the function of increasing the respect for physicians as '[m]ost of the medical works reinforced the establishment view of physic as a complex art demanding learning and judgement, and attacked the amateur tamperings of untrained and illiterate practitioners' (Slack 1979: 257).

On the other hand, works originally intended for professionals were also read by interested laypeople, as is demonstrated by the case of Elizabeth Freke, whose notebook from 1684 contains 'nearly three hundred medical recipes, as well as extensive reading notes from John Gerard's herbal, Nicholas Culpeper's *Culpeper's School of Physick*, Moyse Charas's and George Bate's pharmacopoeias, and Nicholas Culpeper's translation of the *Pharmacopoeia Londinensis*' (Leong 2008: 150–1).

## 8.2 Materials used

The material for this study comes from nine seventeenth-century recipe collections included in a preliminary version of the corpus of *Early Modern English Medical Texts* (*EMEMT*), consisting of 10,000-word extracts of each collection – or the whole text if shorter. These nine collections are divided into two categories based on their overtly stated target audience. Six collections explicitly claim to be aimed at laypeople, or 'the poor and plain men', 'householders in the country' and 'every family', while three are English translations of authoritative collections directed at medical practitioners.

### 8.2.1 Recipe books explicitly directed at laypeople

*The Poore-Mans Plaster-Box* (Hawes 1634) does not mention its author but was entered into the Stationer's Register as written by R. Hawes.[2] The collection is a cheaply printed six-sheet quarto volume of forty-six pages in blackletter type, with roman type used for headings and for highlighting special terms. According to its author,

> What is written in this booke, is written to the poore, and plaine man, not for the rich or learned; nor to instruct gadding women, that they might leave their callings, and turne Chirurgeons, to the destruction of many poore men: to none of these purposes, was this published, but for an instruction, for poore householders to help their Children, and Servants in their nede. Vale. (*EMEMT*; Hawes 1634: 44)

As has been pointed out by Nagy (1988: 25), Hawes does not claim to be writing for the poorest illiterates such as vagrants, almsmen and social outcasts of his era but rather for the reasonably respectable, albeit poor, householders with no access to professional medical services, which is in fact much more plausible as a target audience than the interpretation of Slack (1979) and Fissell (2007) quoted above.

*An Alphabetical Book of Physicall Secrets* (Wood 1639) is attributed on the title page to Owen Wood, of whom no further information is given, making his identification difficult. This extensive collection contains 238 numbered pages of recipes organized alphabetically according to the disease to be cured, printed in roman type and in octavo format. The intended audience is again stated explicitly on the title page as 'House-holders in the Country' and 'Ladies and Gentle-women' who have no access to a learned physician (*EMEMT*; Wood 1639: title page).

*A Pretious Treasury* (Winter 1649) is a short, cheaply printed leaflet of twenty pages, allegedly authored by Salvator Winter and Francisco (or Francis) Dickinson, who claimed to be 'expert operators of Italian background' but who could more accurately be described as quacks (Hull 1996: 79). According to the title page, the work contains '70. approved Physicall rare Receits' and simultaneously serves as an advertisement for the authors' services, on several occasions telling the reader that further secrets are available upon personal consultation. Many of the recipes in this joint publication also appeared in shorter pamphlets published individually by the two authors during the same year.

*Approved Medicines of Little Cost* (Elkes 1651) by Richard Elkes is a slim volume of forty-four octavo pages in roman type, especially tailored 'For

[2] This work has been attributed in the *English Short-Title Catalogue* to 'Hawes, Richard, writer on popular medicine' (citation no. S118752), who in turn has been associated with clergyman Richard Hawes (1603?–68) (see *Oxford Dictionary of National Biography*), but there does not seem to be evidence to support this.

the Souldiers Knap-sack, and the Country mans Closet' (*EMEMT*; Elkes 1651: title page). Little is known of the author, who styles himself a gentleman and 'Student in the Art of Physick, living at Bagshot in the County of Surry' (*EMEMT*; Elkes 1651: title page). In the narrative passages found in between remedies and offering more general health advice, he does, however, claim some familiarity with the military life, if only from having spent time with soldiers.

*The Countrymans Friend* by Abraham Miles (1662) promises to be 'No circumventing Mountebanck But a rare method of Chyrurgery and physick, teaching the country people excellent cures, the like was never laid open in any age before' (*EMEMT*; Miles 1662: title page). Little is known about the author, except that in addition to this collection of recipes, he published a number of ballads on various subjects during the latter seventeenth century (see the *English Short-Title Catalogue*). The work itself is a slim 40-page octavo volume in roman type containing cures for various diseases, along with horse remedies and other agricultural 'arts'.

Hannah Woolley (b. 1622?, d. in or after 1674) was one of the first Englishwomen to make an income as an author (Considine 2004). She published a number of works on cookery, medicine and household affairs.[3] *The Compleat Servant-Maid* (Woolley 1677) is a small, posthumous collection of medical, culinary and household medicines in duodecimo format and roman type. Woolley's name is not mentioned on the title page, but the work was based on material from her earlier works.[4] It has been included in preference to the more authentic works published in her lifetime because it was explicitly 'Composed for the great benefit and advantage of all young Maidens' (*EMEMT*; Woolley 1677: title page) in order to help them to qualify as servant maids.

### *8.2.2 Recipe books explicitly directed at professionals*

In 1649, Nicholas Culpeper translated the learned and authoritative *Pharmacopœia Londinensis* into English for the benefit of Englishmen who 'are led by the noses (worse than beasts, as though oppression had already made them mad) by a company of proud, insulting, domineering Doctors' (*EMEMT*; Culpeper 1649: A1v). The Latin original was strictly a professional reference work, intended for 'the learned only, and to the nurslings of Apollo, for the health, not the understanding of the vulgar' (*EMEMT*; Culpeper 1649: B2r). Although Culpeper's English version makes the work more accessible to the layman, it is clearly not his intention

[3] Woolley's medical writings can be taken to reflect a distinctly female and domestic strain of medicine. Apparently, she had no formal medical training, but she does mention in her writings that 'her mother and elder sisters "were very skilled in Physick and Chirurgery," and she learned a little about medical practice from them and more under the patronage of a noblewoman, almost certainly Anne, Lady Maynard (d. 1647)' (Considine 2004).

[4] This is by no means unusual; many of her works reused material from her earlier books.

to enable laypeople to use it. As Culpeper himself points out, his intention is rather to inform them about medicines of the learned tradition and thus to make them less prone to be deceived by doctors or apothecaries (*EMEMT*; Culpeper 1649: 77) and more likely to prefer learned medicine to folk remedies:

As for Apothecaries they have least reason of all to complain, because it tends to the advancement of their trade, If they have not wit enough to know, that private men cannot make up most of these compositions themselves, but knowing the vertues of … them, will resort the more to them for physick, they deserve the name of a company of Dunces. (*EMEMT*; Culpeper 1649: A2v)

While the *Pharmacopée royale Galenique et chymique* (1676) of Moyse Charas (or Moses Charras) did not enjoy the official status of the *Pharmacopœia Londinensis*, this 1,000-page compendium of recipes was one of the largest published in the seventeenth century, combining traditional Galenic pharmacy with the modern chemical one (Coste 2008). It was a thoroughly scholarly work, being characterized as 'very advantageous to those who have any insight in Physick' (*EMEMT*; Charas 1678: A2v) and 'very necessary for all those persons that give their minds to the study and exercise of Physick' (*EMEMT*; Charas 1678: A3r). Charas himself was a well-known figure, a pharmacist who taught chemistry at the Royal Gardens and who served as the Apothecary to the Duke of Orleans and who also attended Charles II of England and Charles II of Spain at various times (Debus 2002: 130). His pharmacopoeia became an international success and was translated into many languages; the English translation was published two years after the original French publication.

The third professionally oriented text is also a translation from a Latin original by George Bate (1608–68), one of the most prominent physicians of his time: 'one of the greatest Masters of his Art in the Universe' (*EMEMT*; Salmon 1700a: A4r). An Oxford graduate and a fellow of the College of Physicians from 1640, he served as a physician both to Lord Protector Cromwell and to the monarchy after its restoration. After his death, his personal collection of remedies was edited as the Latin *Pharmocopœia Bateana*, a sizeable collection of medicinal waters, spirits, oils, salts, electuaries and infusions (Furdell 2008). An English translation of this collection was published in 1700 by William Salmon 'for the Benefit of all the Lovers of this kind of Learning' (*EMEMT*; Salmon 1700a: A4v). Although Salmon also makes the usual apologies for bringing such learned knowledge within the reach of 'the Vulgar' (*EMEMT*; Salmon 1700a: A5r–v), a later passage in his apology indicates that 'the Vulgar' simply means the non-Latinate and that his intention is not to educate the masses but merely to promote equality among the students of medicine:

It is my Opinion, that the Art of Physick is not any particular Man's or Societies proper Right, more than anothers; but that every Man has an equal share in the same. But 'tis like Gold and Silver, he that wins it, or takes pains for it, shall have it. And as in one, every Man has a Right to study Physick if he pleases; and having once made himself Master of the Knowledge of it, has as great a Right to use it as we. (*EMEMT*; Salmon 1700a: A5v)

## 8.3 Interpersonal reference in the recipe collections

In order to study personal reference, an open-ended linguistic category, in the nine recipe texts selected for scrutiny from the *EMEMT* corpus, a list of all words that could refer to a person in the texts was first created, based on an automatically generated word list and a close reading of the texts. This list included both personal and relative pronouns, nouns referring to human agents (e.g., 'physician', 'patient', 'woman') and nominal forms of adjectives referring to human agents (e.g., 'the sick', 'the wise'). A concordance of these words was then manually cleaned of all false hits and duplicates, leaving only unique instances of personal reference.[5] Each occurrence of personal reference was then manually labelled for person (first, second or third) and the role(s) of the referent: patient, healer, author, reader or authority (subdivided into modern medical, classical medical, general public, lay and divine authority).

### *8.3.1 Overt reader reference*

The most obvious indication of a writer's awareness of his or her audience is overt reference to the reader, which introduces him or her as a real participant in the discourse rather than merely an implied observer (cf. Hyland 2001: 552). It serves to engage the reader in the discourse and to create an intimate and personal relationship of trust with the reader.

A quantitative analysis of overt personal reference in the nine recipe collections in Figure 8.1 shows that the texts explicitly intended for lay readers refer to the reader more frequently than the professional texts (highlighted in Figure 8.1), except for Wood (1639), which resembles the professionally oriented texts in this respect.

Miles (1662) and Winter (1649) stand out especially as referring to the reader much more frequently than do the others. This is partially explained by their habit of frequently replacing the definite article with the possessive second-person pronoun, as in Examples 1–4.[6]

[5] For example, the phrase 'those wise Greeks' would be counted as a single reference, although it would appear as three hits in the concordance.

[6] The frequency of possessive second-person pronouns in these texts is 2.80 and 3.14 per 1,000 words against an average of 0.91 per 1,000 words across the whole material.

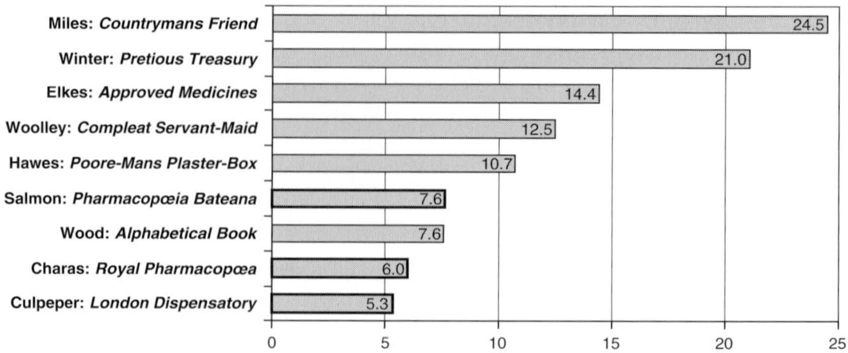


Figure 8.1 Frequency of overt reader reference (per 1,000 words).

(1) and when **your** honey is dissolved (*EMEMT*; Miles 1662: A4v)
(2) then take **your** Flax cloath, and spread it on a board (*EMEMT*; Miles 1662: B2r)
(3) then stop **your** Vessell very well, that the Odour go not forth (*EMEMT*; Winter 1649: 16)
(4) then take **your** wine, and boyl all together (*EMEMT*; Winter 1649: 17)

In addition to the quantitative difference between the professional and lay texts, there is also a qualitative difference in the ways of referring to the reader. The texts aimed at laypeople consistently (97.5–100 per cent of cases) refer to the reader in the second person, whereas the professional texts, excepting Salmon (1700a), also make use of the third person and the inclusive first-person plural, even though the second person is still clearly dominant. In the professional texts, the third person is used in metatextual contexts where the reader is given advice on using the recipe collection, as shown in Examples 5 and 6.[7]

(5) I would not have **the Reader** build to much confidence upon the degrees of temperature (or more properly intemperature) neither of this, or any other simple, because most of them are quoted by Outlandish-Authors; (*EMEMT*; Culpeper 1649: 4, marginal note)
(6) I could insert here several Examples, but I refer **the Reader** to the Decoctions of the preceding Chapter, which may be call'd Apozems. (*EMEMT*; Charas 1678: 57)

The 'inclusive we' is the most common form of reader reference in Present-Day English scientific writing (Hyland 2001: 551). In the recipe collections, it occurs almost exclusively in the professional texts by Culpeper and Charas, apart from a single instance in Elkes, and even in these texts

[7] Third-person reference to the reader is very rare even in these professionally oriented texts. In the lay texts, all of the few third-person noun constructions referring to the reader are in fact vocatives and have been excluded.

with a very low frequency of 0.71/1,000 and 1.75/1,000 words, respectively. The scope of the 'inclusive we' is often unclear and can often be interpreted as including anything from just the writer and the reader to contemporary society in general, as in Examples 7–10. Charas also uses what Wales (1996) calls the 'workshop we', which could easily be substituted with a second-person pronoun, as is actually done in Example 10.

(7) the common Chalke which **we** have in England (*EMEMT*; Elkes 1651: 3)
(8) Celondine the lesser is that which usually **we** call Pilewort, (*EMEMT*; Culpeper 1649: 7)
(9) And yet **we** gather very carefully, purchase very dear, and use to good advantage these pretended Excrements, as Myrrh, Bdellium, Tacamahacca, Storax, Benjamin, Natural-balsom, and several others (*EMEMT*; Charas 1678: 53)
(10) Generally **we** bruise in a Marble-Mortar, or made of some hard-stone, with a Pestle of Wood, the Herbs, the Flowers, the Fruits, the Seeds, out of which **we** intend to draw the Juices, and then put them into a strong Cloth, or Bag, and squeeze out the Juice, either with **your** hands, or in a Press between two flat-pieces of Tin, Iron, or Wood. (*EMEMT*; Charas 1678: 53)

Based on the above observations, the professional recipe collections seem to employ a more versatile and varied strategy of dialogic interpersonality where the reader is invoked less frequently and in a more varied and oblique manner, in contrast to the lay texts employing a more direct second-person approach redolent of spoken communication.

### *8.3.2 Reader as patient*

In recipe texts, the reader is assumed to be the recipient of the instruction, i.e. the healer. Some recipes also refer to the reader as the patient, implying that the reader is medicating him- or herself instead of treating a patient in a professional capacity. Setting up this kind of a scenario in the text would be consistent with the claims of the authors about writing for householders and other laypeople caring for themselves and their neighbours.

Looking at Figure 8.2, the difference between the lay and professional texts is clear; while the professional texts never identify the reader with the patient, it is very common in the collections intended for laypeople. The figure also shows that the two texts that stand out as having an unusually large frequency of overt personal references (Miles 1662; Winter 1649) also have the highest proportion of references to the reader as patient, together with Wood (1639), which has the least reader references of the lay texts.

Changing the viewpoint and looking at all references to patients – reader or not – and the person in which they are referred to, we get the results

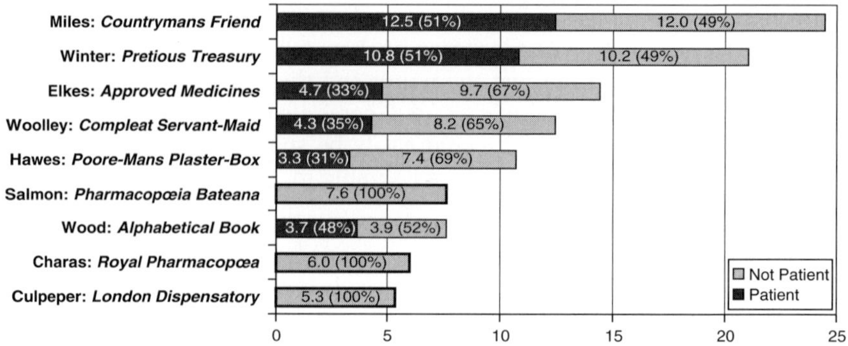


Figure 8.2 Frequency (per 1,000 words) and proportion of references to reader as patient.

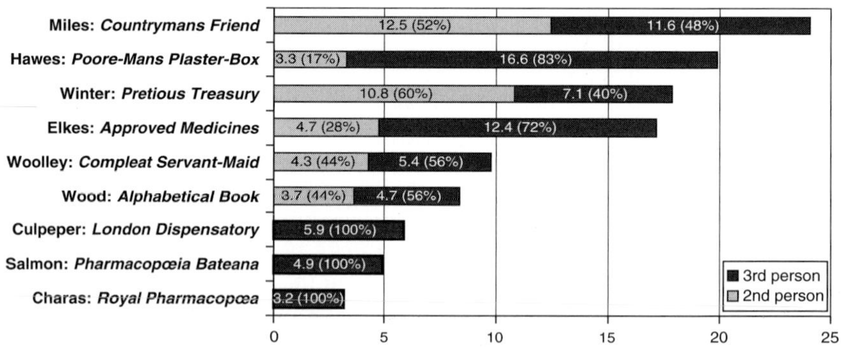


Figure 8.3 Frequency (per 1,000 words) and proportion of patient references in second and third person.

shown in Figure 8.3. In this figure, the texts – ordered by frequency of reference to patients – seem to fall into two clear groups.

Not only are the texts aimed at professionals clearly distinct in not using the second person and in having a low frequency of patient reference in general, two of the lay texts (Woolley 1677; Wood 1639) also have similarly low frequencies, being distinguished from the professional ones only by their use of second-person reference. A qualitative look at the patient references reveals a clear difference in the orientation and attitude of the two groups. While the texts that contain most overt patient references, i.e. Miles (1662), Hawes (1634), Winter (1649) and Elkes (1651), are oriented towards the patient, the professional texts – along with Wood (1639) and Woolley (1677) – focus more on the malady. As can be seen in Examples 11–14, the first group is characterized by instructions not just for preparing and administering remedies but also for helping the patient, who may or may not be the reader, more generally and for restoring his or her health.

(11) A most excellent easy meanes for **those that are hurt** by falls or bruised (*EMEMT*; Hawes 1634: 9)
(12) and in a short time this will **give you ease**, and cure you of that impediment. (*EMEMT*; Miles 1662: A8v)
(13) you may give **the party** of the Antedote before written, the quantity of a Nut in some Scabius water, and cover **him** very warm to sweat an hour, and cool **him** gentlely, it will both **cure and defend him** from it (*EMEMT*; Elkes 1651: 12)
(14) give it **the patient** to drinke in the morning fasting, and at night going to bed, continue this, and it **will make him sound** (*EMEMT*; Winter 1649: 9)

On the other hand, the texts that contain the least overt references to the patient focus less on the patient and more on the malady. In these five texts, the object of the curative action is the ailment instead of the patient and the focus is not so much on helping the patient as on defeating the illness, as can be seen in Examples 15–19 below.

(15) The round, being drunk with wine, **helps** (besides the former) **stuffings of the lungues, hardnes of the spleen, ruptures, convulsions**; both of them **resist poison**. (*EMEMT*; Culpeper 1649: 4)
(16) then strayne it out very close, rub the small of the back therewith, it **helpeth the Stone** as much as a Pease, put into the eare with black wooll, **cureth all griefes** thereof, and **all Aches are cured** therewith. (*EMEMT*; Wood 1639: 7)
(17) It is also a good Collyrium, **curing weeping Eyes**, and strengthning them, **taking away Clouds, Films, Pearls, &c**. (*EMEMT*; Salmon 1700a: 2)
(18) If **Acrimony of humours, boiling of the blood, want of rest and sleep**, accompany **Diseases of the Lungs and brest**, you may add to the Emulsions two drams of white Poppy-seed, and as much Lettice-seed, and change the Syrup of Violets, and Venus-hair into those of White-poppy and Water-Lillies. (*EMEMT*; Charas 1678: 58)
(19) It is good in case of any **Illness or Swouning**, to drive out any **infection and venomous humours**. (*EMEMT*; Woolley 1677: 41)

This focus can be argued to imply a more 'objective' and 'scientific' approach to treatment, orienting the recipes towards a more professional and interpersonally disinterested audience treating patients *ex officio*. In the case of Culpeper (1649), Charas (1678) and Salmon (1700a), this is consistent with the intended audience of medical professionals, but the case of Wood (1639) and Woolley (1677) is somewhat different. For Woolley (1677), this kind of target audience could have been household servants, who were not medical professionals but who were nevertheless expected to render medical services in a professional capacity. In the case of Wood (1639), these characteristics could be considered to reflect the intended audience of 'such Ladies and Gentlewomen, who of charity labour to doe good' (*EMEMT*; Wood 1639: title page), but it seems more likely that the text is actually rooted in a more learned tradition and has not been adapted to a lay audience in this regard.

While the professional texts consistently refer to the patient in the third person, the lay collections vacillate between the second and third persons, with Hawes (1634) and Elkes (1651) resorting to the second person much less than the others. This variation is manifest not only between recipes, with consecutive recipes switching between second and third person, but also within individual recipes, as is seen in Example 20 below.

(20) TAke halfe a handful of Mugwort, and heat it between two tilsors in a fire Showel and lay it as hot all under the throat, as **the party** can suffer it, ... then lay on the Mugwort as hot as **you** can suffer it; do this at a night when **you** go to bed, then wash and gargle the mouth and throat with a little Romanviteral, called the Celestial stone, and this will cure **you** in two or four hours space, keeping **your self** warm. Probatum est. (*EMEMT*; Miles 1662: B1r–v)

Based on the above, writers of texts aimed at laypeople seem more concerned with establishing a personal relationship with the reader by frequently referring to him or her in the second person. Considering that laypeople, unlike university-educated doctors, would not have been able to evaluate the efficacy of recipes on theoretical grounds, the apparent reliability and familiarity of the source would have been important in their evaluation of recipes. The frequent use of personal pronouns and other features of oral communication serves to mimic oral transmission and the direct personal contact associated with it, while the emphasis placed on the reader as patient implies concern for his or her well-being and thus also serves to portray the author as benevolent and trustworthy.

## 8.4 Persuading readers with references to authorities

As Wear (2000: 85) points out, '[m]uch of the discourse about remedies was concerned with convincing readers that they worked'.[8] It is known that compilers of manuscript recipe collections placed great emphasis on the source of a recipe in evaluating its reliability (Leong and Pennell 2007: 139). Authors of printed recipe collections seem to have recognized this, as they frequently

[8] This is also indicated by the prevalence of various types of efficacy phrases (see Mäkinen, Chapter 9, this volume).

refer to a variety of medical authorities as the sources of their remedies and advocates of their therapeutic principles in order to convince their readers.[9] Since quoting unfamiliar authorities would be unlikely to convince readers, these authority references can be expected to reflect the intended audience and its level of knowledge. As authors are known to have borrowed remedies both from earlier printed works and 'from other physicians, from well-known cunning women, and especially from their more eminent patients' (Slack 1979: 257–8), the authorities referred to cover a wide range from simple country people to classical medical authorities.

Using the classificatory labels assigned to personal reference in the text, the instances where the different texts overtly refer to an authority figure was calculated and categorized into the following seven types:

1. classical medical authorities;
2. modern medical authorities;
3. the writer him- or herself;
4. the reader and his or her presupposed knowledge;
5. the inclusive 'we';
6. the general public or ordinary laypeople;
7. divine authority, i.e. God.

As can be seen in Table 8.1, the total frequency of authority reference does not seem to correlate with the stated target audience. Apart from Culpeper (1649), where authority references are radically more frequent than in any other text, and two of the lay texts, which have few authority references, the total frequency of authority reference is quite similar for all of the texts. Although the type of authorities referred to correlates neither with the total frequency of authority reference nor with the stated target audience, the results do reveal some patterns. Reference to classical authorities occurs only in the professionally oriented collections by Culpeper (1649) and Charas (1678), which may imply either conscious audience design or a lack of formal education on the part of the lay authors. The lack of classical reference in Salmon (1700a), on the other hand, could be explained by its later date, by which time classical authorities had already lost much of their relevance in the face of the new experimental philosophy (Wear 1995a: 340–3, Taavitsainen 2009c). This erosion of classical authority is already visible in Culpeper, who frequently refutes or contradicts classical authorities based on empirical observations:

(21) Of Doronicum, a supposed kind of wolf-bane, **I am of the opinion** that **Serapio** and **Avicenna** and **other Arabian Physitians** did not

[9] For earlier studies on reference to sources of knowledge in medieval and early modern medical writing, see Taavitsainen and Pahta (1997b, 1998), Valle (1999) and Hiltunen and Tyrkkö (2009).

> intend that root we now use for Doronicum when they wrote so much against it, **I shall adhear** to the **judgment of Gesner**, which is verified by **dayly experience**, (*EMEMT*; Culpeper 1649: 8)

These reflections on and evaluations of received knowledge account for much of the unusually high frequency of authority reference in Culpeper. The high frequency of classical reference is actually not indicative of reliance on classical authority but rather an active and critical engagement with it. Another salient feature in Table 8.1 is the scarcity of references to divine authority. This is surprising as appeals to divine authority were a common feature in medieval medical recipes (see, for example, Alonso Almeida and Cabrera-Abreu 2002), and both the Galenists and Paracelsians still held God to be the originator of the virtues found in plants and minerals (Wear 2000: 86). This absence of the divine could be a symptom of the increasing secularization of medicine in the seventeenth century (Wear 1995a: 340–1), but further study with a more extensive corpus is required to verify this. Reference to the knowledge and authority of laypeople, on the other hand, seems to be relatively common in both lay and professional texts. Although references to eminent lay personages are included in this category, it includes only two references to a royal or aristocratic person. This is slightly surprising, considering the increase in the number of medical works claiming royal authority in the 1650s (Fissell 2007: 119). Instead, appeals to lay authority mostly take the form of anecdotes or example cases where the source of the cure or medical information is a medically uneducated layperson, confirming Wear's observation that 'learned medicine could be receptive to country knowledge' (2000: 56).

As seen in Table 8.1, the overall most frequent sources or validators of information are the writer's own knowledge and that of the contemporary medical community. The writer's personal authority – most often invoked in the form of his or her 'opinion', 'knowledge' or 'experience' (as demonstrated by Examples 22–4) – occurs relatively frequently in all of the texts except for Woolley and Wood, in which the author is practically absent.

(22) Another remedy for bleeding at the Nose which hath helped divers **to my knowledge**. (*EMEMT*; Hawes 1634: 6)
(23) which **in my opinion is** a very difficult thing to cure, although curable (*EMEMT*; Culpeper 1649: 11)
(24) But **I have found by experience**, that Hogs-blood exceeds them all. (*EMEMT*; Salmon 1700a: 3)

Contemporary medical authority is referred to either in the form of individual authorities or more generally as a body of learned people, as is seen in Examples 25–7:

(25) To make **Dr. Stephens his** Famous Water. (*EMEMT*; Woolley 1677: 37)

(26) **Mathiolus** is very large in commendation of this water, for (**quoth he**) four drachms (that is half an ounce) of this water being taken, either by it self or in the like quantity of good wine, (*EMEMT*; Culpeper 1649: 82)

(27) as my approbation of **some of the best Doctors of this Age** shall justifie (*EMEMT*; Winter 1649: 19)

## 8.5 The use of classical terminology in the recipe collections

At a first glance, the use of Latin or Greek in a recipe collection would seem to indicate a learned target audience, but in fact the use of classical terminology in vernacular recipe collections can have several functions (see also Pahta, Chapter 7 in this volume). The first and most obvious of these is a desire for clarity and unambiguity – the established Latin names for ingredients, sicknesses and body parts formed an international lingua franca for educated physicians. A related function would have been associating the author with the learned tradition and emphasizing his or her reliability. In otherwise vernacular texts, the employment of Latin, Greek or even Arabic terms could also serve the function of educating less learned readers and introducing new vocabulary into the vernacular and through the use, translation and explanation of classical terminology (Wear 2000: 84).

In analysing the use of classical scientific terminology, the occurrence of Latin and Greek words in the selected texts has been examined from both quantitative and qualitative viewpoints. Occurrences of Latin and Greek were located using the same method that was used for personal reference (see Section 8.3 above) and then divided into three categories:[10]

1. **set expressions**, which often occur on their own among vernacular text and are familiar and understandable even without any real knowledge of Latin; examples include *Rec.* (or *recipe*, 'take'), *ana* ('of each'), *viz.* (or *videlicet*, 'that is'), *probatum est* ('it is proved'), *secundum artem* ('according to art') and *cap.* ('chapter');
2. **technical terms**, such as names of ingredients, implements, diseases or parts of the body, which usually occur on their own without grammatical clues as to their status, which is consequently often ambiguous;

[10] In the case of loan words and other ambiguous cases, decisions were made on the basis of morphology: if a word retains its original Latin or Greek inflection, it is considered to be a foreign word, but if its morphology has been accommodated to English or if its status is unclear, it is considered English and is excluded. According to these principles, e.g., 'valerian' or 'valeryane' would be considered English, while the form 'valeriana' (or even more clearly 'valerianæ') would be considered Latin.

Table 8.1 *Frequency (per 1,000 words) of direct authority reference by type.*

| Text[a] | Classical medical authorities | Modern medical authorities | Writer him- or herself | Reader | 'Inclusive we' | General public or laypeople | Divine authority | Total[b] |
|---|---|---|---|---|---|---|---|---|
| Culpeper: *London Dispensatory* | **6.32 (30%)** | **7.65 (37%)** | **4.63 (22%)** | 0.62 (3%) | 0.53 (3%) | 1.07 (5%) | 0 (0%) | 20.83 |
| Elkes: *Approved Medicines* | 0 (0%) | **3.46 (50%)** | **1.96 (28%)** | 0.12 (2%) | 0 (0%) | **1.04 (15%)** | 0.35 (5%) | 6.91 |
| Winter: *Pretious Treasury* | 0 (0%) | 0.39 (8%) | **4.32 (88%)** | 0.20 (4%) | 0 (0%) | 0 (0%) | 0 (0%) | 4.91 |
| Hawes: *Poore-Mans Plaster-Box* | 0 (0%) | **1.84 (43%)** | **1.48 (34%)** | 0 (0%) | 0 (0%) | **1.01 (23%)** | 0 (0%) | 4.33 |
| Miles: *Countrymans Friend* | 0 (0%) | 0 (0%) | **2.10 (50%)** | 0.14 (3%) | 0 (0%) | **1.54 (37%)** | 0.42 (10%) | 4.20 |
| Salmon: *Pharmacopœia Bateana* | 0 (0%) | **0.92 (23%)** | **2.36 (58%)** | 0.10 (3%) | 0 (0%) | **0.72 (18%)** | 0 (0%) | 4.10 |
| Charas: *Royal Pharmacopœa* | **0.72 (21%)** | **0.72 (21%)** | **1.34 (38%)** | 0.10 (3%) | 0 (0%) | **0.62 (18%)** | 0 (0%) | 3.49 |
| Woolley: *Compleat Servant-Maid* | 0 (0%) | **0.91 (67%)** | 0 (0%) | **0.45 (33%)** | 0 (0%) | 0 (0%) | 0 (0%) | 1.36 |
| Wood: *Alphabetical Book* | 0 (0%) | 0 (0%) | 0 (0%) | 0 (0%) | 0 (0%) | **0.19 (100%)** | 0 (0%) | 0.19 |

| | | | | | | | | |
|---|---|---|---|---|---|---|---|---|
| **Average across the texts**[c] | 0.78 (6%) | **1.77 (27%)** | **2.02 (35%)** | 0.19 (6%) | 0.06 (0%) | **0.69 (24%)** | 0.09 (2%) | 5.59 |
| **Total across the corpus**[d] | **1.01 (16%)** | **2.04 (33%)** | **2.00 (32%)** | 0.18 (3%) | 0.08 (1%) | **0.75 (12%)** | 0.08 (1%) | 6.16 |

a The frequency of reference to each authority type is presented normalized per 1,000 words, followed by its percentage of the total for that text, rounded to zero decimals. Authority types exceeding 10 per cent of the total for that text have been highlighted in boldface.
b The totals in this column have been calculated directly from the raw total and may differ from the sum of the rounded figures in the preceding columns.
c The averages have been calculated by taking unweighted averages of the normalized frequency and the percentage of each authority type across the nine texts, emphasizing those authority types that occur in many of the texts and giving relatively more weight to the distribution of types in low-frequency texts.
d The totals have been calculated by normalizing the frequencies of the different types across the whole corpus and calculating their percentages from these values, thus giving more weight to the distribution of types in high-frequency texts (i.e. Culpeper).

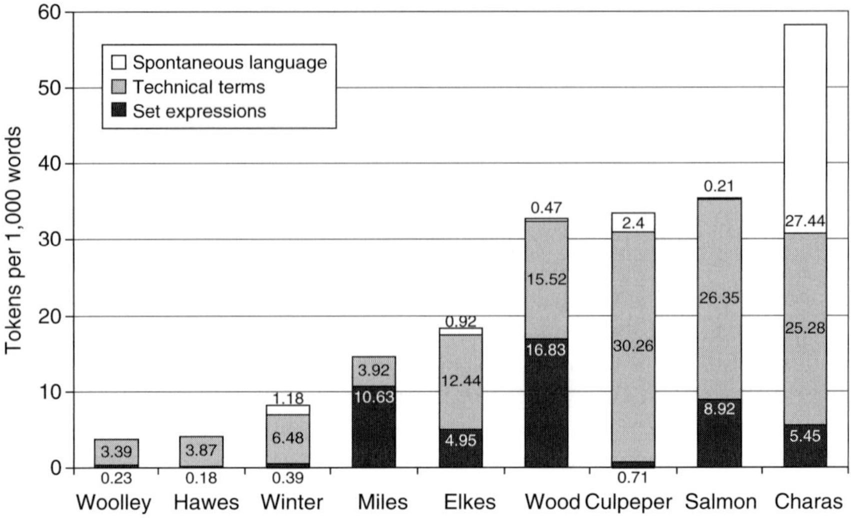


Figure 8.4 Frequency of classical terminology (per 1,000 words).

3. **spontaneous language**, making up whole Latin phrases or sentences with actual grammatical structure.

These three categories can be considered to represent different degrees of classical literacy required of the reader. While the small selection of set expressions could be understood as familiar tokens without any real knowledge of the language, the reader would have to have at least rudimentary command of grammar and vocabulary in order to make sense of Latin or Greek passages representing spontaneous language use. Technical terms, such as names of ingredients, fall somewhere in between these extremes.

As seen in Figure 8.4, the texts seem to fall into three more or less distinct groups based on their use of classical terminology. The first group (Woolley, Hawes and Winter) only uses a small amount of Latin, which mainly takes the form of occasional Latin names used for certain ingredients.[11] These form a rather small set, many of the same terms appearing in all of the three texts. The texts explicitly aimed at professionals are characterized – as expected – by relatively frequent use of classical terminology, consisting predominantly of technical terms. Salmon and Charas also use Latin set expressions quite

[11] The seeming abundance of Latin in Winter (1649) is largely explained by the fact that it contains a single recipe almost entirely in Latin, which accounts for a third of the technical terms and for all of the spontaneous Latin used in the work. This rather unexpected instance of code-switching is most likely due to the recipe in question having been taken directly from a Latin source, highlighting the fact that most seventeenth-century collections were not original works but rather 'Collected out of the most approved Authors both in Physick and Chyrurgery' (*EMEMT*: Winter 1649: title page).

frequently, both as structural markers (the abbreviation for *recipe*) and in listing the amounts of ingredients (*ab* X *ad* Y, *ana*). Culpeper is notably different in this respect, as he insists on expressing the amounts of ingredients in plain English prose instead of the usual Latin-based shorthand.[12] The only text to feature a significant amount of spontaneous Latin is the *Royal pharmacopœa*, which gives the actual recipes – alternating with more general instruction – side by side in Latin and English.

The three texts in the middle form the most interesting group. It is in these texts, especially Miles and Wood, that we find the largest proportion of Latin set expressions, which raises the total frequency of classical terms in these texts above the first group (and, in Wood, to the level of the professional texts). A closer look at the set expressions used in these texts reveals some interesting differences. In Miles, the large number of set expressions is made up solely of the medieval formulaic phrase *Probatum est* used structurally to mark the end of each recipe (see also Mäkinen, Chapter 9 in this volume), the text being otherwise very similar to the first group. The set expressions in Wood, on the other hand, are mostly ones related to the measurement of ingredients, such as *ana* ('each'), *quod sufficit* ('as much as is needed'), *part. aequal.* ('equal amount') and *di.* ('half'), which are the kinds of set expression most used in the professionally oriented Charas and Salmon. Elkes uses both structural expressions (*Rec.* used to mark the beginning of a recipe) and expressions related to measurement (e.g., *ana*).[13]

The use of classical terminology, especially technical terms, thus divides the alleged lay texts into two groups. Woolley, Hawes, Winter and Miles use very few classical technical terms and are quite plausibly accessible even to the relatively unlearned. Wood and Elkes, on the other hand, resemble the professional texts in their use of learned set expressions and also use almost half as many technical terms, making them much less accessible to the unlearned. The frequent use of classical terminology by Wood and Elkes might mean either that these authors are sacrificing accessibility in order to create an impression of professional competence, that many of the recipes contained in them have been taken directly from learned sources, or that the authors were not in fact trying to write for the unlearned. It is also interesting that while the professional texts, especially Culpeper, frequently give the vernacular equivalents of Latin names, Wood and Elkes do so very rarely. One possible explanation for this is that because the professional texts are translations, their translators were consciously rendering the

[12] The same vernacularizing impulse is most likely responsible for the fact that most of the numerous Latin terms – mainly various simple and compound ingredients – in the *London Dispensatory* are accompanied by their English equivalents, reflecting Culpeper's educational aspirations.

[13] The pattern evident in the use of Latin set expressions related to amounts of ingredients is also echoed by the use of apothecaries' symbols, which occur in significant numbers only in Wood, Elkes, Charas and Salmon.

text into English and were thus more aware of the educational aspect of their endeavour, while professional authors writing in English used their customary apothecarial shorthand out of habit without considering its implications for their readership.

## 8.6 Conclusions

Based on the results of the analysis, it is clear that at least some authors of recipe collections ostensibly written for a lay audience do employ various strategies to adapt their text to its intended audience. From the results, two principal strategies emerge for enhancing the appeal of the recipe collections to a lay audience. The first of these involves establishing a familiar and intimate relationship with the reader, while the second relies on ensuring accessibility through the use of simple and clear vernacular terminology and references to familiar authorities.

The first of these strategies is exemplified most clearly by Winter (1649) and Miles (1662), who frequently use second-person references to create the semblance of a personal relationship with the reader. The focus in these collections is clearly on helping and providing relief for the patient, who is the reader most of the time. This gives the texts the feel of a familiar and benevolent person providing advice and help to the reader. A similar focus on the patient is evident in Hawes (1634) and Elkes (1651), but with a lesser degree of second-person intimacy. On the whole, the communicative strategy of these recipe collections resembles the informal and largely oral process of sharing recipes with friends and relatives, which would be familiar to most lay readers.

In terms of accessibility, the texts most suitable to a lay audience are Woolley, Hawes, Miles and, to some degree, also Winter. They contain mostly simple recipes for common ailments, often based on folk medicine, using common household ingredients and providing little theoretical explanation. They are also written in plain English, with little Latin and no apothecaries' symbols or professional formulae. Authority reference is either scarce (as in Woolley) or consists mostly of references to the experiences of the author, his or her friends, common laypeople and, in the case of Hawes, also to certain 'learned men' and doctors of various nationalities.

The degree of interpersonal intimacy is not necessarily tied to the accessibility of the text. Woolley (1677) contains practical and 'non-learned' advice in very accessible English but presents it in a very impersonal manner reminiscent of the professionally oriented texts, pointing out the insufficiency of a one-dimensional distinction between medical professionals and laypeople. While clearly not aimed at medical professionals, Woolley's *The Compleat Servant-Maid* (1677) can nevertheless be considered a professional text, but one aimed at professionals of the service industry, i.e. household servants. This suggests that the two aspects of interactivity examined here may be conditioned by different attributes of the intended audience: the reader's professional relationship to the patient calls for an impersonal style while his or her lack of medical education necessitates the use of lay terminology and avoidance of learned authority reference.

Culpeper's *London dispensatory*, with its extremely learned professional content presented in clear and straightforward English, offers a different kind of example of the multidimensionality of the audience function. It consists of sophisticated Galenic recipes, whose efficacy is based mainly on classical and contemporary medical authorities, including Culpeper's own experience and opinions, which are frequently used to contradict established authorities. The text does not use apothecaries' symbols or other professional formulae, and foreign terminology is frequently glossed or explained. This combination of textual clarity and sophisticated content makes the text simultaneously understandable to laypeople but usable only to readers with medical expertise.

Thus, it seems clear that although the authors' statements about their intended audience should not be taken at face value, they are often backed up by a genuine effort at accommodating their stated target audience and should not be dismissed merely as 'pious hopes or calculated advertisements' (Slack 1979: 237). It seems clear that many – though not all – authors who claimed to be writing for 'ordinary people' did take their audiences into account in various ways. However, instead of a simple division between 'lay' and 'professional' texts, the interpersonal features of early modern recipe collections seem to be conditioned by several different attributes of their intended audiences, the authors employing a variety of different strategies in order to get their message across to the medically uninitiated.

# 9 Efficacy phrases in Early Modern English medical recipes

MARTTI MÄKINEN

## 9.1 Introduction

This article will focus on passages in Early Modern English medical recipes that can be interpreted as validating remedies or as attempts to persuade the reader of their efficacy. Such phrases are usually found at the end of recipes, and there are some set formulae expressing the function of the passage, although free formulation is very common, especially in Early Modern English medical recipe collections. The aim of this article is to discuss earlier definitions of the efficacy phrase and to present variation in the use and formulation of functional passages between 1500 and 1700. The article investigates how advances in medicine and scientific thinking are reflected in the efficacy phrases and why such phrases persisted throughout this period.

## 9.2 What is an efficacy phrase?

Efficacy phrases (EPs) are passages in medical recipes that testify to the value or effectiveness of the end product: the medicine itself. The term *efficacy statement* was first used by Hunt in 1990. Such passages are usually dispensable: the ultimate function of a recipe is not altered by leaving the phrase out (C. Jones 1998: 199). The following example illustrates the form and function of a stereotypical EP (shown in bold type):

(1) A precyous powder for a webbe in the eye.
Take .ii. drammes of Thutie reparate & of Sandradon .i. dramme of Suger .i. dramme & bray the~ them wel togyder tyll it be ryght small & take that powder & cast it into the eye without ony peryll a lytell at ones **for this medycyne is proued**. (*EMEMT*; *Treasure of Pore Men* 1526: 7v)

The recipe in Example 1 begins with a title that indicates the purpose of the recipe, 'for a webbe in the eye'. Then follow ingredients, '.ii. drammes of Thutie'; preparation procedure, '& bray the~ wel togyder'; and administration, '& take that powder & cast it'. The recipe is rounded off by an EP, 'for this medycyne is proued'. This phrase seems detached from the rest of the recipe and immaterial to its purpose, which is to instruct the reader how to prepare the medicine. The EP in the example conveys no information that is necessary for the preparation of the end product; were it deleted, the rest would still be understood as a recipe with all the necessary recipe elements: from purpose to administration.

EPs in medieval texts have been studied or touched upon in several articles and books (Bühler 1961; Stannard 1982; Hunt 1990; Cameron 1993; C. Jones 1998; Taavitsainen 2001c). Their function has been described as 'padding' (Bühler 1961), 'incidental data' ('a curious, almost formulaic use of certain words'; Stannard 1982: 72) and a conventional closing of a recipe that is highly formulaic (Cameron 1993). Jones (1998) was the first to take a closer look at EPs, which she designated as kinds of tag phrases, found at the end of recipes, always attesting to the value of the medicine. As regards the function of EPs, Jones accepts that one of their possible uses might be that of a text-organizing device, but she also points out that as the phrases are still strongly present in Early Modern English texts, they cannot simply be accounted for in this way. The phrase at the end of the example, 'for this medycyne is proued', is an English equivalent of the Latin phrase, *probatum est*. The word 'proued' does not necessarily refer to any systematic testing of the drug, or even to any instance in which it was actually used: some of the EPs may have been derived from scholastic scholarly texts where the proof of the efficacy of a medicine was not a result of a series of laboratory tests but rather a logical outcome of a textual discussion in which contemporary theories of medicine were considered with respect to the recipe in question (C. Jones 1998: 206).

According to Jones, EPs are always recipe-final tag phrases. Among these, she further distinguishes between *specific phrases*, which refer to the ailment in question, and *stock phrases*, which do not (C. Jones 1998: 201, 204; cf. Examples 2 and 3, EPs in bold (author's emphasis)). Within the category of *stock phrases*, Jones further identifies 'proof phrases', one of which occurs in Example 1.

(2) Take shelles that chykyns were hatched in & brenne them & make powder of them & put the powder in his nose **& it shall staunche hym**. [specific] (*EMEMT*; *Treasure of Pore Men* 1526: 14r)

(3) Also, if there be any man that is ramage: take the Flowers and the leaues, a great qua~tytie, and boyle them together in a good quantytie of cleane water, in that, Paciens bulneat: **and it shall heale hym**. [stock] (*EMEMT*; Partridge 1573: F4r)

Examples 2 and 3 are almost alike, except for the fact that the former uses a verb phrase (VP) which identifies the type of ailment in question. General promises of a relief from the malady, such as that in Example 3, fall under the category of *stock phrases*.

EPs in Early Modern English recipe literature still remain an uncharted area; earlier scholarly literature on the topic mentions that EPs seem to continue, but so far no surveys or studies have been made of EP use in Early Modern English. This article will address that issue, and an attempt will be made to answer questions such as: To what extent did EPs vary in Early Modern English? Are there any perceptible trends in the use and functions of EPs from 1500 to 1700? Are new scientific ideas reflected in recipe literature? Why did efficacy statements persist until as late as the eighteenth century?

## 9.3 Medical recipes: context for efficacy phrases

Medical recipes fall within the domain of therapeutic literature, i.e. they are texts whose function is, at least partly, to deal with and to manipulate a person's health medically. In the early modern period, genres that contained or consisted solely of therapeutic passages are theoretical medical treatises, surgical texts, medical journals, regimens of health and remedies and *materia medica* texts. The last two of these genres have been studied for this article.

Remedy literature and *materia medica* encompass texts such as herbals and lapidaries, recipe collections, antidotaries, medical dispensatories, individual recipes, etc. All these texts may contain medical and other recipes. Medical recipes, which are the focus of this article, need to fulfil three criteria: they must have

1. a passage stating the recipe's medical purpose;
2. a passage specifying ingredients;
3. an instance of a VP in the imperative denoting *take* (or a word to that effect) either in Latin or in English. (Mäkinen 2006: 23)

These criteria rule out any recipe-like passages that use the passive voice to convey instructions (common in, for example, Latin remedial literature), or other renderings of recipe information, which have been called *recipe paraphrases* elsewhere (Taavitsainen 2001c: 107; Mäkinen 2004: 148, 2006: 23–5).[1]

Recipes can be divided into several parts, or *recipe constituents*, according to the function of each part. These are: purpose, ingredients, procedure and equipment needed, application and administration, rationale and incidental data (Stannard 1982: *passim*). The first four constituents are deemed necessary for a recipe to be recognized as such: *purpose* indicates the malady or disease for which the medicine is intended; the constituent *ingredients* lists the medical substances required for preparation of the medicine; the constituent *procedure and equipment* indicates what processes and utensils are needed; and the fourth constituent, *application and administration*, contains

[1] The term 'recipe paraphrase' is from Taavitsainen, and the phenomenon has been effectively described in her 2001a article, although the term is not given in the article.

information about the manner, dosage and timing in the administration of the medication.

The two remaining constituents, *rationale* and *incidental data*, are optional and therefore do not contain information necessary for identification of the text type. The rationale gives reasons why the combination of ingredients described in the recipe should be used to cure the disease in question. This constituent seems to be rare in Late Middle English/Early Modern English remedial and *materia medica* literature, although the more theoretical texts seem to employ it occasionally. In his 1982 study, Stannard lists the following different items under the heading of *incidental data*: fables, legends, synonyms, etymologies, amulets, *incantamenta*, anecdotes, medical case reports, names of authorities, prognostications, aetiologies of diseases, folk beliefs, superstitious practices and EPs. In Hunt's corresponding element, *statement of efficacy* (1990: 22–4), he includes not only the formulaic expressions at the end of a recipe, such as *probatum est*, but also recipe-initial formulaic expressions, effects and side effects, case reports and references to sources and authorities. Hunt is thus more or less in agreement with Stannard.

Jones' definition states that EPs 'are those which attest to the value of a recipe, and which are found in this final closing position' (1998: 201). This excludes everything else but the recipe-final formulaic tag phrases. This definition is employed by Taavitsainen in her discussion of the various ways of conveying the medical value of recipes. However, her analysis also includes case reports in the number of efficacy statements. Thus, her definition is similar to those presented by Hunt and Stannard (Taavitsainen 2001c: 104–6).

Medieval EPs have also been discussed in an article by Alonso Almeida and Cabrera-Abreu (2002), whose work focuses on the formulation of promise in EPs and other incidental data from a relevance-theoretical point of view. Also, they make the point that, according to Jones' definition, phrases other than EPs can be interpreted as evaluating the efficacy of a medicine, as long as they are read and interpreted within their context. Thus, in many cases, the passages that Jones would classify as stock phrases could also be interpreted as specific EPs, based on the textual implicature. This approach supports Taavitsainen's view and explains the efficacy phrase-like function of phrases that are found in recipes in non-final positions.

## 9.4 Efficacy phrases: working definition

For the purposes of analysis and in order to ensure compatibility with Jones (1998), this study will adopt the formal definition of EPs given by Jones, with some influence from other authors mentioned above. The EPs collected will be analysed into stock, specific and general phrases. The term 'stock phrase' denotes a phrase that is highly formulaic and that indicates the potency of the medicine without disclosing the type or the name of the malady. The definition of a 'specific phrase' is directly from Jones; thus, a specific phrase will mention the name of the malady, or the vocabulary used will indicate its nature. General phrases are akin to stock phrases in the sense that they do not refer to the malady in question; however, nor are they formulaic. An instance of a general phrase can be seen in Example 4:

(4) To heale the Emorhodes or Piles in a nighte, a rare secrete and verie excellente.

TAke the leaues of grene Elder, … ye must let the patient slepe as moche as he will, **who, in the mornyng shall finde hym self as lustie, and as well disposed as if he had neuer had the disease.** (*EMEMT*; Ruscelli 1562: C.j.)

The purpose of the phrase in the above example is to cast the recipe in a beneficial light, and therefore classification as an EP is justified. It does not follow any particular formula, nor does it directly or indirectly disclose the name or nature of the disease. General phrases are thus thematically detached from the purpose of the recipe, simply attesting to its power to heal the patient.

The present study deviates from Jones' definition where the position of the EPs within the recipes is concerned: recipe-initial and recipe-medial statements of efficacy are also considered in this study. Since there are relatively few of these, the focus tends to be on the recipe-final phrases in the analysis and discussion.

## 9.5 Material and method

The texts used in this study are from the Corpus of Early Modern English Medical Texts (*EMEMT*; see Chapter 2 in this volume; the version used is from January 2008). The study focuses on Category 3 in this text pool (recipe collections and *materia medica*), which, at the time of writing, contained forty-four texts and about 350,000 words.

Internally, Category 3 of *EMEMT* is quite heterogeneous: the texts vary from plain recipe collections such as *Antidotharius* (1530) to more theoretical works that include recipes, such as Richard Elkes' *Approved Medicines* (1651), and to 'pure' medical dispensatories and pharmacopoeias, such as Nicholas Culpeper's *London Dispensatory* (1649). In order to counter the problems posed by this variety, this article differentiates between learned and lay texts. This grouping is data-driven and is based on the extracts at the author's disposal. Therefore, for example, the prefaces have not been considered in the grouping of texts. The main criterion in deciding on a text has been the level of specialized knowledge that is needed to understand the text and the terminology used, i.e. the questions asked of every text have been: 'Would a layperson understand this text?' and 'Would he or she have been able to prepare a medicine according to the instructions given in the recipes?'

The disparate nature of the material also means that not all the texts or text extracts in Category 3 of *EMEMT* contain passages that would meet the criteria set for medical recipes as defined in Section 9.3 above. There are 1,003 recipes in twenty-seven texts contained in Category 3; thus, not all the texts in Category 3 are relevant for the study. This leaves a subcorpus of roughly 250,000 words. The recipes collected provide material for the qualitative survey of early modern usage of EPs in medical recipes and, beyond that, raw figures for a minor descriptive statistical analysis of trends in the centuries in question.

## 9.6 Historical scope of the survey

### *9.6.1 Advances in science*

The period this article deals with witnessed many advances in science. In the sixteenth century, Nicolaus Copernicus' *De revolutionibus orbium coelestium* (1543) challenged the Ptolemaic cosmic model by removing the Earth from the centre of the universe and replacing it by the Sun. Some forty years later, Zacharius Janssen's microscope opened windows into a hitherto unexplored world. Galileo Galilei's *Dialogo sopra i due massimi sistemi del mondo* (1632) reinforced the Copernican heliocentric view of the universe, and, only a few years later, René Descartes published his *Meditationes de prima philosophia* (1641), making Man the measure of everything and thus laying the philosophical foundations for empirical thinking. Robert Boyle's achievements in chemistry (cf., for example, *The Sceptical Chymist*, 1661) were important in both science and medicine. Finally, in 1687, Isaac Newton's *Philosophiae naturalis principia mathematica* established the physical laws of mechanics that explained the motions of celestial bodies and gave the scientific community the impetus to finally abandon the Ptolemaic or Tychonic models of the solar system.

Developments in natural sciences were leading scholars away from the study of ancient authorities and towards first-person observation of nature, i.e. knowledge about a scientific matter no longer relied for its authority on second-hand information in ancient books but rather on the scholar himself, who had first-hand, self-acquired information about the phenomenon in question. This, in turn, led to recognition of patterns in the natural world and eventually to explanations of their mechanical principles. Similar developments can be seen in medicine. In 1530, Otto Brunfels had published a new herbal, with picture plates drawn from live examples of plants: hence the name, *Herbarum vivae eicones*. Andreas Vesalius published his *De humani corporis fabrica* (1543), which departed from established practice in anatomical publications not only by its ground-breaking illustrations of the human body but also by truthfully recording what had been observed. It was thus also a departure from the false assumptions of Galenic medicine.

William Harvey demonstrated the circulation of blood in *Exercitatio anatomica de motu cordis et sanguinis in animalibus* (1628), and Richard Lower drew on Harvey's work when formulating his own ideas about the cardiopulmonary system (published in 1669 as *Tractatus de corde*) and when honing his techniques for performing blood transfusion. Janssen's invention of the microscope, mentioned earlier, was partly instrumental in the discovery of capillaries and bacteria (by Marcello Malpighi in 1661 and Antonie van Leeuwenhoek in 1674, respectively).

### *9.6.2 The clash of medical theories in the early modern period*

The milestones in the advance of medicine briefly mentioned above were all related to phenomena that could be visually observed, and, thus, the advances in medicine mostly took place in understanding the mechanics and the structure of the human body. What was still hidden from physicians were its biochemical processes. Reasoning about the causes of the phenomena observed was accordingly little better than Galenic discussions about the human body: what could not be observed could only be guessed at (Wear 1998a: 297–9).

The above problem had also become apparent in the theoretical rejection of Galenic medicine, both in the sixteenth century in Paracelsian medicine and in the seventeenth century in Helmontian medicine. Both schools promoted chemical medicines, and Helmontians also strongly advocated a departure from the cruel methods of Galenic medicine. The practice of bloodletting especially was to be abandoned. Whereas Paracelsians were still somewhat encumbered by residual notions of magic, Helmontians assumed a rational line of argument: if the foundations of the old world view were in the process of being rejected, then theoretical medicine, which was based on that world view, should likewise be rejected (Wear 2000: 39, 353). However, for the aforementioned reason, the Helmontians had to stop where Galenists had got it wrong: there were simply no ways of obtaining real information about the inner workings of the body at a molecular level, despite the bold Helmontian claims that the new medicine was based on chemistry. In discussions regarding the human body, Helmontians had to resort to existing terminology and ideas for want of a better theoretical apparatus.

Galenists did not remain idle in the face of the new currents of thought in medicine. In the latter half of the seventeenth century, Helmontians noticed that Galenists were giving themselves a 'facelift', by taking a leaf out of van Helmont's book and accepting chemical remedies alongside traditional ones (Wear 2000: 416). This was devastating for the Helmontians, whose doctrine had been at a disadvantage, enjoying less support among the population at large. Any physician would have wanted to appear commercially attractive, and we can only guess at the pains advocates of the new medicine took when trying to persuade patients to accept treatments that deviated from the old ways. Galenists who adopted new methods had less of a challenge: the only thing they needed to worry about was adaptation of the new to the old; their medical orthodoxy was already approved of by the public.

By the turn of the seventeenth and eighteenth centuries there was still support for the Galenic discipline, which must partly explain what can be seen in medical recipes of that period. The paradigm shift in the natural sciences may have changed the foundations of theoretical thinking, but that change could not proceed any further than the eye could see. As far as medical practice itself was concerned, there was little change between 1500 and 1700, despite all the advances in science (Wear 1998a: 296).

## 9.7 Survey of early modern usage of efficacy phrases

This section will present the variety of EPs in English medical recipes between 1500 and 1700, which will be illustrated by examples and comments.

As was mentioned in Section 9.5, there are twenty-seven texts with recipes in the *EMEMT* Category 3. Table 9.1 gives a breakdown of the texts into lay and learned texts, according to the criteria mentioned earlier.

Table 9.1 further contains information about the numbers of recipes found per text and the types of EPs where relevant. This table will be referred to in the further statistical survey of the material.

The division of texts into lay and learned should be taken with a caveat: histories of early modern medicine usually draw a distinction between 'popular' and learned medicine. However, the term 'popular' can be understood in many ways: for example, the word may have a particular meaning when it is used in the context of a largely illiterate society. Other possible groupings for the current material could be texts intended for the use of both upper and lower classes or practical and theoretical medical texts. These groupings are not mutually exclusive: a medical text that would have been most useful to a layperson who worked with the well-being of others would also most likely have been a practical or a non-theoretical text (Wear 1998b: 17–19; Leong 2008: 147; Taavitsainen 2009c: 41–2).

### *9.7.1 Variation in efficacy phrases*

The examples given in this section, from both learned and lay texts, are meant to illustrate the kind of variation in EPs that is difficult to quantify. Even though the statistical survey later in Section 9.7.2 will differentiate between the EP types, the figures cannot fully convey what can be learned from the text.

Stock phrases, such as the one in Example 5, are present in both lay and learned texts throughout the period studied, although they occur in only a small minority of the recipes in learned texts. The example is representative of the learned material in the sense that almost none of the stock phrases

Table 9.1 *Texts, their division and the types of efficacy phrases.*

| Text | Year | Lay/Learned | With EP | Without EP | Stock | Specific | General |
|---|---|---|---|---|---|---|---|
| Anonymous: *Treasure of Pore Men* | 1526 | lay | 17 | 12 | 4 | 12 | 1 |
| Anonymous: *Antidotharius*[a] | 1530 | learned | 3 | 17 | 0 | 2 | 1 |
| Anonymous: *Ten Recipes by Henry VIII* | 1548 | lay | 1 | 9 | 1 | 0 | 0 |
| Braunschweig: *Homish Apothecarye* | 1561 | learned | 20 | 4 | 10 | 10 | 0 |
| Ruscelli: *Secretes of Alexis of Piemovnt* | 1562 | lay | 17 | 1 | 4 | 6 | 7 |
| Gale: *Antidotarie* | 1563 | learned/lay | 5 | 53 | 4 | 0 | 1 |
| Feckenham: *Booke of Sovereigne Medicines* | 1570 | lay | 38 | 5 | 12 | 21 | 5 |
| Partridge: *Treasury of Commodious Conceits* | 1573 | lay | 13 | 23 | 6 | 7 | 0 |
| Partridge: *Widdowes Treasure* | 1595 | lay | 36 | 4 | 13 | 18 | 5 |
| Clowes: *Booke of Obseruations* | 1596 | learned | 0 | 34 | 0 | 0 | 0 |
| Dawson: *Good Huswifes Jewell* | 1596 | lay | 10 | 0 | 4 | 4 | 2 |
| Plat: *Delightes for Ladies* | 1602 | lay | 13 | 0 | 0 | 7 | 6 |
| Hawes: *Poore-Mans Plaster-Box* | 1634 | lay | 73 | 4 | 34 | 35 | 4 |
| Wood: *Alphabetical Book* | 1639 | lay | 26 | 15 | 14 | 9 | 3 |
| Culpeper: *London Dispensatory* | 1649 | learned | 1 | 16 | 0 | 0 | 1 |
| Winter: *Pretious Treasury* | 1649 | lay | 16 | 19 | 2 | 8 | 6 |
| Elkes: *Approved Medicines* | 1651 | learned | 7 | 11 | 3 | 2 | 2 |
| Grey: *Choice Manual* | 1653 | lay | 17 | 68 | 4 | 11 | 2 |
| Paracelsus: *Supreme Mysteries of Nature* | 1655 | learned | 7 | 12 | 0 | 5 | 2 |
| Porta: *Natural Magick* | 1658 | learned | 11 | 8 | 4 | 5 | 2 |
| Palmer: *Recipe Book* | 1659 | lay | 3 | 51 | 3 | 0 | 0 |
| Miles: *Countrymans Friend* | 1662 | lay | 38 | 1 | 38 | 0 | 0 |
| Woolley: *Compleat Servant-Maid* | 1677 | lay | 13 | 29 | 4 | 5 | 4 |

| | | | | | | | |
|---|---|---|---|---|---|---|---|
| M., W.: *Queens Closet* | 1679 | lay | 25 | 63 | 7 | 11 | 7 |
| Salmon: *Pharmacopœia Bateana* | 1700 | learned | 2 | 36 | 0 | 2 | 0 |
| Salmon: *Phylaxa medicinae* | 1700 | learned | 1 | 12 | 1 | 0 | 0 |
| Woolley: *Supplement to the Compleat Servant Maid* | 1700 | lay | 35 | 48 | 33 | 1 | 1 |
| **Total** | | | 448 | 555 | 205 | 181 | 62 |

*Notes:* With EP = a recipe with an efficacy phrase; Without EP = a recipe without an efficacy phrase; Stock, Specific and General = efficacy phrase types.

[a] *EMEMT* versions later than the one used for this chapter (January 2008) give a later date for *Antidotharius*, i.e. 1552. As regards the scope of this text, and the descriptive statistics later, the text would still be counted among the texts of the first half of the sixteenth century.

found are so-called 'proof' phrases (translations or derivations of the Latin *probatum est*). Most of the learned stock phrases refer to the medicine in question, as in Example 5 here, or to the patient, for example 'he will be cured'.

(5) A sure medicin for the toth ake.
TAke a garlyke head pil it beat it in a morter that it waxe soft moisty ... And if thou wilt haue it to heale then take the Walwurt leafe and turne the smoth syde inwardely **and it healeth**. (*EMEMT*; Braunschweig 1561: 12)

However, the proportion of stock phrases in lay texts increases over time, and of these an increasing number are in Latin in the period prior to the eighteenth century. Example 6 shows a stack of two stock phrases in a lay recipe (either one could stand alone), of which the former is a paraphrase of the assertion, 'you will be healed', and the latter corresponds to the Latin *probatum* phrase.

(6) A Medicine for Fevers.
Take Cammomile and Centory, stam them, and wring out the juice, drink it in Butter-milk, Posset-Drink, mingled with Wine, with continuance, **and you shall find perfect Cure: Probatum est**. (*EMEMT*; Woolley 1700: 146)

While the use of Latin seems to increase steadily towards the end of the seventeenth century, the frequency of EPs diminishes. It must also be noted that there are no examples of learned Latin stock phrases in the material studied. The use of Latin in EPs will be further discussed in Section 9.7.2.

Specific phrases, which either mention the name of the ailment or imply it in a VP that specifies the nature of the ailment, cf. Example 2, can be found in the material throughout the period studied. This is true of both learned texts (Example 7) and lay texts (Example 8).

(7) For the swelling of the Gums, beat the Roots and Leaves of Plantaine, and lay them to the swelling when you go to bed; **and in the morning you shall finde your Gums well**. (*EMEMT*; Porta 1658: 222)

(8) Dr. Bassa an Italian. An approued Receipt to break the Stone in the Kidneys.
IN the Month of May distill Cowdung, then take two live Hares, ... **and it will break any Stone in the Kidneys**. (*EMEMT*; M., W. 1679: 7)

As in Examples 7 and 8 above, the specific EP frequently just repeats what has been said in the purpose or the title of the recipe. It may even be argued that specific EPs are a special case of lists of virtues, consisting only of one item. Therefore, it may at times be difficult to distinguish between the two, as will be seen in the case of Example 9, which is analysed as a specific phrase in this study:

(9) Against Driness in the Brain, and other Disease in the Head.
Take of the following Metals, well refined: Of Gold, … **It is of wonderful operation against all Diseases of the Head, and Brain.** (*EMEMT*; Paracelsus 1655: 107–8)

Here too, the EP repeats the contents of the purpose of the recipe. If only one purpose had been mentioned at the beginning of the recipe, it would have been obvious that the function of the final part of the recipe was a list of medical properties. However, the different medical properties listed say something about the efficacy of the medicine or about its main ingredient: the more diseases or ailments can be cured by the medicine, the more potent it must be. This line of thought has also been pursued in Taavitsainen (2001c). However, as this study keeps to Jones' definition of EPs, the lists of medical properties are beyond its scope.

Of the three categories, that of *general phrases* is the least easy to define. The characteristics of this phrase type are that it is usually not formulaic; it does not mention or imply the name of the disease, but it does contribute a statement that casts a beneficial light on the medicine or the recipe. However, this category does exclude passages such as case histories, despite the fact that case histories are sometimes found in the position normally assigned to EPs.

(10) Gracia dei, lyke as mayster Peter de Argelata, set in the boke of the flesshe makynge medycynes.
TAke whyte Rosyn, white wax Armoniacum of eche .xii. ounces … **And the surgyans that nowe be praysed it moche**. (*EMEMT*; *Antidotharius* 1530: A.i.)

(11) A pretty way to stanch bleeding at the Nose.
If the party bleede on the right side, then bow downe the little finger of the patient on the right side; if the patient bleed at the left nostrill, then bend the little finger of the left hand. **I received this as a truth from a friend, if you prove it, you can receive no hurt by it**. (*EMEMT*; Hawes 1634: 6)

(12) A good remedie for one that is deffe.
TAke Mint, Sage, Penniroiall, Rosemarie, … And with the grace of God, he shall find hymself healed in fewe daies, prouided, that the disease be in aniwise curable. **If in case this helpe not, ye neede not seeke any other remedie in the worlde** (*EMEMT*; Ruscelli 1562: C4–Dj)

The examples above are from learned (Example 10) and lay texts (Examples 11 and 12). The phrase from *Antidotharius* is remarkable for the fact that even though the text itself draws on classical sources, the EP can and will be interpreted by its readers to have contemporary referents. Example 11 is not a recipe as such but rather a remedy that involves physical intervention. Nevertheless, even this remedy is tagged with a phrase that attests to its efficacy. The passage is unlikely to be a paraphrase of a classical text, as it identifies a contemporary *friend* as the source of this 'truth'. The author does not go any further in asserting the efficacy of the remedy but leaves it to his readers to try it for themselves (the verb 'prove' should be interpreted as 'try' here). As it is not a recipe for a medicine to be taken internally, the clause 'you can receive no hurt by it' is probably among the truest found in EPs. Example 12 vouches for the efficacy of the recipe through the non-existence of a better medicine.[2] The possibility of failure is not denied; however, according to the EP, among all the medicines that may fail, this is the best.

There are further ways in which the slot for EPs has been used in the early modern period that deserve mention. In Example 13, one can see EPs stacked upon each other:

(13) and this doyng, **you shall see a wonderfull operation, and ye shall not nede to vse Lignum sanctu~, nor any other thing. This remedy onely is sufficiente for all menne, and hath been proued and experimented diuers tymes, and vpon diuers persones.** (*EMEMT*; Ruscelli 1562: B.ij)

The passage in the slot for an EP begins by a stock phrase ('you shall see') followed by a general phrase ('ye shall not nede'). Next comes a stock phrase (a 'proof' phrase), and the whole passage is rounded off by a reference to several cases ('and vpon diuers persones'). Such stacks of EPs are not uncommon, and the effect achieved or attempted, as with, for example, multiple negation, is one of emphasizing the efficacy statement. This may thus indicate a decline in the persuasiveness of EPs or an attempt to combine the first-person authorial observation with the old formulaic expressions. Even the latter would amount to a weakening of EPs because it would mean that the new expressions were encroaching on their slot and taking over their function.

In the following example (14), a free formulation stating the author's experience occupies the slot for EPs:

(14) Sweet and delicate dentifrices or Rubbers for the teeth.
… **And heere, by those miserable experiences that I haue seene in some of my neerest friendes, I am inforced to admonish all Gentlewomen to be carefull howe they suffer their teeth to bee cleansed and made white with anie Aqua fortis, which is the Barbars vsuall water: for vnlesse the same be both well**

[2] This is a rare recipe in the material studied, as the EP is not the final element of the recipe. All in all, there are only twenty-four recipe-medial EPs among the 1,003 recipes studied.

**delayed, and carefullie applied, shee may happen within a fewe dressings to be forced to borrow a ranke of teeth to eate her dinner, vnlesse her gums do helpe her the better.** (*EMEMT*; Plat 1602: H5r)

The passage here is not exactly a case history, even though reference to real cases seems to be made. The passage does not overtly praise the efficacy of the medicine but denies the efficacy of other medicines for the same purpose: the function of an efficacy statement is achieved by pointing out the inferiority of other medicines and methods.

Finally, towards the end of the period studied, one sees one more new use for the slot of efficacy statement:

(15) Aqua Regulata, Our Eye Water.

I. TAke Fennel Water, or White or Damask Rose Water five quarts; Salt of Vitriol half an Ounce. Saccharum Saturni, two drachms and an half: Dissolve, digest ten days, ... and keep it quiet upon the faces for use.

II. **This is inferiour to no Eye-Water extant, but is one of the best Remedies yet known**

[a list of virtues follows]

**Price twelve pence an Ounce.** (*EMEMT*; Salmon 1700b: 4–5)

Example 15 is a recipe that is used as an advertisement, an item in a sales catalogue. The text in question, Salmon's *Phylaxa medicinae*, is a pharmacopoeia aimed at the medicine-buying public. It might be thought that the fact that such texts provide the reader with full recipes would mean that no one would be interested in buying the medical products themselves. However, the opposite seems to be the case: access to instructions was a very persuasive way to show the validity and potency of the medicines. The members of the public who could afford to buy ready-to-use products must have welcomed the opportunity of doing so rather than going through the laborious process of preparing the medicines themselves. The passage here is also an example of the fuzzy border between efficacy statements and lists of medical properties that has already been observed in the case of Example 9.[3]

### 9.7.2 *Distribution of efficacy phrases in lay and learned texts*

The first examples in this chapter, (1–4), have shown the types of stock, specific and general EPs. Examination of Table 9.1 and the variation presented in the previous section show that these types continue throughout the period studied. This section will examine further the temporal aspect of the

[3] Lists of medical properties in general seem to have been an essential part of medical advertising (cf. Furdell 2002: Chapter 7), which provides for a further argument for treating such lists as part of the domain of efficacy statements.

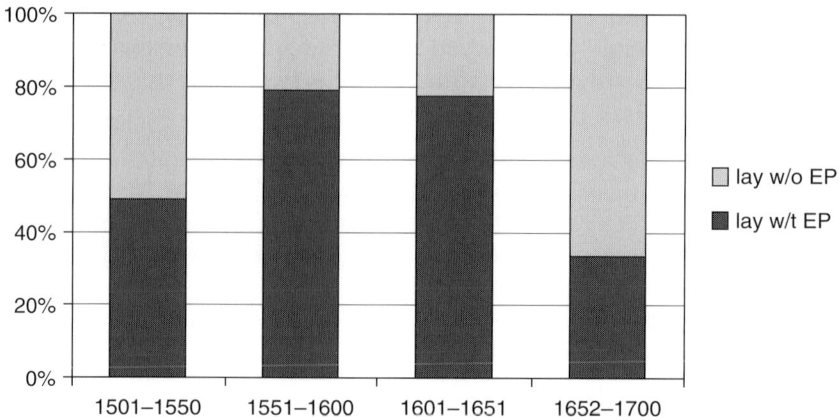


Figure 9.1 Presence of efficacy phrases in lay texts.

distribution of EPs in terms of descriptive statistics, covering the different EP types and texts intended for lay and learned audiences.

Figure 9.1 shows the percentages of recipes in lay texts with and without EPs (all recipes = 100 per cent). The use of EPs in medical recipes aimed at lay audiences shows a growing trend until 1600, after which it stays level for the next fifty years. During the latter half of the seventeenth century, they seem to become rarer. Before 1550, EPs are used in at least half of the recipes, and in the second half of the sixteenth century the percentage is as high as 80. The drop to the post-1650 level is worth noting, and it may be a sign of a new era in medicine. As was previously noted, the latter half of the sixteenth century was a period of the Helmontian controversy, during which Galenic medicine also adopted new methods: recipes of non-classical origin could be published by Helmontians and Galenists alike. If EPs were, as Jones suggests, references to scholastic discussions regarding the effects of medicines, or even simples, then the lack of EPs in the late seventeenth century may indeed be a sign of a paradigm shift.

Figure 9.2 shows the percentages of recipes in learned texts with and without EPs. Changes in the use of EPs in learned texts between 1500 and 1700 are not as dramatic as in the case of lay texts: a slight increase can be seen, but, on the whole, the proportion of such recipes with EPs stays about the same over this period. This discrepancy calls for a closer look at the various types of EPs. Figures 9.1 and 9.2 show that changes in the frequencies of EPs from 1500 to 1700 were mostly confined to texts written for lay audiences.

Figure 9.3 shows how the different types of EPs identified in Section 9.4 are distributed. General phrases seem to hover between 5 and 15 per cent throughout the period. The remaining 85–95 per cent of cases are specific

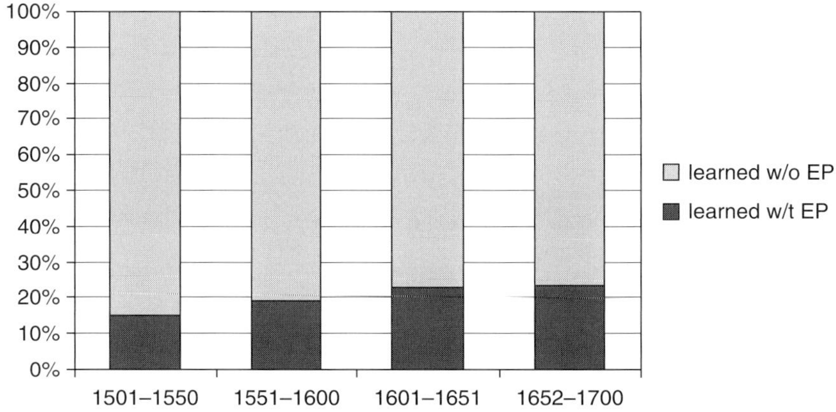


Figure 9.2 Presence of efficacy phrases in learned texts.

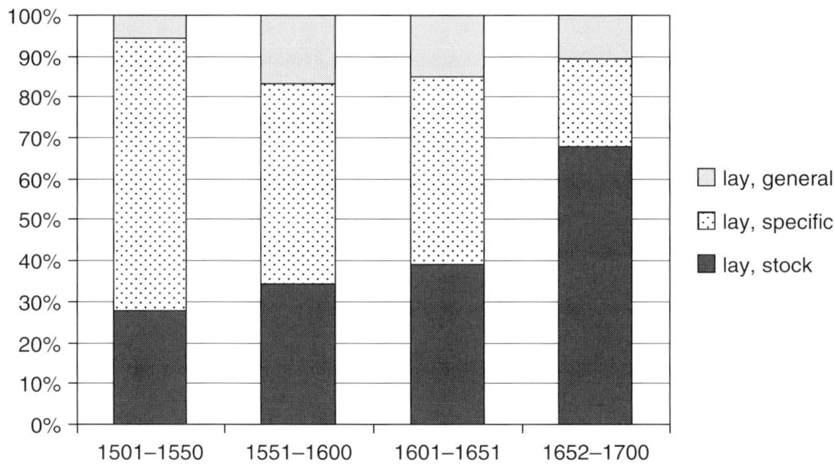


Figure 9.3 Efficacy phrase types in lay texts.

or stock phrases in roughly equal proportions until the latter part of the seventeenth century, when stock phrases increasingly dominate. The figure also shows that the relative frequency of specific and stock phrases becomes reversed in the period between the first half of the sixteenth century and the second half of the seventeenth.

In Figure 9.4, one can see the distribution of EPs in learned texts over the same phrase types as those discussed earlier. The figure should be interpreted with caution, due to the scarcity of data, and therefore the first column may be disregarded, since the absolute number of all the learned

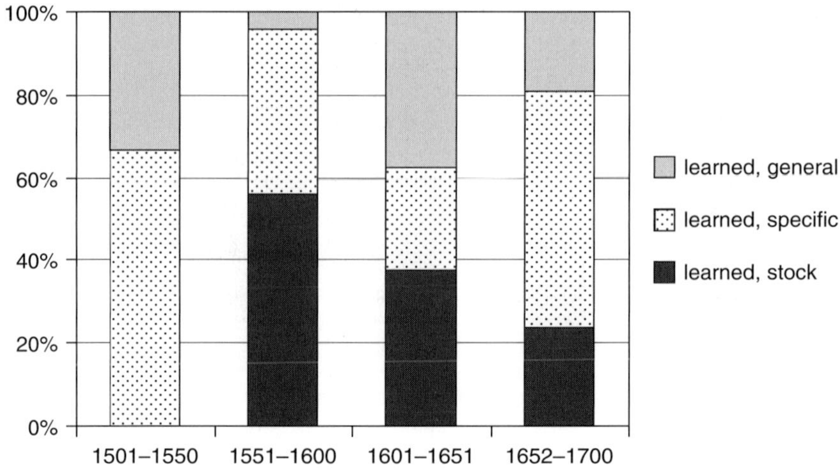


Figure 9.4 Efficacy phrase types in learned texts.

recipes with EPs in that period is only three. However, subsequent periods do show a trend, leading to the one between 1652 and 1700, in which general and specific phrases are much preferred to stock phrases. The change over this 200-year period in the frequency of EPs is minimal (cf. Figure 9.2) but the change in the preferred type is perceptible. Learned medical texts may have been harbingers of a new scientific approach to medicine: stock phrases such as *probatum est*, which reflected the old ways of reasoning and thinking, may have fallen into disfavour for this reason.

The first four figures can be summed up as follows: EPs in lay texts become fewer, and more formulaic; the majority of the EPs used in the latest period of the study are stock phrases. However, EPs in learned texts become slightly more frequent, and, at the close of the seventeenth century, specific and general phrases are preferred to stock phrases.

The final figure that deserves attention is Figure 9.5, which shows the division between languages in the lay EPs (interestingly, there are only English EPs in the learned texts). The trend is clear: by 1650, Latin EPs are almost obsolete; however, the second half of the seventeenth century sees a revival of the use of Latin. As previously indicated, this development is only observed in the lay texts. The growth in the use of Latin corresponds closely to the growth in the use of stock phrases, *probatum* being the most frequently used. In the material used for this chapter, roughly half of the Latin stock phrases in the period 1652–1700 can be ascribed to one text only, Miles' *Countrymans Friend* (1662), where all but one of the thirty-nine recipes sampled have an EP, all of which are stock phrases in Latin. Miles' text does make a difference in Figure 9.5, but even if it were to be excluded from the list, the period would stand out from the rest because of its abundance of Latin stock phrases.

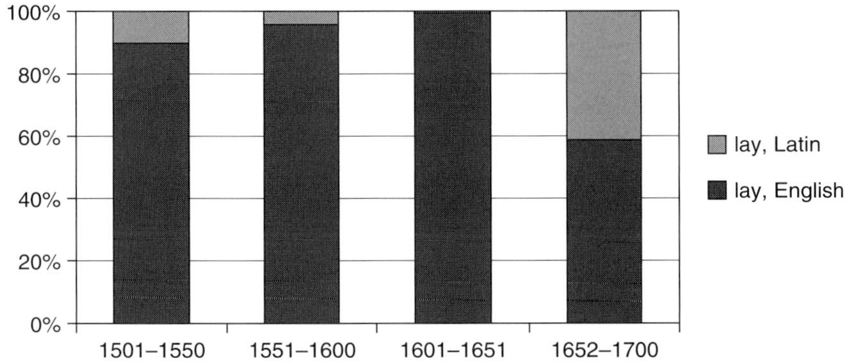


Figure 9.5 Distribution of efficacy phrases between Latin and English in lay texts.

## 9.8 Discussion

As has been demonstrated, EPs persist throughout the 200-year period studied in this chapter. The slot and the function of EPs are still needed in 1700, although the variation in their use and form indicates that they have been affected by changes in scientific thought and in ways of perceiving the world. Thus, despite being a persistent element in medical recipes, EPs do show some signs of change.

One possible reason for change which has already been mentioned is the fact that EPs whose origins were in classical texts and scholastic medicine were inconsistent with the new ways of thinking. Others were the lessening of the effect of EPs and the need to use the existing slot for something else. Examples of new uses of the slot were advertising the medicine (cf. Example 15) or marking the end of a recipe by a text-organizing device, to which Miles seems to have reduced the *probatum est* phrase in *Countrymans Friend.*

Empiricism was permeating into the methods used in medicine, especially in the seventeenth century, but, as Andrew Wear (2000) has pointed out, the reasons underlying symptoms were still hidden. The new thinking can be seen in the methods by which physicians tried to arrive at diagnoses, but empiricists and humoralists alike were still unable to explain their remedies or to account for the effects that these might bring about. The language and the terminology used by both seems to have been the same, perhaps because there was no reason to abandon the old as long as there was nothing new to adopt.

The variation in the use of EPs in the seventeenth century may be due to the ideological shift towards empiricism, but, as was pointed out earlier, the new science was not reflected in all the recipes published in the latter half of the period studied. Also, Galenists demonstrated willingness to reform or, at least, determination to oppose the Helmontian movement, even if that meant taking a leaf from their opponents' book. 'The new philosophy did not, and could not, alter traditional rational ways of thinking about illness and the effects of medicines – although the terms in which the explanations were couched, of course, did change radically' (Wear 1998b: 319).

One thing that has not been looked at yet is contemporary appreciation of EPs. Example 16 below is from Thomas Dekker's satirical pamphlet, *The Guls Hornebooke*:

(16) Fear not to taste it; a caudle will not go down half so smoothly as this will; you need not call the honest name of it in question; for antiquity puts off his cap, and makes a bare oration in praise of the virtues of it: **the receipt hath been subscribed unto, by all those that have had to do with simplex, with this moth eaten motto, *probatum est*.** (Dekker 1609/1904: 17)

Even though Dekker's text may not reflect the views of the majority of his contemporaries, it is probably quite true that 'proof' phrases had been overused by the beginning of the seventeenth century. Dekker's attitude to the phrase is very telling, and it bears out the view that EPs underwent an inflationary process, leading to them being heaped upon each other in an attempt to maintain their original effect. If what Dekker says about traditional EPs was generally accepted, they seem to have become hollow and are no longer fulfilling their purpose. There was a need for new, creative and non-formulaic uses of the EP slot since the old phrases no longer had the desired effect. All this may have also been due to a gradual departure from Galenic thinking.

The old phrases still had their uses, however. The early modern physicians were keenly aware of their patients' psychological needs, and, in that respect, EPs were still as useful as ever:

(17) For bleeding at the nose.

Let the party lye on his backe, and let him have a wet cloth to receive the blood in, that his cloathes may be kept cleane: then bathe his Temples with cold water, and lay a double napkin wet in water and vinegar in his necke, and hold your two fourefingers hard on his Temples, **and tell him also that it is stanched, though it bleede still; for that will worke strangely on his imagination and I have often found, so that he will gather strength suddainly, and the bleeding will cease.** (*EMEMT*; Hawes 1634: 5–6)

The example above is not a recipe but rather a remedy to staunch nose bleeding. It is a 'textbook example' of suggestion, which may have been the best that any physician could have offered his patients in the early modern period. It has been suggested that physicians in the Middle Ages were already aware of the importance of patients' attitudes (McVaugh 1997: 216). Seen in this light, the theoretical framework behind EPs may be of secondary importance: the need to have some means by which to influence the patient's frame of mind may have been an overriding reason for the continued use of EPs in practical medicine.

Like many historical corpus studies, this survey would have benefited from the consultation of more texts. While the number of recipes in lay texts may be adequate for the purpose, more learned texts would have been useful. Sadly, texts are scarcest where the need is greatest, namely for texts from the first half of the sixteenth century. The material issues may handicap the trends perceived and the generalizations made but, acknowledging the shortcomings of the material, the questions raised in this chapter can still be discussed.

Other issues surrounding the material are related to the nature of textual variation itself. The heterogeneous texts within a corpus category would benefit from comparison with other genres. This survey has used only the recipe and *materia medica* literature, but these are not the only medical genres that contain recipes. Comparison with, for example, surgical recipes would yield tools to differentiate between genre-internal and genre-external variation, a possibility that may be pursued in further studies. Other questions that have not been addressed in this chapter include the use of EPs in recipe paraphrases and the role of lists of virtues, case histories and similar elements which were usually present in recipes and designed to aid assessment of their efficacy.

## 9.9 Conclusion

This survey of efficacy statements in the early modern period English recipe literature from 1500 to 1700 has shown that EPs were still established elements in medical recipes at the end of that period, even though the element itself underwent some changes. The first-person observation that characterizes the centuries in question is sometimes evident in efficacy statements. In addition to attesting to the value of a recipe, EPs may have gone on to perform several additional functions simultaneously. Typical of these are text-organizing devices and, at a later stage, new functions such as advertisement and suggestions for inducing positive frames of mind.

Despite the advances in science, especially in chemistry, the theoretical foundation of medicine seems to have changed slowly: in 1700, English medicine was still strongly Galenic; consequently, there was no need for the form of the recipes to change. However, there is some evidence that less importance was being attached to EPs and of a departure from Galenic thinking: the Helmontian controversy seems to have been sowing new ideas even among adherents of Galenic medicine.

The differences in the development of lay and learned recipes are fairly clear. In lay recipes, EPs become rarer, more formulaic and, by the second half of the seventeenth century, the use of Latin phrases increases. The use of EPs in learned recipes increases slightly, but steadily, as time passes, but by 1700, formulaic EPs are becoming outnumbered by specific phrases. During the latter part of the period studied, it becomes more common to stack EPs and to use the slot more creatively. These developments may signal a decline in the importance attached to EPs, when compared to that in the Middle Ages, and a gradual retreat from Galenic thinking. However, there is also evidence that some need was felt for a slot in recipes in which to express other things better suited to the new scientific insights. This seems to be one of the reasons that EPs were still in use in 1700.

## Acknowledgements

The author wishes to acknowledge the support of the Middle English Grammar Project, Department of Cultural and Language Studies, at the University of Stavanger, under the auspices of which this article was written. The Middle English Grammar Project is funded by the Norwegian Research Council.

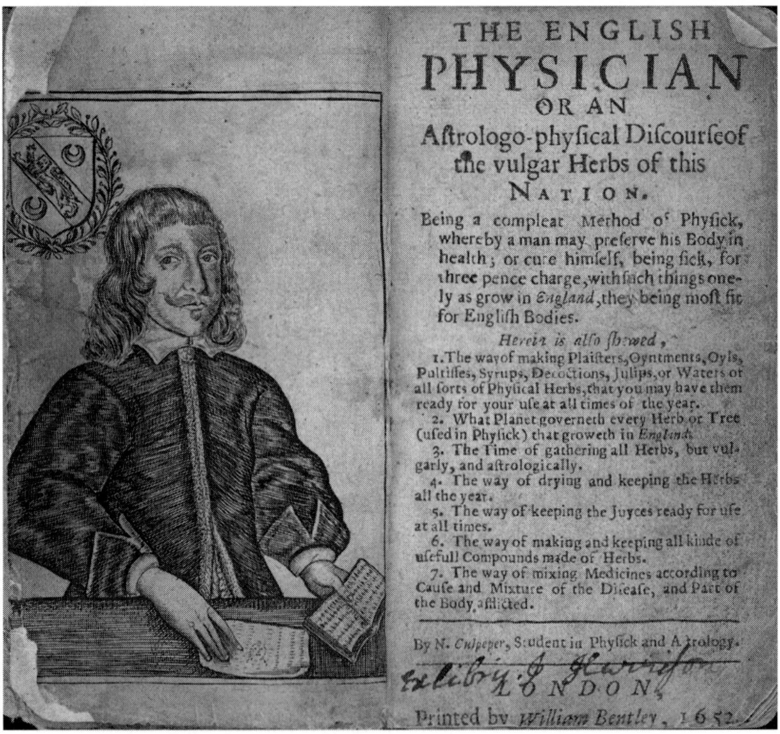


Plate 9 Frontispiece and title page, *The English Physician; or, an Astrologo-Physical Discourse of the Vulgar Herbs of This Nation – Being a Compleat Method of Physick* by Nicholas Culpeper, 1652

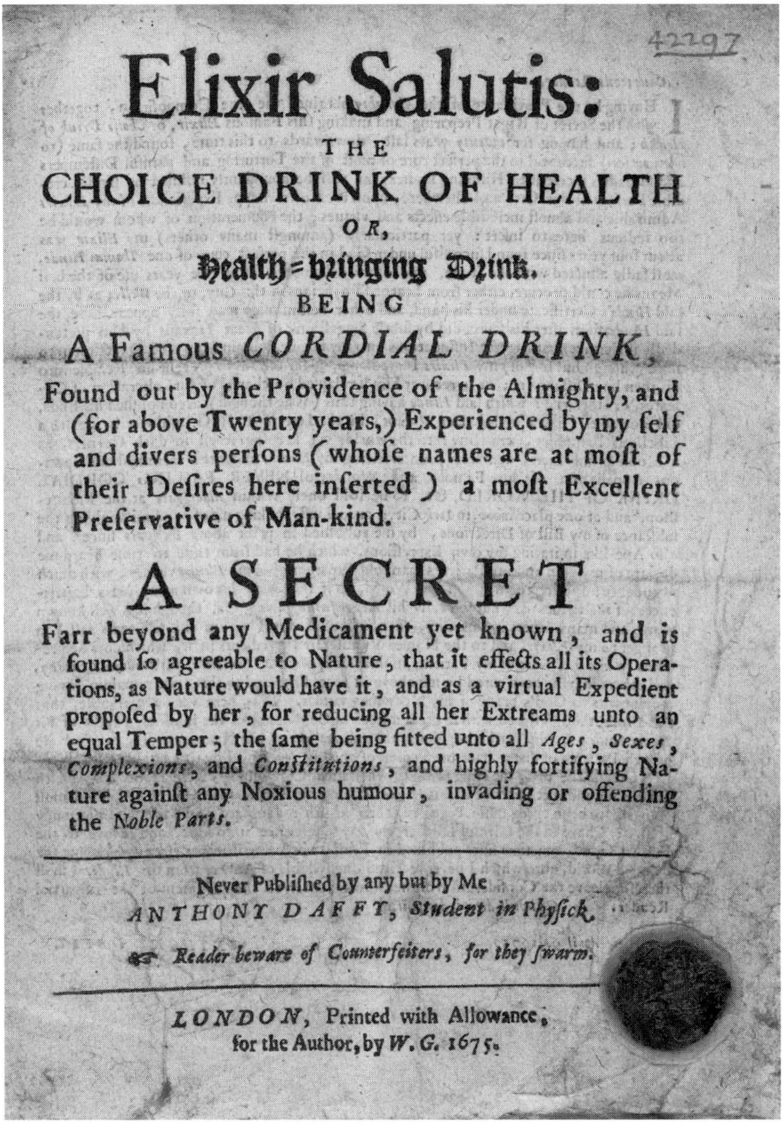



Elixir Salutis:

THE

CHOICE DRINK OF HEALTH

OR,

Health-bringing Drink.

BEING

A Famous *CORDIAL DRINK*,

Found out by the Providence of the Almighty, and (for above Twenty years,) Experienced by my ſelf and divers perſons (whoſe names are at moſt of their Deſires here inſerted) a moſt Excellent Preſervative of Man-kind.

A SECRET

Farr beyond any Medicament yet known, and is found ſo agreeable to Nature, that it effects all its Operations, as Nature would have it, and as a virtual Expedient propoſed by her, for reducing all her Extreams unto an equal Temper; the ſame being fitted unto all *Ages*, *Sexes*, *Complexions*, and *Conſtitutions*, and highly fortifying Nature againſt any Noxious humour, invading or offending the *Noble Parts*.

Never Publiſhed by any but by Me

*ANTHONY DAFFY*, *Student in Phyſick*.

*Reader beware of Counterfeiters, for they ſwarm.*

*LONDON*, Printed with Allowance, for the Author, by *W. G.* 1675.

Plate 10 Title page of *Elixir Salutis: The Choice Drink of Health* by Anthony Daffy, 1675

# 10 Medical pamphlets: controversy and advertising

MAURA RATIA AND CARLA SUHR

## 10.1 Introduction

Pamphlets were a new genre of ephemeral texts that started to proliferate from the mid sixteenth century onwards. They were cheap and easy to print and distribute, and thus their prices were much lower than those of books. This made them potentially available to people of all social classes, and the practice of reading pamphlets aloud in coffee shops or even on street corners gave even the illiterate access to news, politics and advertisements (Shepard 1973: 13–14).[1] The breakdown of censorship in 1641 caused an explosion in the numbers of printed titles, which can largely be explained by a shift from long folio and octavo works towards shorter quartos and broadsides in pamphlets and other forms of cheap print such as newsbooks (Raymond 2003: 168). Medical topics also multiplied, and while recipe books and general guides to medicine continued to be the most frequently published medical genres, a new genre of pamphlets advertising proprietary medicines became the third-most popular kind of medical publication in the second half of the seventeenth century (Fissell 2007: 114, Table 6.2). Pamphlets participating in medical as well as other controversies were another new genre, developing from the late sixteenth century onwards. These two kinds of medical pamphlets had different audiences: literate controversies had a limited readership of educated medical professionals, whereas advertisements had the widest readership possible and were probably read aloud like news pamphlets.

This chapter will investigate whether the difference in intended audiences of medical controversies and advertisements for proprietary medicines is reflected in the interpersonal strategies aiding reading and/or listening comprehension. We have focused our study on the uses of first- and second-person pronouns as indicators of interpersonality and on discourse deictic markers. Even though both types of pamphlets are from the same register of

[1] A pamphlet is generally regarded as a small printed and unbound book of quarto size or less (or, with single sheets and leaflets, of folio size), between eight and up to ninety-six pages (Fritz 2010; Spencer 1958: 102). Some scholars claim that pamphlets are best defined as a polemical text type (Bach 1997; Fritz 2010) or a publication type (Claridge 2001: 56).

medical writing, we will show that they have quite distinctive styles for taking into account their audiences.

## 10.2 Medical pamphlets in the sixteenth and seventeenth centuries

The following section briefly outlines the socio-historical background of these two types of medical pamphlets and describes the materials used in this study.

### *10.2.1 Medical pamphlet controversies*

Controversies were communicated in writing in sixteenth- and seventeenth-century Europe in the field of politics, religion and science (Gloning 1999). Linguistic research on controversies is relatively new, although written controversies have a long tradition and history, from the philosophical dialectics of antiquity and ancient sectarian controversies to the *quaestiones* and *disputationes* of scholasticism (Bylebyl 1985: 223, 226; Gloning 1999: 86–7; Fritz 2003: 200; Taavitsainen 2004; Weijers 2007). The period from the sixteenth to the eighteenth century has been designated the 'Golden Age' of controversies (Fritz 2010). In the beginning of the era, new approaches and trends to medicine emerged, and conflicting ideas were sometimes contested in controversies. Typically, rather than speaking for themselves, the individuals engaged in a dispute often represented a group or an ideology (Gloning 1999: 87–8). The new medium of the pamphlet was particularly suitable for controversies, as they were fast to print and could reach a wide audience.[2]

It has been claimed that controversies are intrinsic to science (Gil 1985: 362; but see Mendelsohn 1987: 94). Famous scientific controversies of the early modern period are the Copernican controversy (see Moss 1993) and the controversy over the motion of the heart and the circulation of blood (see Bylebyl 1985; Gorham 1994). The tobacco controversy is special among medical controversies because the recreational use of tobacco soon spread and outweighed its medicinal use, ultimately causing a social and cultural crisis in England (Grafton et al. 1992: 161). For this reason, the controversy was of interest to lay audiences as well, although, at the core, the controversy was medico-moral, affected by religious politics and economics – for example, England having to buy expensive tobacco from the Spanish (Harley 1993). The controversy lasted for almost a century before it dwindled.

Two tobacco pamphlets in dialogue with each other were chosen for analysis. The first, *Work for Chimny-Sweepers*, written in 1602 under the

[2] Unfortunately, it is difficult to estimate what proportion of pamphlets participate in controversies (see Engelhardt and Caplan 1987a: 4). In addition to pamphlets, controversies also occurred in letters, in critical reviews and in treatises (Fritz 2010; cf. Ratia 2006).

pseudonym Philaretes, is a crucial text in the controversy because it was the first text to openly attack tobacco use. The second text, a reply to the first called *A Defence of Tobacco*, was written the same year by another anonymous author, later identified as Roger Marbecke (Greenhill 2004). A typical textual strategy in controversies is a list of arguments in the first pamphlet; in the reply, these arguments are quoted again and then refuted one by one with a counter-argument (Fritz 2003: 201–2).

Two texts from the controversy over alkali and acid 100 years later are also examined. Sir John Colbatch was an advocate of the doctrine of acids and alkalis, a theory more popular on the Continent than in England. Colbatch was unorthodox in claiming alkalis to be 'the Cause of all or most Distempers' (1696: title page). He reasserted the theory in a lengthy work, *The Doctrine of Acids* in 1698, which ultimately started 'the debate between the physician and the gentleman', i.e. Thomas Emes and Colbatch himself (Bevan 2004). Emes replied to Colbatch with an equally lengthy essay the same year, claiming his work to be 'A Specimen of the Immodest Self-applause, Shameful Contempt, and abuse of all Physicians, gross Mistakes and great Ignorance of the Pretender *John Colbatch*' (1698: title page).[3] The controversy continued in pamphlets in 1700, when Colbatch anonymously wrote *A Letter to a Physician Concerning Acid and Alkali. Being an Answer to a Late Piece, Intituled, A Dialogue Between Alkali and Acid, Written by a Gentleman.* It seems that hiding behind anonymity enabled Colbatch to freely praise his own work: 'I confess I am amazed to see the Ingenious Author of the Hypothesis of Acids, treated with the utmost Contempt and Scorn' (Colbatch 1700: 4). Emes wrote a reply to Colbatch during the same year: *A Letter to a Gentleman Concerning Alkali and Acid. Being an Answer to a Late Piece, Intituled, a Letter to a Physician Concerning Acid and Alkali.* Emes appears to be ignorant about the true identity of his opponent, but perhaps not so: 'I fancy the Gentleman has learnt Logick of Mr. Colebatch, (altho' he would be thought to converse with him only in an epistolary way) he argues so like him' (Emes 1700: 48). These two pamphlets show how a controversy can build up in treatises and eventually continue in pamphlet format, making the exchange of arguments more precise and focused.

### *10.2.2 Pamphlet advertisements of proprietary medicines*

Pamphlets were also used for medical advertisements aimed at literate and semi-literate crowds, and they were a prominent subgenre of late eighteenth-century medical publishing. Proprietary medicines advertised in newspapers, handbills and pamphlets were probably the earliest extensively marketed branded products and 'those that became most familiar to late seventeenth and eighteenth-century consumers' (Styles 2000: 148–9). The texts were

[3] Throughout the article, italics in the excerpts are original.

meant to be read not only silently but also aloud in coffee shops or on the street, and thus the potential audience of these texts included the uneducated or semi-literate masses as well as the growing middle class. Pamphlet advertisements have been characterized as 'early modern infomercials', 'neither purely informational nor purely promotional but an extremely successful hybrid of the two' (Fissell 2007: 120, 126). The promotional aspect is clear from the extensive use of hyperbole: for example, Nendick's popular pill was advertised as the 'only medicine, which hath had the fortunate success above all medicines, yet found out to be famed for its incomparable Vertues and brought into Universal use by its infallible Operations' (*EMEMT*; Nendick 1674: A1r). The authors of the advertisements were usually also the manufacturers of the advertised products. The kind of information disseminated in these texts is strikingly similar, and one could claim that certain informational elements – such as descriptions of virtues, directions for use and information about prices, packaging and distribution – formed conventional parts of medical pamphlet advertisements. Some of these elements were probably copied from recipes, as many of the elements are very similar (e.g., purpose, application and administration and rationale; cf. Hunt 1990: 16–24; Mäkinen 2006: 87–94; Stannard 1982: 60–5).

The marketing revolution of proprietary medicines has traditionally been placed in the eighteenth century, as that century has been distinguished as the period when publicity (especially in newspapers) and distribution took off on a national level (see, for example, Porter 1989a: 45). In fact, medicine figured prominently in the earliest newspaper advertisements from the mid seventeenth century onwards (R. B. Walker 1973), and more recently it has been argued that the marketing revolution took place in the late seventeenth century in the form of advertisements in more ephemeral forms of print such as almanacs (cf. Curth 2002, 2007). The high numbers of pamphlet advertisements for proprietary medicines seem to corroborate the claim for cheap print as the first locus of large-scale advertising: pamphlets advertising proprietary medicines make up between c. 13 per cent and c. 25 per cent of all new medical titles in each decade of the period 1650–90, with an average of 11 per cent for the period 1640–1740 (Fissell 2007: 116–17).[4] Cheap print travelled quickly across the country in the backpacks of itinerant merchants and thus reached a larger audience than the London-based early newspapers. A significant factor that no doubt contributed to the close link between print and specifically proprietary medicines was that many booksellers and printers also sold medicines (some of which they manufactured themselves), and thus the nationwide distribution network of the book trade overlapped with that of proprietary medicines (Isaac 1998).

[4] The breakdown by decade for this period is as follows: 1650–60: c. 25 per cent; 1660–70: c. 13 per cent; 1670–80: c. 20 per cent; and 1680–90: c. 23 per cent. The percentages have been estimated from Figure 6.3 in Fissell (2007: 117).

Medical pamphlet advertisements have to a large extent been ignored by historical linguists studying advertising as they have focused their analyses on newspaper advertising during the eighteenth century (cf. auf dem Keller 2004; Fries 1997; Gieszinger 2000; Görlach 2002; Gotti 2005). However, in light of their popularity in the latter half of the seventeenth century, it is clear that these early forms of advertising merit closer study.

The advertising material used in this study consists of three medical pamphlet advertisements in the corpus of *Early Modern English Medical Texts* (*EMEMT*), supplemented by nine other texts. Most of the texts are shorter than 5,000 words, and even the longest one does not exceed 10,000 words. The texts range from 1664 to 1690; they are thus from the period when medical pamphlet advertisements formed a significant proportion of all printed medical titles. The medicines advertised in these pamphlets were some of the most well known in the seventeenth century: for example, Anthony Daffy's Elixir Salutis (more colloquially known as Daffy's Elixir) continued to be a household name until the twentieth century (Porter 1989a: 101). Like many other proprietary medicines, Elixir Salutis had several competing manufacturers, for, in addition to Anthony Daffy (and later his heirs), Thomas Hinde, Thomas Witherden and Thomas Woodward all claimed to hold the true recipe for the medicine and pronounced the others counterfeit products. Texts by all four authors are included in the selection of pamphlets used in this study.

## 10.3 Personal pronouns and interpersonality

The relation between author and audience is approached by looking at personal pronouns. They construct and shape relationships between authors and readers and/or hearers, which is crucial in pamphlets.

This study focuses on first- and second-person pronouns including possessive and object forms. Third-person pronouns are omitted from analysis. First- and second-person pronouns are central in interaction because they do not normally refer to the text, but their referents are defined by the speech roles of the speaker and the hearer (Wales 1996: 44). These pronouns 'emphasize the author's role and judgement in shaping or recording knowledge and the recipient's role as a receiver' (Taavitsainen and Pahta 1998: 163). However, the pronoun 'you' is ambiguous because it can be either singular or plural depending on the context. The pronoun 'we' is complicated in another sense, because it seldom means 'more than one *I*', and this complexity cannot be explained by the inclusive and exclusive uses of the pronoun (Lyons 1968: 277; Wales 1996: 58).

The pronoun 'we' is useful in polite interaction between self and another, because in theory it minimizes benefits to self and maximizes benefits to the addressee, but actually the authority of the speaker, subjectivity and egocentricity of viewpoint tend to surface or to be reasserted (Wales 1996: 58).

'We' is a rhetorical convention to distance the speaker from an overt self-reference in order to make the personal source of knowledge more palatable (Mühlhäusler and Harré 1990: 129). Especially in a social and ideological sense, it can mean 'more than one' of the same: the addressee can belong to the same group and share the speaker's views, or the addressee can be excluded from the group ('exclusive *we*') (Wales 1996: 58–9). For example, usage referred to as 'authorial *we*' commonly co-occurs with verbs of saying, showing, thinking, etc., often in the preterite, for example '*We* have already discussed', and with verbs of anticipating, returning, postponing, etc., for example '*We* deal with some such cases below.' In contrast, usage Wales refers to as the 'workshop *we*' could easily be substituted with 'you' and co-occurs with verbs of seeing, looking, etc., and with modals of obligation, for example 'Already *we can see*' and '*we shall* at some stage *need* a term' (Wales 1996: 58, 65–6). Within a larger cultural context, generic 'we' can be used with reference to, for example, *Englishmen* or *physicians* as a group.

For this study, we have analysed all first- and second-person pronouns in the medical controversies and advertisements and have carefully scrutinized their referents. Only the most typical uses in each text are commented on.

### *10.3.1 Interpersonality in controversies*

Interpersonality is a central feature of controversies because of their basis on spoken dialogue (Fritz 2003: 200). The strategies for using personal pronouns in argumentation alternate greatly between the texts because of the individual styles of the authors. The frequencies of first- and second-person pronouns are shown in Table 10.1.

In general, controversies seem to employ the first-person singular frequently and, to a lesser extent, the first-person plural. However, the use of the second-person pronoun varies greatly between the texts. The pamphlet by Philaretes differs from the others most with an overall low frequency of first- and second-person pronouns, the only exception being a slightly higher use of the first-person plural. The style of the text seems distanced with minimal communication with the audience. The text is different from the others because it was the first outright attack on tobacco. At the same time, it was not written directly to anyone, the intended audience formulated thus in the preface: 'many excellent Phisitions and men of singuler learning and practise, together with many gentlemen and some of great accompt' (*EMEMT*; Philaretes 1602: A3r). This is unlike the other pamphlets, whose titles indicate that they were written as replies to an ongoing debate. Colbatch and Emes both employ the same formula typical of controversies: 'Being an Answer to a late Piece', whereas Marbecke writes: 'VVITH A FRIENDLY ANSWER TO THE late printed Booke.' The word 'answer' seems to function as a kind of token in the titles signalling controversy.

Table 10.1 *The frequencies of first- and second-person singular and plural pronouns in two controversies.*

| Controversies | Text | Word count[a] | First-person singular/1,000 (N) | First-person plural/1,000 (N) | Second person/1,000 (N) | *Total/1,000 (N)* |
|---|---|---|---|---|---|---|
| Tobacco | Philaretes (1602) | 10,566 | 3.5 (37) | 7.6 (80) | 0.4 (4) | **11.5 (121)** |
| | Marbecke (1602) | 20,766 | 18.1 (376) | 5.8 (121) | 21.3 (442) | **45.2 (939)** |
| Acid and alkali | Colbatch (1700) | 11,108 | 18.2 (202) | 5.0 (55) | 7.1 (79) | **30.2 (336)** |
| | Emes (1700) | 21,653 | 21.4 (463) | 4.6 (100) | 1.2 (27) | **27.2 (590)** |
| | **Total** | **64,093** | **16.8 (1,078)** | **5.6 (356)** | **8.6 (552)** | **31.0 (1,986)** |

*Note:* (a) The word counts for these texts are, in fact, to be expected with the replies being twice as long as their antecedents, resulting from the typical textual strategy in pamphlets (see Section 10.2.1).

The first-person singular 'I' is used by Philaretes in authorial phrases, sometimes neutrally but also to assert authority, as in '*I am not ignorant*.' Some expressions clearly denote caution, as in Example 1:

(1) and to come to those which are of perfect health, **I take it** very dangerous and hurtfull for them often to vse this Tabacco feume: (*EMEMT*; Philaretes 1602: C1r)

Similarly, caution can be implied with '*I hold it*' and 'if *I be not deceiued*'. In addition, personal pleas, '*I pray you*' and '*I assure you*', are used to persuade the reader. The caution implied in this pamphlet makes it stand out from the rest.

Marbecke writes with strong authorial focus in epistemic phrases, for example, '*I thinke/me thinke*', '*I know*', '*I trow*' and '*I beleeue*', enforcing the idea of the process of experimentation as a personal experience (Taavitsainen and Pahta 1995: 524; see also *mental verbs* in Palander-Collin 2009). Authority is further enforced with expressions such as '*I am sure*'. The expression '*I* thinke' differs from the other epistemic verbs in its function because it can express either certainty or uncertainty. With reference to the author in this text, it does not convey uncertainty but is used as an evidential expression (see Palander-Collin 1999: 31, 35–3; cf. Aijmer 1997). However, the most common usage refers to something that the author believes his opponent might believe, as indicated in Example 2:

(2) But yet thus much **I do know**, and **I thinke** your selfe also will not deny. (Marbecke 1602: 24)

Here periphrastic 'do' is used together with epistemic 'know' to assert authority; *do*-periphrasis does not occur in other texts except Marbecke's (a total of sixteen instances).[5] As a contrast to affirmative 'I do know', 'I thinke' suggests uncertainty. In comparison to the other authors, the possessive pronoun 'my' is used a great deal by Marbecke, the most frequent expressions being '(I) for my part', 'in my opinion' and 'in my iudgement', creating a contrast with the opponent.

In the controversy over alkali and acid, Colbatch uses epistemic phrases moderately: 'I think', 'I know' and 'I believe'. By the time the pamphlet was published, Colbatch had already been admitted as a licenciate to the Royal College of Physicians and had published several books (Cook 2004). Colbatch's style represents the formal type of argumentative writing where the persuasion is not overt but subtle.

Colbatch's opponent Emes uses the following epistemic phrases, also in the negative: 'I think/thought', 'I believe' and 'I know/knew'. But the main function

[5] Unlike today, periphrastic 'do' was frequent in affirmative statements in the sixteenth and seventeenth centuries (Rissanen 1991: 324). For *emphatic use*, see Rissanen (1991: 338) and Nurmi (1999: 27).

of verbs connected to the first-person pronoun is to indicate dialogue, 'answer' being the most frequent of these (thirty-nine instances), shown in Example 3:

(3) **I answer**, the Gentleman has so often, unbecoming a Gentleman, made me say what I never said, that I now can hardly believe he is indeed a Gentleman, but rather some little Medicaster, or very small Surgeon. (Emes 1700: 56)

'I answer' stands out, since it always occurs at the beginning of the sentence in Emes' pamphlet. Interestingly, the opponent is always a noun, usually 'the Gentleman', which differs from the direct dialogue in the tobacco pamphlets between 'I' and 'you', the two authors. In addition, a speech-act verb 'say'/'said' occurs often, being the most frequent verb following after the first-person pronoun (forty-two instances), also occurring as 'I did not say' (six instances) and 'I never said' (four instances). The possessive pronoun 'my' is used to refer with self-importance to 'my Dialogue', 'my Assertion', 'my Experiments' and 'my Arguments'.

The differences in the use of the first-person plural between the texts are mostly qualitative. Philaretes uses persuasive 'we' in his tobacco pamphlet, as seen in Example 4:

(4) **We see** this thing confirmed by Galen himself, in his second booke and second Chapter, De temperamentis, and also by Auicen. (*EMEMT*; Philaretes 1602: E2v)

Workshop 'we' is indicated by the verb 'see' involving the reader in the argument. The possessive 'our' is often used, for example, with reference to '*our* bodies', '*our* norishment' and '*our* spirits', to create an idea of unity (see Lee 1992).

Marbecke makes use of the neutral, authorial 'we', but the possessive 'our' with generic references is used in a similar way to Philaretes, to create common ground with the reader, for example, '*Our* bodies/body', '*Our* countrie', '*our* blood' and '*our* temperature'. In these references, the pronoun still includes the opponent, unlike in Example 5:

(5) and seeing **our poore friend Tabacco**, hath a good and a speciall property, to resist, that professed great enemy, the cold: me thinke, it were a reasonable sute, to intreate, that Tabacco, might rather be esteemed as a friend, then a foe, euen to old age also. (Marbecke 1602: 42–3)

The reference to 'our friend Tabacco', with the emotive adjective 'poore', is to propagandists of tobacco, excluding Philaretes. The opponent is similarly excluded when the persuasive 'let us' is used, for example, 'now *let us* weigh your argument', which invites the reader to participate in the argumentation.

Colbatch uses 'we' as a generic reference to people in general. The possessive 'our' is used almost exclusively with connection to '*our* Author' or '*our* Bodies'. The repetitive use of '*our* Author', the opponent, can at times be interpreted as disparaging, as in Example 6:

(6) Sir, **I** am of opinion that **our Author** cannot produce a Catalogue of Medicines equally efficacious in the cure of Diseases. (Colbatch 1700: 50)

There is also a humorous reference to '*our* Alkali man' meaning the opponent Emes. 'Sir' is the patron of the pamphlet, referred to a few times in the text. In fact, there is no direct dialogue between the two writers, unlike in the tobacco pamphlets. Emes persuades the reader differently from Colbatch, using, for example, workshop 'we' with modals of obligation, especially 'will' and 'must'. The generic 'we' refers to 'us colleagues', often excluding Colbatch. Colbatch was radical in his views, whereas Emes seems confident of having his colleagues' support, also seen in Example 7:

(7) If the Disease was caus'd by Alkalies and cur'd by Acids, it was caus'd by Alkalies and cur'd by Acids; a Wit! But there's an If in the case, which makes the Argument worth nothing: For if this cannot be found (as **I** am sure it has not yet by any certain Experiments the **Acidists** have given **us**) **we** are never the better for the Supposition. (Emes 1700: 15)

Binary opposition is created between 'Acidists' and 'us', and there is an intriguing widening of reference from 'I' to 'we' in the same sentence. There are some references to '*our* Bodies' and '*our* Food', also to '*our* Gentleman/ Gent.', referring to the opponent, but these references are neutral.

'You' is very seldom used by Philaretes. However, the author sometimes addresses the reader with formulaic expressions 'I pray *you*' and 'I assure *you*', which can also have emotive value. The comparison to the reply by Marbecke is striking, because 'I' and 'you' are used repeatedly in the reply, which signifies involved discourse. There are instances of 'I pray *you*', which refer to the reader, but they are an exception. Most often, 'you' refers to Philaretes – the opponent. Similarly, 'your selfe' occurs often and clearly points to the opponent. Expressions such as 'I can tell *you*' and 'as *you* see' influence the reader to believe in the harmlessness of tobacco. It appears that the author is constantly referring to Philaretes instead of appealing to the audience as well.

In the controversy over acid and alkali, there is no direct dialogue between the opponents, only between the authors and their patrons. Colbatch refers to his patron as 'Sir' and 'you' many times (see Example 6). When 'Sir' is not used, 'you' also invites readers, as in Example 8:

(8) **He** says, the Doctor's preparation of Steel with Sal Armoniac is not made with an Acid. **I** think it is; and to prove it to **you**, if **you** make

> this Preparation in a Retort and a strong Fire, **you** shall find nothing but an Alkali Spirit to arise, and the Acid will remain with the Steel. (Colbatch 1700: 46)

Here both Colbatch and Emes refer to the opponent as 'he' instead of 'you'. Emes, unlike Colbatch, refers to his patron as 'Sir' only twice. Also, the second-person pronoun is infrequent in his pamphlet, most occurrences being generic: for example, 'if *you* take' is the most common and does not actually signal interaction but is similar to a passive-like construction.

Overall, the four pamphlets share a similar kind of use of the first-person plural, which can be taken to indicate their argumentative function. These persuasive uses of the pronoun were employed in all the texts to include the audience in the argumentation. However, there were great differences in the use of the first-person singular and the second person between the texts, from almost non-existent use to abundant. Especially the lack of the second-person pronoun in the pamphlets by Philaretes and Emes is marked, making the discourse less involved.

### *10.3.2 Interpersonality in medical pamphlet advertisements*

Since medical pamphlet advertisements were often intended to be read aloud, thus simulating the situation of a proprietary medicine manufacturer hawking his product, the expectation is to find strong authorial presence. But how do these texts interact with their audiences?

Table 10.2 below shows the frequencies of first- and second-person pronouns in medical pamphlet advertisements.[6] Combining the results for individual texts with close readings shows that there were several different strategies for dealing with the readers and/or listeners of these texts.

First-person pronouns are much more frequent than second-person pronouns, and they are used in several contexts, as shown in Examples 9 and 10. The authors often emphasize their own importance in the discovery and successful administration of the advertised medicines. In addition, authors stress their ownership of the medicines by the use of the possessive form – '*my* elixir', '*my* pill', '*my* drink' – to distance themselves from their competitors' products. Example 10 also shows how authors comment on the structure of the text.

(9) And **I** do in the presence of the Almighty Searcher of hearts, faithfully promise, that this **my** *pleasant inoffensive Drink*, is with much carefulness and integrity duly prepared by **me**; so that **I** have (through the Lord's goodness) successfully given the same unto **my** wife (*lying in*) and unto *Babes* in the *Moneth*), (so qualifi'd as in **my** *Directions* for taking the same is particularly exprest.) (*EMEMT*; Daffy 1673: 7)

[6] The counts for first-person singular and plural were combined, because the plural cases were very few: less than 1/1,000 words (forty-one hits).

Table 10.2 *Frequencies of first- and second-person pronouns in medical pamphlet advertisements.*

| Text | Word count | First person/ 1,000 (N) | Second person/ 1,000 (N) | Total/1,000 (N) |
|---|---|---|---|---|
| Daffy (1673) | 2,884 | 20.1 (58) | 0 (0) | 20.1 (58) |
| Elixir (1670–80) | 3,208 | 1.6 (5) | 1.2 (4) | 2.8 (9) |
| Fletcher (1677) | 2,447 | 11.9 (29) | 1.6 (4) | 13.5 (33) |
| Hinde (1673) | 2,558 | 29.7 (76) | 2.3 (6) | 32.1 (82) |
| Lockyer (1664) | 7,259 | 28.7 (208) | 5.4 (39) | 34.0 (247) |
| Lomax (1680?) | 4,451 | 9.2 (41) | 3.4 (15) | 12.6 (56) |
| Maynwaringe (1684) | 9,168 | 23.3 (214) | 9.9 (91) | 33.3 (305) |
| Nendick (1674) | 6,046 | 17.5 (106) | 0.8 (5) | 18.4 (111) |
| Tablets (1680) | 1,903 | 6.3 (12) | 9.5 (18) | 15.8 (30) |
| Winter (1664) | 3,776 | 35.0 (132) | 19.1 (72) | 54.0 (204) |
| Witherden (1679) | 2,715 | 36.5 (99) | 1.5 (4) | 37.9 (103) |
| Woodward (1690?) | 3,403 | 0 (0) | 20.0 (68) | 20.0 (68) |
| **Total** | **49,818** | **19.7 (980)** | **6.5 (326)** | **26.2 (1,306)** |

(10) **I** shall give those Directions that were communicated to **me**, together with the description of the Cordial, and which **I** have found by experience to be most beneficial upon several persons that have had it of **me**, as **I** could give an Instance by setting down the Names of hundreds. (Witherden 1679: 4)

The highest frequencies of first-person pronouns are found in texts that use the pronouns for all of the above three purposes: Hinde, Lockyer, Maynwaringe, Winter and Witherden.

The authors' anxiety to assert their rights to the medicines as their own inventions and to distinguish themselves from the competition thus clearly influences their choice of singular over plural. Authorial 'we' is used in a few instances, as is the case with workshop 'we'. There are also some instances of generic 'our' or 'us', as in 'our Bodies' and 'our Microcosmal Sun', but on the whole the texts are strongly author-centred and only occasionally include the audience as participants in the discourse. The difference is great in comparison to controversies, which consistently use first-person plural in argumentation.

By placing themselves in the text in these various ways, the authors create a rather one-sided relationship with their audience that serves to emphasize the role of the author as the source of information and, indeed, the ultimate source of the medicine. As the pamphlet was often the only connection between the manufacturer of a medicine and its buyer, the text functioned as the voice of the seller. In a situation where the text was read aloud, it was more persuasive and convincing when, through the use of first-person pronouns, it seemed as if the author was present himself.

There is only one text with no first-person pronouns at all, Woodward, where the author consistently refers to himself in the third person, even though he is identified as the author on the title page. Woodward is the only author to distance himself from the audience in this way. Anonymity seems to play a role in the frequency of first-person pronouns, as the two anonymous texts – *Elixir* and *Tablets* – have markedly lower frequencies for these pronouns than the other texts. *Elixir* has a remarkably low frequency for both first- and second-person pronouns, making it stand out among the other advertisements. By writing in an impersonal style, the author is perhaps aiming to sound scholarly and that way convince his audience of the worthiness of his medicine.

Second-person pronouns are most frequent in the sections that give directions on the proper use and dosage of the medicines. Thus, the two texts that do not have such sections, Daffy and Fletcher, have very low frequencies of second-person pronouns.[7] Conversely, the extremely high frequencies of second-person pronouns in Winter and Woodward are explained by the fact that the directions for use take up most of the texts. Second-person pronouns alternate regularly with imperatives – where a second person is implied – and passive forms, and in some cases with the third person. The choice of structure for giving directions has repercussions for the closeness or distance of the author and audience. Second-person pronouns and imperatives are the more interpersonal strategies, whereas the use of the passive and of words like 'patient' or 'person' instead of 'you' creates a distance between author and audience. Compare, for instance, Examples 11 and 12 below.

(11) **It has been found by experience** to be a most incomparable Remedy in the highest *Feaver*, even when **they** Rave: **It may be taken** at any time, according to the **persons** strength, for it immediately quiets the Spirits, and cheers and comforts **them**. (*Elixir* 1670–80: 6)

(12) But if **your** Body be weak or laxative, **take** not above two or three *Pills* at the first, **you** may increase or diminish the number as occasion requires, and in that **you'l** be a *Physician* to **your** self. (Woodward 1690: 4)

The use of the passive and 'person' rather than a personal pronoun in Example 11 makes the text impersonal and places the focus on the medicine rather than the reader/listener, whereas the use of the second person makes Example 12 more dialogic and brings the focus to the audience.

There are some cases when second-person pronouns are used as tools in argumentation, for example to voice possible objections that the author can refute. However, admitting even the possibility of doubting a medicine's infallible cure of diseases is not good policy in advertisements, so this argumentative technique is rare. Another strategy of argumentation that

[7] Both texts refer the reader/listener to separate sheets of directions which are obtained together with the medicines from the suppliers.

makes use of second-person pronouns is addressing the reader to make the discourse more dialogic, as shown in Example 13:

(13) **I** know, **your** chief Desire is to see what *Extraordinary*, this Medicine hath, and can do; and **I** shall satisfie **you** therein; for it were a Crime to conceal what this Medicine hath effected, and what *Help* it affords to *Nature*, distressed and languishing, above the power of any other Medicine; which **I** shall shew **you**, as followeth. (Maynwaringe 1684: 7)

Argumentation is not a significant feature in medical pamphlet advertisements, however, so first- and second-person pronouns are very rarely used for this purpose; in fact, Maynwaringe is exceptional in this respect, for the text argues for the virtues of the 'catholic medicine' at a sophisticated theoretical level that uneducated readers and listeners would probably not have been able to follow. Giving directions remains the primary use for second-person pronouns in medical pamphlet advertisements.

Imperatives and passive forms, and to some degree also the distancing third person, seem to be on an even footing in the repertoire for giving directions in pamphlet advertisements.[8] In some cases, notably Woodward and *Tablets*, it is possible that second-person pronouns are preferred over the other ways of formulating directions in order to compensate for the low frequency of first-person pronouns and the resulting lack of interpersonality. However, as second-person pronouns are so rare in functions other than giving directions, it is apparent that the relationship between the author and the audience in medical pamphlet advertisements was not dialogic. Instead, the author's role as the source and owner of information imparted was emphasized by the use of first-person singular pronouns.

## 10.4 Discourse deixis

If personal pronouns give an indication of the interpersonality of texts, the use of discourse deixis shows how authors took their readers and/or listeners into account by aiding their comprehension of the texts. Discourse deictic markers support the processing of a text by its readers and/or listeners by making explicit the links between parts of a text or by telling them where they are in the text. Discourse deixis can be divided into two types on the basis of function: direction signs and information signs. Direction signs, such as 'earlier' or 'following', tell the reader/listener that something has been mentioned previously or will be taken up later in the discourse. Backward-referring deictic markers can serve as reminders or emphasizers of important points as well as indicators of where to look up the point

[8] As the precise ratios of these features were not calculated for this paper, this is necessarily an impression based on close readings.

discussed. Forward-referring deictic markers can be used to circumvent possible objections by telling that the point will be discussed more fully later or to sustain the readers' or listeners' interest. Direction signs can also be precise, referring to a recognizable layout feature such as 'article' or 'page'. Information signs, on the other hand, refer to the text as a whole or a specific point in the text ('this pamphlet', 'here'), or comment on the progress of the text ('I will now turn to') (Claridge 2001).

Deictic features have been found to be register- and text type-sensitive (Kurzon 1985: 194). The use of discourse deixis in the different registers of the pamphlets of the Lampeter Corpus of Early Modern English Tracts has been analysed previously in order to assess the reader-friendliness of the texts and also to find out if texts planned to be read aloud (sermons, speeches and real or fictional dialogues published as pamphlets) contain deictic markers as guides for comprehension for potential listeners. The use of discourse deixis in the different registers of the pamphlets of the *Lampeter Corpus of Early Modern English Tracts* has been compared to assess the reader-friendliness of the texts and also to find out if texts were planned to be read aloud. The frequency of backward-referring deictic markers does indeed seem to be register-specific, as the frequencies of these markers are different in different registers, while forward-referring deictic markers and informational deictic markers are more evenly spread. Interestingly, the more oral texts have less discourse deixis than the more literate ones even if they are contrived speech rather than actual speech (Claridge 2001).

Accordingly, our assumption was that the more literate controversies would have more discourse deixis than the planned-to-be-spoken advertisements, even though all the texts are from the same register of medical writing. For this empirical study, word lists of deictic markers were supplemented by close readings. As these words often have multiple functions, we used concordances to check that the words were actually used as deictic markers rather than as, for example, discourse particles. The following words (in their various spellings) were identified as backward-referring deictic markers: 'above', '(a)fore', 'before', 'former', 'last' and '(the) said'. Forward-referring deictic markers were 'after(wards)', 'ensuing', 'hereafter', 'hereunder', 'following', 'as followeth', 'further', 'next' and 'now'. Precise deictic markers were 'argument(s)', 'chapter(s)' and 'page(s)'. Finally, the following words were informational markers: 'here', 'in this place', 'next', 'now' and 'this'.[9]

[9] In this material, 'now' was seldom used as a deictic feature; most instances acted as discourse particles. It can also function as both a forward-referring deictic marker and an informational marker. 'Before' can also have two functions: backward-referring and forward-referring.

### *10.4.1 Deixis in controversies*

Deictic features are something to be expected in learned medical controversies because of their often complex structure, where one needs to take heed of the different arguments and claims that have been made in order to follow the argumentation. Table 10.3 below shows the frequencies of the various kinds of deictic markers in the two controversies studied here.

However, a thorough search of the deictic markers revealed that the majority of them are atypical in that they refer to other texts of the controversy, in this case always to the other counterpart of the dispute, helping the reader to follow the plural voices of the controversy. This kind of intertextual deixis is shown in Table 10.4 below, partly to show that according to the traditional view, it would not be considered deixis but also to stress that this type of deixis is central in controversies and can provide us with essential information about their structure. For example, the number of intertextual deictic markers used by these authors suggests that once the controversy proceeds, more of these are needed to keep track of different arguments.

The total number of deictic markers in pamphlet controversies, excluding intertextual deixis, is only slightly lower than the number found in the scientific register of the Lampeter Corpus.[10] The difference emerges with the density of intertextual deixis in controversies; this type of deixis was rare in the Lampeter Corpus. Precise and informational deixis seem essentially intertextual in light of this material. The precise deictic markers 'page(s)', 'argument(s)' and 'chapter(s)' (in the order of frequency) are almost solely intertextual, as shown in Example 14:

(14) The Gent. saith, **pag. 14**. That from the **24 page** of my Dialogue to the **29**, there's nothing but scurrility. (Emes 1700: 19)

In the tobacco controversy, the word 'argument(s)' is sometimes surprisingly used as a precise deictic marker. It meets the criterion of being a 'recognizable layout feature' (Claridge 2001: 65), as Philaretes' pamphlet starts with a list of numbered arguments organized as separate entities to be dealt with one at a time. The organization of these arguments is structurally similar to chapters. Marbecke, in his reply, first restates the argument verbatim before he confutes it, often in a verbose manner, as in Example 15:

(15) But for that the proofe of **this your fifth reason**, hangeth vpon the proofe of your fourth **argument**, as your selfe saith, and for that cause, your selfe also is willing to referre vs ouer, to that fourth part of your Discourse. (Marbecke 1602: 39)

[10] For comparison's sake, here are the results (per 1,000 words) for each register of the Lampeter Corpus: politics 0.85 (backward), 0.2 (forward) and 0.4 (informational); religion 0.3, 0.16 and 0.3; economy 1.2, 0.2 and 0.4; science 0.9, 0.4 and 0.5; law 3.0, 0.3 and 0.2; miscellaneous 0.6, 0.3 and 0.4 (Claridge 2001).

Table 10.3 *Frequencies of deictic markers in two medical pamphlet controversies.*

| Text | Backward-referring deixis (N) | Forward-referring deixis (N) | Precise deixis (N) | Informational deixis (N) | Total (N) | Total/1,000 |
|---|---|---|---|---|---|---|
| Philaretes (1602) | 21 | 0 | 3 | 5 | 29 | 2.7 |
| Marbecke (1602) | 20 | 10 | 0 | 14 | 34 | 1.6 |
| Colbatch (1700) | 6 | 7 | 0 | 1 | 14 | 1.3 |
| Emes (1700) | 4 | 5 | 2 | 1 | 12 | 0.6 |
| **Total (N)** | **41** | **22** | **5** | **21** | **89** | |
| **Total/1,000** | **0.6** | **0.3** | **0.1** | **0.3** | | **1.4** |

In Example 15, there is also an informational deictic marker: 'this your fifth reason'. Many different nouns occur with the intertextual informational deictic marker 'this' in Marbecke's pamphlet: 'argument', 'chapter', 'point', 'reason', 'accusation', 'assertion', 'discourse' and 'question'. Their use can be classified as deictic, because they all refer to one of the eight arguments laid out by Philaretes and replied to meticulously, one by one, by Marbecke. Informational deixis is, on the whole, typical for Marbecke, who uses all four types occurring in the texts: 'here', 'in this place', 'now' and 'this'. A clustering of deictic markers can be seen in Example 16:

(16) as hath alreadie partly bene shewed **before** in your second **Chapter**, and shall **hereafter** more at large be declared. (Marbecke 1602: 33)

Here, 'before' is a backward-referring deictic marker, 'Chapter' is a precise deictic marker and 'hereafter' a forward-referring deictic marker. These clusters describe well Marbecke's highly structured style of writing.

Forward-referring deictic markers are used by everyone except Philaretes. Colbatch, for example, uses 'following', 'further', 'after', 'next', 'now', as in the 'following Observations' and 'following Experiments', after which a detailed description follows. These types of markers seem to give a learned touch to the text and are influenced by the author's need for clarity rather than the wish to aid reading comprehension. Similarly, informational deictic markers help the author to position himself in the text, whereas precise deictic markers clearly aid the reader to follow the argumentation.

Philaretes stands out with his infrequent use of deixis, with the exception of backward-referring deictic markers and especially with the word 'before', which occurs often, as in Example 17:

(17) The venemous and poisoned substance and nature of Tabacco, is manifested and prooued by this, that it is daily experimented, and **before** was prooued by **vs**, to be a violent and most forceable purge. (*EMEMT*; Philaretes 1602: E3v)

Table 10.4 *Frequencies of intertextual deictic markers in two medical controversies.*

| Text | Backward-referring deixis (N) | Forward-referring deixis (N) | Precise deixis (N) | Informational deixis (N) | Total (N) | Total/1,000 |
|---|---|---|---|---|---|---|
| Philaretes (1602) | 0 | 0 | 0 | 0 | **0** | **0** |
| Marbecke (1602) | 11 | 4 | 22 | 38 | **75** | **3.6** |
| Colbatch (1700) | 2 | 2 | 29 | 4 | **37** | **3.3** |
| Emes (1700) | 2 | 3 | 91 | 14 | **110** | **5.1** |
| **Total (N)** | **15** | **9** | **142** | **56** | **222** | |
| **Total/1,000** | **0.2** | **0.1** | **2.2** | **0.9** | | **3.5** |

These backward-referring deictic markers remind the reader of what has been dealt with before. There is also an example of authorial 'we', referring to a part earlier in the text which mentions the author with the first-person singular. There is no intertextual deixis in Philaretes' pamphlet, which can be explained by the fact that the text is the only one in the group that was not directed to a single person, or even to a clearly defined audience.

The number of deictic markers in medical controversies is thus exceptional with regard to intertextual deixis, covering the majority of instances. Precise deictic markers are prominent, but informational deictic markers are also used. The latter have been classified as author-centred, although when they are used as intertextual deictic markers they aid the reader rather than the author. The tendencies to favour backward- or forward-referring markers seem to be individual preferences by authors, and these types of deictic markers are not prominent in controversies.

### *10.4.2 Deixis in medical pamphlet advertisements*

It could be assumed that, in comparison to controversies, discourse deixis will not feature prominently in the fairly short medical pamphlet advertisements; after all, short texts do not need to comment on the structure of the texts or remind readers or listeners of what has been said earlier (Kurzon 1985: 198). The texts in the Lampeter Corpus range from 3,000 to 25,000 words in length, whereas the advertisements considered here are mostly only between 2,000 and 4,000 words long. As mentioned above, a study of the Lampeter Corpus found that the more orally oriented texts (i.e. texts originally spoken, meant to be spoken or to mimic speech) contained fewer deictic markers than other kinds of pamphlets; thus, the most audience-oriented register in that study, religion, had the lowest frequencies of deictic markers (Claridge 2001). As medical pamphlet advertisements were often intended to be read aloud, it would therefore not be unexpected to get low frequencies of deictic markers. However, this turns out not to be the case.

Table 10.5 *Frequencies of deictic markers in medical pamphlet advertisements.*

| Text | Backward-referring deixis (N) | Forward-referring deixis (N) | Informational deixis (N) | Total (N) | Total/1,000 |
|---|---|---|---|---|---|
| Daffy (1673) | 11 | 1 | 8 | **20** | **6.9** |
| *Elixir* (1670–80) | 4 | 1 | 2 | **7** | **2.2** |
| Fletcher (1677) | 5 | 2 | 1 | **8** | **3.3** |
| Hinde (1673) | 0 | 0 | 5 | **5** | **2.0** |
| Lockyer (1664) | 6 | 4 | 12 | **22** | **3.0** |
| Lomax (1680?) | 3 | 3 | 9 | **15** | **3.4** |
| Maynwaringe (1684) | 5 | 1 | 14 | **20** | **2.2** |
| Nendick (1674) | 4 | 2 | 6 | **12** | **2.0** |
| *Tablets* (1680) | 4 | 1 | 2 | **7** | **3.7** |
| Winter (1664) | 4 | 1 | 3 | **8** | **2.1** |
| Witherden (1679) | 0 | 2 | 1 | **3** | **1.1** |
| Woodward (1690?) | 0 | 3 | 2 | **5** | **1.5** |
| **Total (N)** | **46** | **21** | **65** | **132** | |
| **Total/1,000** | **0.9** | **0.4** | **1.3** | | **2.6** |

*Note:* Results for deictic markers for precise references are not included in this table, as only one text has them (Winter, five hits). Intertextual deictic markers are also so scarce (two hits) that they have been omitted from the table.

Table 10.5 shows the frequencies of deictic markers found in medical pamphlet advertisements, broken down into backward-referring, forward-referring and informational deictic markers.

The frequency of all discourse deictic markers in medical pamphlet advertisements is higher than of the pamphlets in the Lampeter Corpus except for those in the legal register. Medical pamphlet advertisements have much more informational deixis than the texts in the Lampeter Corpus, whereas the results for forward- and backward-referring discourse deixis in medical pamphlet advertisements are almost exactly the same as for the register of scientific writing in the Lampeter Corpus (Claridge 2001). If a lower frequency of discourse deixis is taken to be a characteristic of more orally oriented texts, the results for medical pamphlet advertisements thus seem to indicate that these texts did not take a listening audience into consideration. Analysing the contexts more closely reveals, however, that the use of discourse deixis in medical pamphlet advertisements does not cater exclusively to a reading audience but to some extent also takes into account a listening audience.

Backward reference is most commonly done with the temporal deictic markers '(a)fore' or 'before'. 'Afore', the more literate of the two terms, usually occurs in combination with the verbs 'say' and 'mention'; these are also the verbs most commonly occurring with 'before'. Examples 18–20 show three uses:

(18) To carry away all congealed and fixed humors, take some of my Purging Spirit, as **afore** directed. (Winter 1664: A4v)

(19) It is found a most certain Remedy for the *Collick* and any *Griping* of the *Guts*, and stayeth *Vomiting*; which Virtues have been successfully experienced by **the aforesaid** *Benjamin Hope* of *Camerwell*, Mr. *Layton* of *Chick-lane*, *London*, Cordwainer, Mris *Petit* in *Curfiters Alley*, and my own Family. (*EMEMT*; Daffy 1673: 5)

(20) And I do conclude in the *Affirmative* it is good for *any* Disease (as I said **before**) Curable by *Physick*. (*EMEMT*; Lockyer 1664: 13)

In the first example, the reference is to a place several pages earlier in the text where detailed instructions have been given on the use of Winter's purging spirit; this reference is not very helpful to someone listening to the text, as it is unlikely that they can remember the instructions from when they were mentioned earlier. The second example shows the formulaic use of *the aforesaid* + [name], which together with *(the) said* + [name] is typical of the legal register.[11] Daffy is the only text in which this use is found, because he refers to cases several times in the course of his text; this is the reason he has such a high frequency of discourse deictic markers in

[11] The high frequency of 'the said' and 'afore' is the reason why the legal register has a much higher frequency of backward-referring discourse deictic markers in the Lampeter Corpus (Claridge 2001: 60–1).

comparison to the other texts. Though this use is characteristic of a more literate register, it does not require a listener to actually remember anything that has been mentioned previously but functions rather as a reminder of a previous statement.

The majority of backward references in medical pamphlet advertisements are of the kind found in Example 20: general reminders of important points, where the author wishes to reiterate and emphasize the fact that the medicine cures all diseases (except those that cannot be cured with the help of medicines). These kinds of backward reference are often sprinkled throughout the text, drawing attention to the fact that the point is important enough to be repeated (several times) in the discourse. Thus, it would seem to be especially helpful for listeners if a text is read aloud.

Forward referencing is not common in medical pamphlet advertisements and is usually found before lists of diseases or symptoms or, most often, lists of distributors of the medicine, as in Example 21:

(21) Lastly, those that are desirous to enjoy these *Pills*, they may repair to the *Discoverer* thereof, and to these places **following**, Where they are to be had, and no where else, unless you will be cheated. [A list of forty-four distributors and their directions follows.] (*EMEMT*; Lockyer 1664: 14–15)

Forward referencing is almost exclusively done with the deictic marker 'following' (the more formal 'as followeth' is only found in three instances). The lists announced by forward-referring deictic markers are long, especially the ones giving the names and directions of distributors, and they would therefore probably have been hard to remember for a listener. However, marking an upcoming list with a deictic marker alerted listeners to be ready to note the listed items in case one or more applied to them or, in the case of distributors, to listen to who was the closest one if ever the medicine were needed. With such a small sample of texts it is impossible to draw any comprehensive conclusions, but it does seem that the function of forward-referring deictic marking is to signal a list following directly rather than to sustain a reader's interest or to prevent criticism, which are the more usual functions of these markers (Claridge 2001: 62).

There is a striking difference in results for informational deixis in medical pamphlet advertisements and in the Lampeter Corpus, as the frequency of informational deictic markers is much higher in the advertisements than in the Lampeter Corpus. The frequencies of the different registers of the Lampeter Corpus vary between 0.2 and 0.5 per 1,000 words, whereas in the pamphlet advertisements the frequency is 1.3 per 1,000 words. Two terms, 'here' and 'this', predominate, with 'this' being the only deictic marker that occurs at least once in every text. Deictic 'this' is combined with a noun that refers to the text as a whole (e.g., 'pamphlet', 'book', 'narrative') or to a part of it (e.g., 'preface', 'receipt') and is often used to explain the authors' motivations for writing the pamphlets or to outline their contents, as in Example 22, or to show the function of the text, as in Example 23:

(22) therefore desiring after a full and clear perusal, that it may satisfie, I have undertaken in **this Small Tract or Method**, Confirmed by certain knowledge, evident Cures and credible relations, to give general satisfaction to all persons concerning the particular proofs of the Use, Vertues, Operations, and safety of this only Medicine (*EMEMT*; Nendick 1674: To the Reader)

(23) And to prevent all errors and mistakes whatsoever in taking of them, be careful to observe the *Rules* given in **this Book**, which bids you begin with *Two* Pils, and *three* the next day, and *four* or *five* the next day, if those which you took before do not *work* to your mind, and then rest one or two daies (*EMEMT*; Lockyer 1664: 14)

Note that Lockyer not only reminds the reader/listener that the directions for taking his medicine are to be found in the book, but he repeats the rules to ensure that they are followed, which is especially helpful to someone listening to the text being read aloud and thus unable to flip back in the text to find the rules.

The fourth function of informational deictic markers found in medical pamphlet advertisements was to tell the readers and hearers what had been omitted from the texts. This was done in the interests of keeping them from becoming too long (and thus too expensive). Testimonials were clearly expected in these texts, since not including them had to be justified, as in Example 24:

(24) I have set forth **this**, to inform the wonderful Effects that have been wrought by this Cordial Spirit, and abundantly Testified at large by many, which **this Bill** cannot contain, to give all sorts of Persons full satisfaction of its Innocent and wonderful Operation in the whole Body of Man; but for brevity sake I have **here** omitted. (Hinde 1673: 1)

Even when testimonials have been included, authors are at pains to emphasize that many more have been left out to spare the reader from getting bored. Anonymous testimonials are explained, just as the inclusion of named testimonials is justified. In some cases, the descriptions of all the wonderful virtues of a medicine are also cropped short in the interests of holding the audience's interest. Clearly, omissions were addressed to pre-empt possible objections by readers (or listeners).

In contrast to controversies, deixis is used for marking precise references in only one text, Winter, and there are only two instances of intertextual deictic markers, both referring to the authors' own texts rather than to someone else's, even though the existence of other texts is acknowledged by naming the authors. Unlike controversies, however, medical pamphlet advertisements do not address specific points in other texts but argue in very general terms over the merits of the opponents' claims. As space was very limited, the competition only gets a passing mention, and the focus of the text is kept on the value of the advertised medicine and the authors' right to ownership of the medicine.

The authors' concern to avoid misunderstandings by explicitly stating their motives and aims for writing the texts and by addressing what is included in the text and what is left out emphasizes the role of the author. The conspicuously frequent use of informational deixis is thus evidence of the author-centredness of medical pamphlet advertisements, as was the case with the use of first- and second-person pronouns. However, outlining the contents of the texts also tells the audience what to expect – and thus helps to avoid misunderstandings – and addressing possible objections to omissions indicates that authors were aware of their audience, especially when they claim to leave things out in consideration of the audience. While informational deictic markers function just as well for readers and listeners, the ways in which directional deictic markers are used in medical pamphlet advertisements seem to show that authors took pains to include listeners in their intended audience as well as readers.

## 10.5 Discussion and conclusion

In this study, we have investigated how two types of the new genre of pamphlets differ in their strategies for interpersonality and aiding reader/listener comprehension. The intended audiences of medical controversies were limited to educated medical professionals, whereas medical advertisements were read aloud to semi-literate masses, and this difference plays a significant role in their use of first- and second-person pronouns and discourse deictic markers.

Both types of medical pamphlets are strongly author-centred, but medical controversies have more variation in their strategies of interpersonality, including various ways of using the complex plural 'we' that is almost non-existent in medical advertisements. The emphasis on the author is further enhanced by the scarcity of addresses to the intended audience: *you* can refer to the opponent in the controversies or even to the patron of the work, whereas in advertisements the pronoun is mostly only found in directions for use, when imperatives or passives are just as likely alternatives for the more interpersonal pronoun.

Both controversies and advertisements have surprisingly high frequencies of discourse deictic markers, but their uses are very different and show the influence of the different audiences. Medical controversies had very complex structures that required heavy use of intertextual and precise deictic markers to help point to exact places in an opponent's text. These are not necessary in medical advertisements as they are much shorter and did not interact with other texts as controversies did. Informational deixis is used frequently and in various ways by different authors in both controversies and advertisements to structure the arguments. Where a listening audience may have been taken into account is in the use of backward- and forward-referring deictic markers in advertisements, though they aid in reading comprehension just as well. A comparable use is not evident in medical controversies.

Our study has revealed that detailed information can be gained from examining the use of personal pronouns and discourse deixis in different kinds of pamphlets. Both linguistic features tell about the use and purpose of these texts – how the relationship between the author and the reader/hearer was formulated and how the audience was taken into account. The subgenres of medical controversies and advertisements, if they can be called that, developed quite distinctive styles. These could be looked into further in other pamphlets as well, to get a more thorough picture of early modern pamphlets and their strategies of argumentation.

# 11 The development of specialized discourse in the *Philosophical Transactions*

MAURIZIO GOTTI

## 11.1 Introduction

An important milestone in the history of English scientific and medical writing is the foundation of the Royal Society, 'the institutional embodiment of the new science' (M. Hunter 1981: 48), which took place in 1662, after a period in which its members had met in an informal manner (Hartley 1960). In their preliminary meeting on 28 November 1660, the founders of the Royal Society determined that the purpose of their gathering was 'a designe of founding a Colledge for the promoting of Physico-Mathematicall Experimentall Learning' (quoted in Hall 1991: 9) and chose the phrase *Nullius in verba* ('On the words of no one') as their motto. These new researchers were convinced that many natural philosophers in the past had been anxious to provide explanations and theories before having enough evidence on which to base them and emphasized therefore the need for an experimental approach so as to collect abundant data from which correct generalizations could be derived.

On 6 March 1665, the first issue of the *Philosophical Transactions* of the Royal Society of London (henceforth *PT*) was published, evolving from the communal correspondence which was common among its members (Gotti 2006a). As the practice of exchanging information by means of correspondence through unofficial networks was proving more and more difficult to carry out, due to the increasing number of specialists and research groups working in the field, it was decided to create a new journal devoted to specialized matters and mainly addressed to those really interested in them, imitating the French scientific periodical *Le Journal des Sçavants*, which had appeared on 5 January 1665 under the editorship of Denis de Sallo de la Coudraye.

The main aim of the *PT* is well expressed in the full title of the journal: *Philosophical Transactions: Giving Some Accompt of the Present Undertakings, Studies and Labours of the Ingenious in Many Considerable Parts of the World.* The *PT* was meant to serve as a newsletter, to favour the spread of news within the Royal Society and other learned circles. Further aims were made clear by the editor, Henry Oldenburg, in his introduction to the first issue of the journal: the new publication had not merely been designed as a channel of information for those working in this particular field but also had a proselytizing function as it was meant to arouse the interest of new minds in specialized matters and to promote their involvement in scientific research according to the criteria shared by the members of the Royal Society.

As can be seen in its full title, the *PT* had been designed to make known not only the ideas and discoveries of British specialists but also of 'the Ingenious in Many Considerable Parts of the World'. Indeed, foreign contributions to the first volumes amounted to as much as 40 per cent of the total (Heilbron 1983), several foreign researchers – such as Antonie van Leeuwenhoek and Marcello Malpighi – contributing to the journal on a regular basis by reporting their experimental findings. This universality of readership is also reflected in the decision of a few authors to write their contributions in Latin; indeed, in the first volumes, contributions in Latin represented about one-fifth of the total (Atkinson 1999: 93), which confirms the important role played by that language as a lingua franca in the scientific community of that period. Although most of its parts were written in English, the *PT* also became very popular outside Britain, and its copies circulated in various countries on the Continent. Some issues were translated into French, which confirms how relevant they were considered in that country; illicit translations into Latin also existed, a testimony of the widespread international popularity that this journal had acquired.

## 11.2 Inadequacy of contemporary discourse

The innovative decision of the Royal Society to publish its journal primarily in English involved extensive use of new specialized lexis and novel forms of communication, as existing vocabulary and expository forms (the aphorism, the essay, the dialogue and the treatise) were inadequate for the purposes of the new discourse community (Gotti 2006b). The decision of the Royal Society was in line with the heated debate in sixteenth- and seventeenth-century England, as the adoption of other languages (Latin, in particular) was felt to be no longer sufficient for this purpose. These centuries were very important for the development of English medical discourse, as 1500–1700 marked a remarkable period of increasing use of the vernacular for medical and scientific writing.[1] Indeed, at the beginning of this period Latin still had a dominant role. Moreover, an analysis of the combination of Latin and English in late medieval English medical manuscripts reveals code-switching as a widely exploited discourse strategy, one that implies a century of bilingual readership (Voigts 1996). At the end of this period,

[1] On the process of vernacularization of English medical discourse, cf. Taavitsainen and Pahta (2004), especially Chapter 3 (Taavitsainen 2004).

English prevailed, and the process of vernacularization can be described as largely completed by 1700, when we can find a full range of sophisticated university treatises on medicine in English where Latin played little or no role. Indeed, of the 238 medical books published in 1640–60, 207 were in English (Webster 1975: 267).

Great epistemological and methodological developments took place in that period, in both medicine and surgery: old scholastic thinking began to be replaced by new patterns of thought and new methodologies based on observation and interpretation of physical phenomena (cf. Vickers 1987; M. Hunter 1989; Jardine 1999; Shapiro 2000). These developments determined the need for corresponding changes both in the ways of communicating the new discoveries attained by means of innovative procedures and apparatus and in the expressive tool to be used to describe and argue about the new phenomena observed and analysed. The evolution of the methods adopted in the study of medicine and the development of new medical and surgical procedures implied a change not only in the approach to the interpretation of the issues analysed but also in the way in which phenomena ought to be described and opinions expressed.

Criticism was made both of how language was employed in the various processes of medical research and, in particular, of the suitability of the tool itself for an accurate, precise expression of the concepts reported. Those specialists who intended to use the native language in the expression of medical phenomena often pointed out its deficiencies and inaccuracies. For example, Andrew Boorde often inserted Latin quotations in his work 'for [he] nor no man els [could] not in theyr maternall tonge expresse the whole termes of phisicke' (*EMEMT*; Boorde 1547: 38v). Similarly, Christopher Langton complained of the limited number of vernacular anatomical terms:

I can do no lesse then count the negligence of our Phisitions to be the cause of [the lack of English anatomical terms]: for yf they had written of theyr arte in theyr mother tunge, as they do in other places, why shulde we lacke englysh names, more then we lacke eyther Latyn names or Greke names? and yet to saye the truthe, it is better for vs English men to haue English names, then eyther Latyn or Greke. (*EMEMT*; Langton 1545: 27r)

Another criticism often made by specialists was the polysemy characterizing many words, which often made texts ambiguous. The remedy suggested consisted in the coining of new terms providing a stricter delimitation of meaning. Indeed, the coining of native terms – particularly frequent in the case of translation – is often explained as a desire for greater clarity; this is the motivation provided by Boorde for his translation of 'obscure wordes and names into Englyshe':

For as muche as olde, auncyent, and autentyke auctours or doctours of Phisicke in their bokes doth wryte many obscure terms, geuinge also to many and dyuerse infyrmities, darke termes, dyffycyle to vnderstande, some and mooste of all beyng Greeke wordes, some and fewe beynge Araby wordes, some beyng Latyn wordes, and some beyng Barbarus wordes. Therfore I haue translated all soche obscure wordes and names into Englyshe, that euery man openlye and apartly maye vnderstande them. (*EMEMT*; Boorde 1547: Av$^r$)

The realization that the English language was inadequate for the needs of expression of men of science led to its gradual amelioration, from both a quantitative and a qualitative point of view. British scientists made great efforts to increase the number of specialized terms and to improve the exactness of their meanings (cf. Gotti 2008: 153–69).

## 11.3 Lexical innovations

The field in which the English language proved to be particularly inadequate was that of 'names of art', that is, of the technical terms that made up the basic lexis of a subject. This lack of specialized terms often made the translation of works into English an arduous task or made it difficult for English specialists to write essays in their native tongue. Two main principles were followed in coining new terms: that of using the resources of the native tongue, either to give a specialized meaning to an existing word or to form a new one, or borrowing a similar term from a foreign language. In defining a new concept, the specialist sometimes employed a word already existing in the language, adding a specialized meaning to its usual one(s). However, the most frequent policy adopted to increase the English medical lexicon was the borrowing of terms from other languages, particularly from Latin.[2] Latin and Greek were endowed with large and respected specialized lexicons, as too was – although less extensively – Arabic. This process of borrowing involved the adoption of not only single words but also prefixes and suffixes, which were used more and more often to create new terms. For example, if we consider combining forms of classical origin such as *-ology* and *-meter*, we can see many new English words created in the seventeenth century including these suffixes: 'pathology', 'ichthyology', zoology', 'osteology', 'psychology', 'micrometer' and 'thermometer'.

Native and classical elements were usually mixed in texts. Indeed, the existing native terms commonly referred to general parts ('ankle', 'arm', 'knee', 'shoulder', 'elbow', 'hip') while the new terminology (mainly derived from classical sources) defined the component elements of these general parts

[2] This was part of a more general tendency. As Barber's (1976: 166–95) analysis has pointed out, a great number of the new words that became part of the language in the seventeenth century were made up of Latin loan words, with a considerable proportion belonging to specialized fields of discourse. This is confirmed by McDermott (2002: 216–18). Previous studies on early medical terminology include Norri (1992, 1998, 2004), McConchie (1997), French (2002) and Furdell (2005).

(e.g., 'ulna', 'radius' and 'humerus' as components of 'arm'). Some native terms experienced a semantic transition from one referent to another, scientifically more appropriate: 'womb', for instance, passed from generalized 'stomach' to exclusively feminine 'uterus'. In some cases, two forms (general and medical) were neo-Latin; in these cases, the former was already present in the language, having been borrowed during the Middle English period, while the latter appeared in the language in the Early Modern English period; some examples of these doublets are 'gender' and 'genus', 'prove' and 'probe', 'spice' and 'species' and 'palsy' and 'paralysis'. Moreover, once a loan had been introduced, it was frequently used as a root from which further words could be formed by means of affixation. Examples are: *parenchyma* > *parenchymatic*, *anatomy* > *anatomical* > *anatomically*. Some neologisms were obtained from existing words (either native or loan words themselves) by means of compounding: for example, 'lung sick' ('sick of a pulmonary complaint'), 'pine-glandule' ('pineal gland'). Several quotations taken from the *PT* show the author's consciousness that he was coining neologisms, and this awareness was often explicit (Examples 1 and 2):

(1) All Placentiferous Animals (if I may assume this word) he affirms to have three Membranes, and Sows, Mares, and Women also; (*EMEMT*; *PT*, 2, 1667: 509)
(2) That it hath been observed to be dangerous, to have a vein opened at once in both arms, or leggs, which is here called a Neronian Venaesection (*EMEMT*; *PT*, 7, 1672: 5106)

Although he thought he was right in borrowing terms from other languages, the writer was aware of the difficulties of interpretation that readers might meet when they encountered the new terms. Therefore he not only took care to point out the novelty of a term or its origin but was very keen to specify its semantic value. This attitude reflects the particular importance that specialists placed on the fact that their words should be decoded easily and correctly by their readers. In these explanations, the author made use of different encoding techniques. On some occasions, he clarified the meaning of a certain expression by providing a synonym for it (Examples 3 and 4):

(3) concerning the use of that kernelly substance, call'd Pancreas (in English, the Sweetbred) (*EMEMT*; *PT*, 1, 1665–6: 178)
(4) into which the Animalcle has entred as its Punctum or place of nourishment; (*EMEMT*; *PT*, 16, 1687–8: 482–3)

On other occasions, instead of providing a concise synonym or antonym of the new term, the author gave a full paraphrase of it or an exemplification, as in Example 5:

(5) Then he proceeds to the description of the Allantoides (the Membrane immediately encompassing that skin wherein the Foetus is wrapped) (*EMEMT*; *PT*, 2, 1667: 509)

## 11.4 Creation of new genres

Also from the textual point of view, there was a great development in this period: the early printed works mainly consisted of translations of treatises and new compositions of general guides to health and handbooks of medical instructions, often including accounts of illustrative and typical cases (Bennett 1969). The normal mode of publication for scientific work was in a separate treatise, and men of science kept abreast of the times through private manuscript correspondence. The eighteenth century showed a greater variety of genres, with the addition of new forms such as anatomical observations, book reviews, journal articles (LeFanu 1984) and experimental essays (Gotti 2001).

As regards the *PT*, in addition to influencing the overall balance of languages used for specialized purposes (Latin versus the vernacular), thus increasing the lexical resources available for scientific and medical writing in England, this journal greatly contributed to the textual development of specialized discourse by giving rise to a number of new genres in English. The various issues of the journal consist of a variety of text types, referred to in the journal itself by several different titles: for example, 'accounts', 'calculations', 'comparisons', 'descriptions', 'essays', 'experiments', 'explanations', 'extracts', 'inquiries', 'investigations', 'letters', 'observations', 'proposals', 'remarks' and others. The same titles were often used to introduce very different types of texts, and similar text types were often referred to by different names. Indeed, at this time, textual forms were still very loosely structured, and there were not yet any clear conventions and codifications concerning them. For the purposes of our analysis, the texts published in the *PT* will be grouped into four categories according to their main textual form and function: news items, experimental accounts, letters and book reviews.[3]

### *11.4.1 News items*

News items were not real 'articles' in the modern sense of the word, mostly consisting of brief reports and short observations resembling the news items published by contemporary newspapers. The main difference was that the news of the *PT* concerned topics relating to the natural sciences and other specialized disciplines, including medical matters. The variety of these news items and brief reports depends on the fact that the main contributors and addressees of the early issues of the *PT* were not only those scientists involved in the systematic observation and description of natural phenomena

[3] In their chapter in this volume (Chapter 12), Gray, Biber and Hiltunen identify three categories of texts in the *PT* (reports, book reviews and letters). These greatly coincide with the last three categories listed by me. I have added, however, a fourth category (that of news items), which includes the articles mainly giving news about 'strange' facts and observations from real life rather than reporting one's own experimental accounts.

and in experimental activity but also the larger category of the 'virtuosos' (M. Hunter 1981), mainly interested in curious facts and in the unsystematic collection of specimens of various kinds. The composite nature of this early scientific community reflects that of the membership of the Royal Society, as is well described by Valle (1999: 111):

It consisted of an inner 'esoteric' core of committed Baconian experimental philosophers, above all Boyle, Hooke and Desaguliers, whose aim was the creation of new knowledge ... Around this inner circle was a larger concentric zone of the exoteric community, the bulk of the Society: men who were capable of taking an informed interest in what was happening, and of contributing to it on a more minor level. Surrounding this again was a sizeable penumbra of the genteel London public, who went to the weekly meetings of the Society for entertainment, and because it was the fashion, but who had no clear understanding of what they were hearing or witnessing; men, in fact, very like Pepys.

This composite nature of the readership explains why some news items, especially in the first issues of the *PT*, referred to curious facts, such as the stillbirth of a monstrous calf. Here are a few titles: 'Observables upon a Monstrous Head' (*EMEMT*; *PT*, 1, 1665: 85–6), 'An Extract ... concerning some Natural Curiosities of those parts, especially a very strange and very curiously contrived Fish' (*EMEMT*; *PT*, 5, 1670: 1151–3). These monstrous accounts were often made more reliable by mentioning the names of witnesses and their professional qualifications, for example, 'A Narrative of a Monstrous Birth in Plymouth, Octob. 22, 1670; together with the Anatomical Observations, taken thereupon by William Durston, Doctor in Physick, and communicated to Dr. Tim Clerk' (*EMEMT*; *PT*, 5, 1670: 2096–8); 'A Relation of a Monstrous Birth, Made by Dr. S. Morris of Petworth in Sussex, from his Own Observation: and by Him Sent to Dr. Charles Goodall of London: Both of the Colledge of Physicians, London' (*EMEMT*; *PT*, 12, 1678: 961–2). As can be seen from the titles, although the reason for presenting these facts was not merely to surprise or attract readership, the language used was rich in adjectives denoting exceptionality and unnaturalness such as 'curious', 'dreadful', 'monstrous', 'odd', 'strange' and 'unusual'. Descriptions, however, tended to be sober and neutral, as can be seen in the case of a monstrous birth in Sussex (Example 6):

(6) It had two heads. Both the Faces very well shap'd. The left Face looked Swarthy; and never breathed. And the left Head was the bigger; and stayed longer in the Bearing ... The Breast (and Clavicles) very large; about seven Inches broad. But two hands. And but two feet. (*EMEMT*; *PT*, 12, 1678: 961–2)

These news items about monstrous facts were published not only to arouse interest, but also to stimulate research in fields concerned with them

(Daston 1998).[4] Moreover, many of these news items were reported following a well-organized structure, resembling that of an experimental account. For example, the structure of 'Observables upon a Monstrous Head' consists of a brief introduction to the topic, outlining the main contextual elements of the account, followed by the section describing the strange aspects of the news reported, organized in a very orderly way (Example 7):

(7) The Head being opened, and examined, it was found.
First, That it had no Sign of any Nose in the usual place,
Next, That the two Eyes were united into one Double Eye,
Lastly, That just above the Eyes, (*EMEMT*; *PT*, 1, 1665: 85–6)

These monstrous accounts were written mainly for an informative purpose, but the specialized nature of the writer is reflected in the highly precise terminology often used in them. However, even when the writer was a specialist, he was aware of the different degrees of specialization of his readership and often provided a paraphrase or a common equivalent for the specialized terms he was using. In Example 8, the writer uses specialized terms such as 'Optick Nerve', 'Membrane', 'Sclerotis', 'Cornea', 'Iris' and 'Crystalline Humours', but he also accompanies the latter two with their common language equivalents ('Rain-bow-like Circle' and 'Balls') probably as an aid to comprehension for readers who were non-specialists in medical matters:

(8) the two Eyes were united into one Double Eye, which was placed just in the middle of the Brow, the Nose being wanting, which should have separated them, whereby the two Eye-holes in the Scull were united into one very large round hole, into the midst of which, from the Brain, entred one pretty large Optick Nerve, at the end of which grew a great Double Eye; that is, that Membrane, called Sclerotis, which contained both, was one and the same, but seemed to have a Seam by which they were joined, to go quite round it, and the fore or pellucid part was distinctly separated into two Cornea's by a white Seam that divided them. Each Cornea seemed to have its Iris, (or Rain-bow-like Circle) and Apertures or Pupils distinct; and upon opening the Cornea, there was found within it two Balls, or Crystalline Humours, very well shaped; (*EMEMT*; *PT*, 1, 1665: 85–6)

### *11.4.2 Experimental accounts*

In the first issues, only a minority of the papers were devoted to experimental activities, and only after the eightieth issue did the percentage reach

[4] As Shapiro (2000: 87) aptly remarks, 'The vogue for marvels, a Europe-wide phenomenon, influenced art, drama, and natural philosophy as well as the new news media. Both the "marvelous" and the "news" emphasised novelty and rarity, the bizarre and the strange. The history of "news" and "facts" cannot be separated from the "wonders" and "marvels" of the age.'

about 40 per cent (Bazerman 1988: 65). Some of these experimental accounts were solicited by the Fellows of the Royal Society, who often invited colleagues to report on the results of their activities, especially if these had not yet been published. Experimental accounts usually contained no abstract but had very long titles, describing the contents of the papers themselves. They were often preceded by an introduction written by the editor, meant to contextualize the accounts and to present the author in a very positive way, in line with the polite tone of 'civil' communication (Shapin 1994; Gotti in press), as in Example 9:

(9) These Experiments, made by that Indefatigable Benefactor to Philosophy, the Honourable Robert Boyle in order to bring some more Light to the Doctrine of RESPIRATION, as well as to minister occasion to Inquisitive Naturalists to make farther Researches into the same, were by their Noble Author communicated to the Publisher of these papers; (*EMEMT*; *PT*, 5, 1670: 2011)

Bazerman's analysis (1988) of the first ninety volumes of the *PT* has shown that in the first period (1665–1700) articles consisted of mere reports of events, and only later did they tend to argue over results and offer claims and experimental proof. The brevity of many of the contributions to the *PT* confirms that these had been mainly conceived as informative reports. Particularly in the first volume, articles tended to be short (one or two pages long) and focused on a single experiment. Experimental accounts usually started from the observation of natural phenomena which had aroused the curiosity and intervention of the researcher. The voice commonly used in experimental essays is active, often putting the researcher in a thematic position and usually conferring on it the grammatical function of the subject, so as to parallel his active role in the experimental activity (Example 10):

(10) I took a Calf and a Sheep … and having prepared a Jugular Vein in each, I planted my Pipes and Quills … both in the Jugular Vein of the Calf … Then I took out of the Sheep 49 ounces … of blood … : I stopp'd the Vein of the Sheep, and unstopp'd the Pipe in the Calf (*EMEMT*; *PT*, 2, 1667: 449)

The active presence of the scientist is emphasized not only when he is performing some operation but also when the behaviour of the animal or object used in the experiment is being described. In many cases, indeed, such behaviour is reported as perceived by the researcher, as if to underline the fact that what is being narrated is not happening spontaneously but as a result of the experimenter's actions, whose role therefore remains central in all the parts of the report. Although the active voice is quantitatively predominant in the narration, there is also appropriate use of the passive form. This is usually employed in reporting how certain procedures (usually involving the utilization of equipment) have been carried out. The shift from the active to the passive voice in these cases underlines the passing from the active role of narration of events to the description of procedures that are becoming standardized in the experimenter's repertoire or in that of scientists in general (Example 11):

(11) There was taken a considerable quantity of Man's Urine ... Then this Liquor was distilled with a moderate Heat ... ; after which the Superfluous Moisture was also abstracted (or evaporated away) till the remaining Substance was brought to the consistence of the somewhat thick Syrup, or a thin Extract. (*EMEMT*; *PT*, 17, 1693: 583)

Evidentiality (Chafe and Nichols 1986) was usually attained by means of observation and perception, two processes which were deemed basic and preliminary to induction (Taavitsainen 2001b). The actions regarding observation and perception were usually expressed by verbs having a first-person pronoun subject, as in Example 12:

(12) I found ... all my endeavours were destructive to my purpose; ... And though the Portion were never so small, yet my bare eye could make this discovery; much more could I, when assisted by a Microscope, perceive, I had destroyed more Vessels, than preserved, in despite of the exact care, I was capable to use. (*EMEMT*; *PT*, 1, 1666: 316)

Similarly, results were reported as the product of an observation or experimentation process (Example 13):

(13) And by many tryals upon my hands ... I was perswaded, that in long droughts, and lasting dry Frosts, those waters were more effectually and more speedily healing, than at other times. (*EMEMT*; *PT*, 1, 1666: 358)

The researcher usually described the object of his observation with great care and caution as he had perceived it, reporting events faithfully and sincerely and expressing his opinions and conclusions with the degree of positiveness corresponding to the certainty of the facts described, availing himself of the various modal and hedging expressions that the English language offered in order to suit the different degrees of certainty of the facts reported. Example 14 illustrates this attitude:

(14) It seems not irrational to guess afore hand, that the exchange of bloud will not alter the nature or disposition of the Animals ... The most probable use of this Experiment may be conjectured to be, that one Animal may live with the bloud of another; (*EMEMT*; *PT*, 1, 1666: 357–8)

This careful attitude prompted the author to use modal expressions and verbs such as 'seem' and 'appear' to report with caution the actions as he perceived them and to speculate about the implications of his observations, as can be seen in Example 15:

(15) The Figure of the third sort, I could not well discover, sometimes they appeared oval, and at other times round, they were so small that I could not discern them greater than as at E. (*EMEMT*; *PT*, 17, 1693: 646)

The same prudence is shown by hedging expressions, usually parenthetical (Example 16):

(16) We have found it but twice that the recipient Animal pissed blood after it, and, as far as I can judge, I believe I have infallible ways of preventing all such disorders; (*EMEMT*; *PT*, 2, 1667–8: 623)

In taking this cautious attitude, not only did the experimenter show his professional correctness but he also proved himself to be a reliable and faithful witness to the events that he was reporting. Moreover, in order to make his narration more reliable, the author carefully inserted the testimony of his collaborators. Such witnesses were sometimes named in an explicit way, and titles were often added to make the testimony appear more reliable (Example 17):

(17) To the truth of these Relations, not onely the said Joseph Shute and Maria Stert, have put the one his name, the other her Mark, the third and seventh of January 1666, but also Sir William Strode, and Mr Colepresse have subscribed the same, as believing the Relation to be true. (*EMEMT*; *PT*, 1, 1666: 381)

The confirmation provided by the presence of esteemed and reliable witnesses proved particularly useful in cases in which innovative or expensive apparatus was used to carry out the experiment. Although not able to repeat the experience in his own laboratory, the reader – reassured by the presence of reliable spectators – was nevertheless able to scrutinize the contents of the report, and – by means of this process of 'virtual witnessing' (Shapin 1984: 491) – to make a correct evaluation of them. The very detailed way in which experimental accounts were reported was also meant to give the reader the opportunity to witness the event in a virtual manner. Moreover, the minuteness of detail and the accuracy of the narration were meant to make repetition easier and thus encourage the growth of empirical practice in the community of scientists. A further reason that justifies the experimenter's recourse to this detailed narrative technique is his need to acquire official recognition of his results. Indeed, the detailed and accurate description of his personal scientific experience was considered one of the requisites for transforming a personal account into an official protocol to be submitted to the broad community of men of science. The careful and objective narration of experiments could provide the basis of proper scrutiny and reliable judgement and thus permit the transformation of personal results into facts widely accepted by the scientific world. Having thus obtained the consensus of a wider public, experimental data could become 'matters of fact' and part of scientists' shared culture (Taavitsainen and Pahta 1995).

The great number of details provided can also be explained by their usefulness in the interpretation of the success or failure of the experiment. The data were usually reported as they were observed, without the writer being required to accompany them with hypotheses or comments. This allowed the researcher to report all the details of his experimental activity, even those he was not able to explain, thus reducing his theoretical responsibilities and the risk of being criticized. His experimental accounts provided the identification of useful superstructures on which other scientists might be able to build appropriate theories. The same principle also enabled writers to report experiments that had been unsuccessful, as the analysis of these experiences might help the reader not to make the same mistakes as those reported or enable him to draw interesting conclusions. Moreover, the tone was often humble; the author usually avoided extolling his achievements and often used devices that played down their importance, such as the expression 'if it may deserve that name, and not rather that of a Trifle' in Example 18:

(18) I am to acquaint you of an Experiment, if it may deserve that name, and not rather that of a Trifle; the matter of which is known to many, but unapplied (for ought I know) to such use as it affords. (*EMEMT*; *PT*, 3, 1668: 727)

The tone was always 'civil', even in disputes. Criticism was expressed in an objective way, avoiding a direct attack on the opponent but rather acknowledging his efforts to demonstrate his point of view. At the end of the dispute, the 'challenger' usually emphasized his confidence in the evidence provided and expressed the hope that his findings would not only convince his 'opponent' but could also be accepted by the whole scientific community.

### *11.4.3 Letters*

As seen above, the original communal correspondence gradually evolved into the news-item and experimental-account text types. However, letters continued to thrive and to be published in specialized journals. Many of these letters were meant to spark off readers' intuitions and explanations and had as their starting point the observation of some curious facts. In some cases, the writer would take advantage of the publication in the journal to seek for explanations or information, as in the following example (19):

(19) SIR,

Since my coming to this place I have with a very strange Case. An Icterial discontented Woman having a desire to dye, wholly rejected the help of Medicine, and within three Months being well nigh her end, there happened an Eruption of Blood out of the Glandula Lachrymalis of one of her Eyes, without any External Injury: There was an evacuation of lbij. of Blood within the space of Thirty Hours. About a Week after the same Sluce was opened again, and she bled till she dyed. Now, I would fain to know what Blood-Vessels come to that Gland, from which such a vast quantity of Blood should be cast forth in so short a time. (*EMEMT*; *PT*, 18, 1693–4: 51)

A few of these letters aroused strong reactions and criticisms and thus started somewhat long and controversial exchanges. Indeed, the letter format was considered an ideal means to defend oneself quickly and publicly from opponents' criticisms and to put forth one's own. This 'dialogic relationship' (Atkinson 1999: 92) is visible in most of the letters and contributions published in the *PT*, which can be seen as complementing each other. Indeed, many contributions were written as a reaction to a previous one, either to confirm or to contradict its contents.

Interactivity within the community was mainly expressed at a personal level rather than through citation in the modern sense, as reference was made to individuals rather than to published texts. However, the number of people quoted was low, which confirms the opinion that in the seventeenth and eighteenth centuries 'persuasive communities' were relatively small (Allen et al. 1994).

Letters were a constant feature of the *PT*. Indeed, in the first volumes they correspond to the majority of items. Atkinson (1999: 81) estimates that 51 per cent of the contributions published in the 1675 volume appeared in letter form. Letters were not always published in their complete form; sometimes only an 'extract' was printed. In some cases, the letters were interspersed with the editor's comments. These comments were often preceded by expressions such as 'Thus far the author' or the words 'So far these Assertions', as in Example 20:

(20) *So far these Assertions*; which we thought fit to insert here to give the Curious and Learned amongst us the opportunity to consider them, and to give-in their thoughts upon them; which we are perswaded will be very welcom to the Author. (*EMEMT*; *PT*, 10, 1675: 387)

Letters were easily distinguishable from news items and experimental accounts as they opened with a salutation and were frequently followed by a polite reference to the editor or to the Royal Society. First- and second-person pronouns were often used to refer to the writer and to the addressee. The tone was polite and the style in line with the 'civil' style used also in the other types of contributions. In this, the letter was facilitated by the fact that this text type was the one that most resembled conversation in highlighting politeness values (Klein 1994). Another reason for the use of this 'civil' style was the fact that the members of this community knew each other either directly or indirectly. Moreover, there was a lower degree of competition compared to contributions to the journal in subsequent centuries.

### *11.4.4 Book reviews*

In each issue of the *PT*, there were one or more book reviews. These were few in the first issues, but later they increased in number and appeared in a section at the end of the journal, indicated in the table of contents by the title 'An Account of Some Books, Lately Published' or simply 'An Account of Some Books'. At first, most reviews were written by Oldenburg himself, apart from those concerning mathematical books, which instead were undertaken by John Wallis. Book reviews took up a smaller part of the *PT* compared to other publications. For example, in the period 1680–9, 1,243 reviews appeared in *Le Journal des Sçavants*, 1,332 in the *Acta Eruditorum* and only ninety-two in the *PT* (Barnes 1947; quoted in Kronick 1976: 79). The majority of contributions to the journal was represented by experimental accounts; indeed, the 1665–1700 issues of the *PT* contained 1,898 experimental accounts against 600 accounts of books (George 1952). Most book reviews consisted of a summary of the contents of the book with some evaluation on the part of the reviewer. Sometimes this evaluative part was scanty or almost absent (see Example 21):

(21) The Title of this Curious piece, is, Diatribae Themae Willisii Med. Doct. & Profess. Oxon. De Febribus Vindicatio, Authore Richardo Lower, &c. In it are occasionally discussed many considerable Medical and Anatomical inquiries, as, … [detailed listing of contents]. It is also inquired into, what the uses of the Lungs are in hot Animals? And many other such material disquisitions are to be found in this small, but very Ingenious and Learned Treatise. (*EMEMT*; *PT*, 1, 1665: 77–8)

Some of the early reviews were not meant to take particular books into consideration but rather to deal with a specific theme that the editor considered highly topical, as was the case with blood transfusions (Example 22):

(22) Whereas there have lately appeared in publick some Books, printed beyond the Seas, treating of the Way of Injecting Liquors into Veines, in which Books the Original of that Invention seems to be ascribed to others, besides him, to whom it really belongs; It will surely not be thought amiss, if something be said, whereby the true Inventor's right may beyond exception be asserted and preserved; To which end there will need no more, than barely to represent the Time when, and the Place where, and among whom it was first started and put to tryal. (*EMEMT*; *PT*, 1, 1665: 128)

In his contribution, the reviewer usually provided information about the author's descriptions and opinions, using a variety of reporting verbs: 'intimates', 'observes',[5] 'maintains', 'concludes', 'endeavours to justifie', 'endeavours to answer', 'undertakes to shew', 'explicates', 'adds', 'pretends', 'treats', 'proves', 'examines', 'defines', 'conceives', 'affirms', 'professes', 'teaches' (*EMEMT*; *PT*, 1, 1666: 301–10). The position of the reviewer as a reporter of the author's views was clearly confirmed by the frequent use of expressions such as 'according to the Author' or 'saies he' in the passages conveying opinions and interpretations of the facts described. However, although the aim of the reviewer was mainly to report the contents of the book examined, his attitude towards the author or his work can sometimes be deduced by his use of evaluative expressions such as 'he *easily* gives an account why', 'he *frankly* pronounces', 'understands *clearly* that' (*EMEMT*; *PT*, 1, 1666: 303–7, emphasis added). Sometimes a very positive evaluation of the book was explicitly expressed by the reviewer, as in Example 23:

(23) What this excellent Author formerly promised of the whole Pathology of Brain and Nerves, he gives in this Book a very considerable Specimen of. (*EMEMT*; *PT*, 2, 1667: 600)

Similarly to some of the contributions to the *PT*, reviews were published anonymously, as this choice enabled the author to extol his works or to criticize those by his opponents with little risk of unpleasant consequences. There were several other reasons for this anonymity: fear of political repercussions, religious persecution, financial loss or ostracism by the scientific community (Kronick 1988). Through the review of the literature, the journal greatly contributed to the advancement of specialized disciplines as it favoured the establishment of widely shared experience and knowledge within the scientific community, providing it with a common empirical and methodological approach.

## 11.5 Evolution of these genres

The seventeenth century was a very important period in the development of specialist knowledge – both in England and all over the European continent – not only for the great epistemological and methodological developments that took place in existing disciplines and in newly created ones but also because it favoured the elaboration of suitable linguistic tools for the expression of specialized concepts. As has been seen, the *PT* provided a great contribution to the propagation of new information regarding specialized facts or events among the wide and varied readership of this journal. Its communicative

[5] According to Gray, Biber and Hiltunen (this volume, Chapter 12), '"observe" is used frequently in the book review category as a means of reporting what the author of the book being reviewed found in his investigations or wrote about in the book.'

role, however, was not limited merely to the fulfilment of goals linked to socialization and solidarity but also included the reform of existing means of discourse and the development of new ones. Indeed, the propagation of discourse conveying new information about specialized facts or events to a social group sharing intellectual and professional interests implied the adoption of various textual forms, each with its own specific pragmatic aim so as to carry out different communicative functions and to meet the expectations of a large number of non-homogenous addressees.

Its considerable importance as a means for the spread of scientific information is demonstrated by the growth of specialized publications and by the increasing number of journal titles in the following centuries. Specialists, both in England and abroad, soon realized the value of scientific journals as a means of communicating news concerning their discoveries and opinions. In the period between 1665 and 1790, about 100 different scientific and technical periodicals appeared (Kronick 1976). A few decades after the issue of the first scientific publications, some discipline-related journals were produced, whose aim was to deal with news pertaining to specific branches of knowledge or specialized disciplines (Garrison 1934; Colman 1999). A further evolution was the creation of publications devoted to specific genres, such as journals mainly concerned with the printing of abstracts, summaries or reviews so as to keep up with the increasing number of books and journal literature available.

The textual innovations made available by the *PT* were widely accepted by the scientific community of the eighteenth century. The various advantages they offered caused them to become very widespread, and their popularity became even greater with the increase in circulation of scientific journals. The new genres became conventionalized in the last decades of the seventeenth century and continued in use for a long time, forming the basis of nineteenth- and twentieth-century scientific reports. The early models influenced subsequent examples of specialized news genres enormously. As Bazerman (1988) notes in his analysis of the first 135 years of the *PT*, the basic narrative structure of early scientific experimental accounts was retained well into the nineteenth century. His conclusions have been confirmed by further research. For example, on the basis of his review of selected research articles published in the *Edinburgh Medical Journal* (*EMJ*) between 1735 and 1985, Atkinson (1992: 359) comes to the conclusion that 'original articles in the eighteenth-century *EMJ* were typically narrative reports of single cases, often presented in epistolary form'.

In particular, the innovative characteristics of the experimental essay made it very popular in the medical field also. To appreciate the importance of this genre, we should consider the fact that, in the following centuries, while some forms of specialized writing – such as the dialogue – almost disappeared, the experimental essay survived and became an essential part of specialized literature, as the rapid diffusion of scientific journals made it an established genre commonly used by men of science. Of course, in the following centuries, important changes concerning this genre took place. Early essays showed frequent use of the active form, reports of unsuccessful experiments and less emphasis on theoretical conclusions than nowadays; moreover, they were characterized by first-person narration and subjective point of view. Later essays, instead, showed a gradual shift from an 'author-centred' to an 'object-centred' rhetoric, expressed linguistically in more-or-less 'involved' terms. While early journal accounts were not considered definitive publications but mainly in-progress reports, later articles acquired the status of final expression of concluded experimental activity, usually implying some theoretical innovation. Moreover, in the course of time, experimental accounts evolved and found a more cohesive structure, commonly consisting of the following steps: stating of purpose, description of the apparatus, account of the phenomena to be investigated, narration of the experiment(s), record of the results and expounding of any theoretical implications. As can be seen, most of these steps were constant parts of early experimental accounts. However, some of the features of early articles have changed throughout the centuries. For instance, there is a more frequent use of the passive form, and the report of unsuccessful experiments has been abandoned, while greater emphasis is commonly laid on the theoretical conclusions to be drawn from the experiments. But many have remained, and these testify to the seminal role that the reflections and writing practices of the contributors to the *PT* have had in the widespread adoption of this important means for the dissemination of specialized news.

# 12 The expression of stance in early (1665–1712) publications of the *Philosophical Transactions* and other contemporary medical prose: innovations in a pioneering discourse

BETHANY GRAY, DOUGLAS BIBER AND TURO HILTUNEN

## 12.1 Introduction

Language users, regardless of register, employ a variety of lexico-grammatical markers to express their attitudes towards, evaluations of and level of commitment to what they speak or write. The linguistic marking of attitudes and assessments has been investigated under a variety of labels, such as *evaluation* (Hunston 1994; Hunston and Thompson 2000), *hedging* and *boosting* (Hyland 1996, 1998), *evidentiality* (Chafe 1986) and, perhaps most widely, *stance* (e.g., Biber 2004a, 2006; Biber and Finegan 1988, 1989; Biber et al. 1999; Hyland 2005; Precht 2003). Stance research has investigated stance markers in a variety of registers and includes detailed investigations of particular stance devices (e.g., Lindemann and Mauranen's 2001 investigation into 'just'), studies on a class of items (e.g., Swales and Burke 2003 on evaluative adjectives) and studies that document the ways in which multiple grammatical and semantic classes of stance features interact (e.g., Biber 2004a, 2006).

In spite of once-held perceptions that academic writing is largely free of overt markers of the writer's attitudes and opinions, recent scholarship has demonstrated that stance is an important aspect of formal written prose. This scholarship has emphasized the role of stance in creating and maintaining relationships between the writer and his or her audience as well as reflecting the value system of writers and their discourse communities (Hyland 1999, 2001, 2002; Thompson and Hunston 2000). Although the overt expression of stance occurs more commonly in conversation than in written registers, stance features also occur relatively frequently in written registers (Biber et al. 1999: Chapter 12).

Most investigations of stance in academic prose have focused on contemporary texts (e.g., Biber 2006; Charles 2003, 2006; Hyland 1996, 1999, 2001, 2002, 2005; Hyland and Tse 2005; Swales and Burke 2003; Thompson and Ye 1991). However, there have also been several studies describing the expression of stance in historical registers. For example, Biber (2004a) tracks stance use from 1650 to 1990, focusing on four historical registers (drama, personal letters, newspaper reportage and medical prose). This study reveals changing patterns of stance use throughout the time periods represented by the corpus, with most of the features increasing in use across time (with the exception of modals, which decreased).

As a key journal in the development of scientific prose in English, the *Philosophical Transactions* (*PT*) of the Royal Society, has been analysed in several studies (e.g., Atkinson 1996, 1999; Gross et al. 2000, 2002; Valle 1999). Although not often the main focus of analysis, stance features frequently arise in the discussion of *PT* texts. For example, Atkinson (1996, 1999) presents an analysis of the evolving nature of articles published in the *PT* from 1675 to 1975, using the complementary methods of rhetorical analysis and multidimensional analysis. Atkinson's rhetorical analysis of *PT* texts finds shifts in how the authors place themselves in the texts. In earlier *PT* texts (1675–1775), Atkinson found that texts were typically 'author-centred', with frequent use of first-person pronouns, active-voice verbs and, key for our purposes, 'the use of language to portray the affective states and psychological processes of the author' as well as a variety of stance markers 'by means of which researchers showed their own diffidence and caution in the interpretation of natural phenomena' (Atkinson 1996: 339). Likewise, Gotti (Chapter 11, this volume) alludes to stance use by authors in the *PT*, claiming that authors of *PT* articles express 'opinions and conclusions with the degree of positiveness corresponding to the certainty of the facts described'. Gotti mentions authors' use of modal verbs, verbs such as 'seem' (a verb which shows a degree of uncertainty) and the inclusion of the experimenter's reactions – all aspects of stance. Gotti claims that hedging allowed the writer to gain confidence from his audience, convincing them he had reliably recounted what he had observed or witnessed.

The views put forth by Atkinson and Gotti are in line with Hyland's ideas regarding the role of hedging in modern academic prose. Hyland (1996: 433) claims that hedging (limiting the strength with which an author commits to a proposition) arises because 'the need to present unproven propositions with caution and precision is essential'. According to Hyland and others (e.g., Meyer 1997), incorporating strategies that weaken statements make the arguments presented in academic prose more credible by anticipating and mitigating the effects of overstatement (Hyland 1996, 1998), which, in turn, allows the author to gain the audience's trust. On the other hand, markers of certainty can position a claim or statement as 'consensually given' (Hyland 1998: 353), i.e. as information accepted as true or correct by the audience.

In this chapter, we investigate the overt expression of specific attitudes or specific assessments of epistemic status in medical prose from the mid seventeenth century to the early eighteenth century, considering three lexico-grammatical structures used to construct stance: modal and semi-modal verbs, adverbials and *that*-complement clauses controlled by stance nouns, verbs and adjectives. Our goal in this analysis is to locate and describe patterns of stance use in the earliest period (1665–1712) of the *PT*. In particular, we focus our analysis on three types of articles published in the *PT* during this early period: reports, letters and book reviews.

We contrast the patterns of stance in these three *PT* text categories to the use of stance features in traditional medical texts from the same period. That is, there was a relatively large number of medical texts in circulation during the sixteenth, seventeenth and eighteenth centuries, including treatises, recipes, regimens and health guides. Against this background, it is possible to describe the ways in which the *PT* texts were innovative, adopting new communicative purposes and directed towards a different primary audience. The linguistic focus of the present study is to document the innovative use of stance features associated with these new communicative purposes.

In the following section, we briefly introduce the typical communicative purposes and audience of *PT* articles, contrasted with those of other seventeenth-century medical texts. Sections 12.3 and 12.4 are methodological, first summarizing the lexico-grammatical stance features included in the analysis (Section 12.3) and then describing the analytical procedures (Section 12.4). Then, in Sections 12.5 and 12.6, we present and interpret the results of our analysis, showing that the early publication types of the *PT* employ distinct patterns of stance that correspond to the new communicative purpose of the *PT*, particularly in the use of *that*-complement clauses.

## 12.2 Audience and communicative purpose in seventeenth-century texts from the *PT* and other traditional medical writing

The *PT* represented a significant innovation in medical prose in the seventeenth century, contrasting with other types of medical writing such as surgical treatises, regimens and remedy books. These categories of medical prose were well established, having a long history in the vernacular. In many cases, these texts can be traced back to classical languages (Taavitsainen and Pahta 2004). The *PT*, in contrast, was a novel venue for the circulation of medical knowledge – and an important one, since medical practitioners were the largest and most active single occupational group among the members of the Royal Society at the time as they collectively pursued topics such as anatomy, respiration, generation, blood, muscle physiology, organic chemistry and animal experimentation (Porter 1989b: 272–3).

It is difficult to verify the exact readership of the traditional medical texts, in part due to the range of individuals interested in medical topics. Along with university-trained physicians, medicine was practised by laypeople (e.g., women members of the family, relatives, friends, charitable gentlewomen and clergymen). Moreover, there were many other kinds of practitioners, including empirics, mountebanks, herbalists, uroscopists and astrologers, who moved from one place to another and offered their services in exchange for money (see Wear 2000: 21–8). In general terms, however, the text categories can be placed along a continuum of learned versus popular knowledge corresponding to the likely audience of the texts. General treatises, treatises on special topics and surgical/anatomical treatises exist on the 'learned' pole of the continuum, typically being written by university-trained professionals for other professionals. On the 'popular' pole of the continuum, recipes were likely aimed at laypeople and professionals alike, and regimens were targeted towards the upper and middle classes, not limited to medical professionals (Wear 2000: 47–8, 154).

In contrast, texts in the *PT* were much more dialogic, often representing a kind of extended interaction among researchers. As a result, positive relations between writers and their audiences were particularly important for contributors to the *PT*, as contributors interacted with the scientific community through publishing in the journal. Atkinson (1996, 1999) notes that the highly dialogic nature of writing in the early years of the *PT* was due to the fact that many contributions to the journal were written in response to other recent publications in the *PT*. The differences from traditional texts with respect to audience and interactivity are related to innovations in communicative purpose. Letters were a frequently occurring text category in the *PT* and, as Gotti notes, were often the mode of transmission for criticizing others and for authors to address criticisms brought against them. In addition, many articles were observational reports or experimental studies (see Atkinson 1996; Bazerman 1988).

In fact, three major categories of texts can be identified in the early issues of the *PT*: reports, letters and book reviews. Reports offered detailed accounts of both experimental and observational research. Reports served as venues through which authors could put forth conjectures and remarks on a variety of scientific topics, including comments regarding methodological issues in the advancement of scientific inquiry. In contrast, letters were submitted by members of the scientific community and were written in a typical letter format. Letters were edited and then published in both extracted and full forms and were typically introduced with a short comment from the editor of the journal. The final category within the *PT*, book reviews, summarized books of interest to the scientific community and typically offered evaluation of the books' contents.

Texts published in the *PT* differed from traditional medical texts with regard to several other contextual characteristics. For example, *PT* texts are relatively short (but complete) communications that were published in a scientific journal, while traditional medical texts are usually longer books (the texts in the non-*PT* subcorpora used in this study are excerpts from these longer works). Importantly for our purposes here, *PT* articles include frequent references to other contemporary scientists working on the same topics, in contrast to traditional texts which less frequently acknowledge other studies.

Important differences in audience and purpose exist between the *PT* texts and non-*PT* texts. While texts in the five categories of non-*PT* texts studied here instructed readers about established doctrines of medical theory and practice, articles in the *PT* provided information about new theories and results, based on empirical evidence. Corresponding to this difference in communicative purpose is a difference in intended readership. Gross et al. (2000: 372) point out that the readership of the *PT* was varied in comparison to the French counterpart of the Royal Society. The community of the Royal Society consisted of both famed and talented natural philosophers and amateurs who were merely interested in medical matters, and the early volumes even included letters from people who were not actual members of the community (Gross et al. 2000: 389). Despite this, the audience of the *PT* texts was quite specialized in comparison to the readership of texts in the five categories of non-*PT* texts. While *PT* readers included both professional and non-professional scientists, the *PT* audience nonetheless consisted of educated, informed readers. In contrast, the traditional medical texts were addressed to a broader, less specialized audience consisting of researchers, practitioners, educated laypeople and even non-educated laypeople.

Thus, to fully understand the characteristics of early texts published in the *PT*, it is important to describe them by comparison to the other categories of traditional medical writing. While other kinds of medical texts had been in circulation for quite some time, publications in the *PT* represented an innovation for the advancement of scientific knowledge. With this innovation came new ways of communicating and interacting with the discourse community. In this chapter, we extend previous research by systematically focusing on a comprehensive description of stance features in texts from the earliest period of the *PT*, considering differences and similarities across the three major types of publications, i.e. reports, letters and book reviews. In addition, we compare these three text categories from the *PT* with five other categories of Early Modern English medical prose represented in the Early Modern English Medical Texts (*EMEMT*) corpus. First, however, a discussion of the lexico-grammatical markers of stance is needed.

## 12.3 Lexico-grammatical markers of stance

In this chapter, we focus on the most overt way a language user can mark personal stance: through lexico-grammatical structures that explicitly express an attitude or evaluation. These stance features can be categorized along two parameters: (1) grammatical category/structure and (2) semantic associations. In the *Longman Grammar of Spoken and Written English*,

Biber et al. (1999) identify three major grammatical structures that convey stance:

1. modal verbs (e.g., 'can', 'could', 'may', 'might');
2. stance adverbials (e.g., 'possibly', 'kind of', 'surprisingly');
3. *to-* and *that-*complement clauses controlled by stance verbs, nouns and adjectives (e.g., 'I argue that …', 'The claim that …', 'It's remarkable that …', 'He is likely to go …').

Within each of these grammatical categories, linguistic items can be classified according to semantic association (i.e. the general meaning being expressed by the stance feature). For the present study, we adopt the basic categories of stance used by Biber (2004a), with some changes in labelling.

For modal and semi-modal verbs, three major semantic distinctions are typically made, and we use these same distinctions in the present study:

- possibility, permission or ability (e.g., 'might', 'may');
- logical necessity or obligation (e.g., 'must', 'should');
- prediction or volition (e.g., 'will', 'would').

Four types of stance adverbials are identified in Biber (2004a):

1. attitudinal;
2. factive (we adopt the term 'certainty');
3. non-factive (we adopt the term 'communication')
4. likelihood.

Attitudinal adverbials portray affective states or reactions (e.g., 'curiously', 'surprisingly', 'humbly'), while likelihood adverbials either express doubt or show a level of commitment less than that of absolute certainty (e.g., 'perhaps', 'possibly', 'largely', 'usually'). Factive or certainty adverbials express a higher level of commitment to the proposition or, in other words, acknowledge a high level of certainty towards the truth of the proposition (e.g., 'always', 'certainly', 'indeed', 'obviously', 'surely'). Non-factive or communication adverbials show point of view or manner of speaking or indicate the source of information (e.g., 'confidentially', 'honestly', 'reportedly', 'in general').

As we focus on *that-*complement clauses in the analysis presented in this chapter, we discuss only *that-*clauses here, although *to-*, *wh-* and *-ing-*clauses are also used to construct stance. *That-*complement clauses can be further divided according to the grammatical category of the controlling word. For verb-controlled complement clauses, verbs controlling the matrix clause can be non-factive (our 'communication' verbs), factive (certainty), likelihood or attitudinal. The meanings of attitudinal verbs (e.g., 'admire', 'complain', 'dream', 'fear'), likelihood verbs (e.g., 'appear', 'believe', 'doubt', 'seem', 'suspect') and certainty verbs (e.g., 'affirm', 'certify', 'know', 'prove', 'understand') correspond to the general meanings of the corresponding adverbials above. Non-factive, or communication, verbs have been further classified in the present investigation into three types. Communication 'declare' verbs indicate a relatively neutral stance (e.g., 'add', 'declare', 'mention', 'say', 'tell') while 'argue' verbs indicate a stronger level of commitment to the propositions introduced (e.g., 'argue', 'claim', 'insist', 'swear'). On the opposite end of the continuum, 'suggest' communication verbs indicate a meaning of hesitancy or lack of certainty (e.g., 'advise', 'hint', 'imply', 'suggest').

Stance nouns controlling *that*-clauses can be categorized in similar ways, and we recognize attitudinal (e.g., 'amusement', 'fear', 'hope', 'wonder'), certainty (e.g., 'argument', 'assertion', 'doctrine', 'evidence', 'fact') and likelihood (e.g., 'belief', 'contention', 'opinion', 'possibility') nouns in the present study. Adjectives controlling complement clauses can also be categorized semantically; however, the meanings are less clear for adjectives. For this reason, we analyse the semantic function of the adjectives only for the frequently occurring adjectives a bit later in the chapter.

## 12.4 Method

In the present study, we seek to document the various ways in which stance is expressed in the earliest periods of the *PT*. We also aim to describe patterns of variation for the expression of stance in the *PT*, considering the three types of articles published during this period. In addition, we compare the patterns of use for a set of stance features for the *PT* categories with five other types of medical texts from this time period. In this section, we outline our procedures for accomplishing these goals.

### *12.4.1 Corpus*

Six categories from *EMEMT* are analysed in this study. Texts from the *PT* (grouped together in the corpus) have been categorized into the three article types for our study.[1] Reports encompass accounts not embedded in a letter format that report on experimental research, observations, conjectures and comments. Reports may also deal with methodological considerations. Letters were published in full or as extracts and were written by members of the society or others hoping to pursue natural knowledge. These letters were typically edited before publication in the journal and were preceded by a short comment introducing the letter. Book reviews summarized medical books and offered evaluation of the books' contents. The remaining five

[1] Gotti's chapter (Chapter 11, this volume) identifies four categories of texts in the *PT*. Because the text categories in the early years of the *PT* had not yet become conventionalized, some variation inherently exists in classifications of the articles within the *PT*. For example, Atkinson (1996, 1999) singles out two genres (letters and experimental reports) while Valle (1999) suggests that the book review is the only genre that stands out as distinctive in the early *PT*. However, for the purposes of our study, we have identified three article types that correspond to the major content and format varieties found in the corpus.

text categories from *EMEMT* are general treatises or textbooks, treatises on specific topics, recipe collections and *materia medica*, regimens and health guides, and surgical and anatomical treatises. Table 12.1 displays the year span represented by the texts used in this analysis, along with the number of texts, the total number of words in the subcorpora and the mean number of words per text.[2]

### *12.4.2 Data analysis and methodological considerations*

The first step in the study was to categorize the texts in the *PT* subcorpus of *EMEMT* into the three text categories. For the present study, we chose to focus on three grammatical structures used to express stance: modals and semi-modals, adverbials and *that*-complement clauses controlled by stance nouns, adjectives and verbs. Within these three grammatical categories, we investigated several semantic groupings, as displayed in Table 12.2 below. Appendix C provides a complete list of the forms (with most variant spellings) used in the analysis. Adjectives were often difficult to categorize in terms of semantic groupings prior to the analysis. Therefore, we analysed the semantic meanings of only the most frequently occurring adjectives controlling *that*-clauses, and these are listed in Table 12.2.

All texts were converted to text files and automatically 'tagged'. However, the accuracy of the automatic tags was not sufficient for many stance features. In particular, *that*-complement clauses were problematic because the *that*-clause often occurs at a distance from the controlling stance word. Examples 1 and 2 below illustrate two of the issues that hindered the automatic identification of complement clauses based on grammatical tags. The first issue is that a single stance item often controls more than one complement clause (Example 1). The second issue is that the controlling word and the complement clause are often separated by punctuation and/or additional clauses or phrases (Example 2). Both of these issues result in the complementizer *that* being separated from the controlling word with many intervening words and punctuation marks, making an automatic analysis unreliable. Thus, we additionally employed interactive coding, described below.

(1) As there have been Remedies found out against excessive Heat, and Means of cooling Meat and Drink; so **it was** lately, on the occasion of the sharp Season, **suggested**, [<u>That Remedies might be thought on against Cold</u>]; and [<u>that particularly it might be inquired into</u>] (*EMEMT*; *PT*, 1, 1666: 379–80, report)

(2) Between 21 and 22 of her age, going down stairs she heard a frightful jolking in her Breast; which she then made known to the rest of the house, who when she shewd them the manner of it by shaking her

[2] Our study was conducted with a pre-release version of *EMEMT*, which contains fourteen texts from volume 27 of the *PT* (1710–) not included in the final version of the corpus.

Table 12.1 *Corpus material for this study.*

| Text category | Years | Number of texts | Total number of words | Mean number of words per text |
|---|---|---|---|---|
| Reports (from *PT*) | 1665–1712 | 64 | 81,371 | 1,271.42 |
| Book reviews (from *PT*) | 1665–1710 | 46 | 52,781 | 1,147.41 |
| Letters (from *PT*) | 1665–1712 | 47 | 51,699 | 1,099.98 |
| General treatises and textbooks | 1652–1700 | 7 | 64,524 | 9,217.71 |
| Treatises on specific topics | 1651–1700 | 22 | 175,467 | 7,975.77 |
| Recipe collections and *materia medica* | 1650–1700 | 13 | 124,738 | 9,595.23 |
| Regimens and health guides | 1656–96 | 5 | 33,772 | 6,754.40 |
| Surgical and anatomical treatises | 1652–98 | 10 | 92,393 | 9,239.30 |
| **Total** | **1650–1712** | **214** | **676,745** | **3,162.36** |

Body, joynd all with her in the wonder, **concluding** (as most would have done by the noise) [that her Breast was almost full of Water]. (*EMEMT*; *PT*, 2, 1667: 546–51, report)

We undertook an iterative process in order to include as many stance items as possible and thus obtain a more robust view of stance use than what would have been possible considering only the stance items and spellings used in previous studies. Starting with the features/lexical items used in Biber (2004a), we added to the stance features in three steps, the first two of which are discussed here. First, we used corpus analysis of the texts to identify additional adverbials and stance adjectives controlling *that*-clauses by examining word lists generated from the tagged *PT* subcorpus for those two grammatical classes.[3] Second, we generated a word list of all words in the *PT* subcorpus to identify the possible spelling variants for all forms in our analysis (nouns, verbs, adjectives, adverbials and modals). This analysis turned out to be especially important because spelling was highly variable in these texts. For example, this preliminary analysis revealed the following possible forms for the verb 'appear': 'appear', 'appeare', 'appears', 'appeares', 'appeared', 'appeard', 'appear'd', 'appeareth' and 'appearing'.

To locate occurrences of stance features in the corpus, a computer program was written to count the words in each text, to identify the selected stance features and to output coded keyword-in-context (KWIC) entries

[3] We did not search for additional nouns and verbs controlling *that*-clauses because there seemed to be less variation in these two classes.

Table 12.2 *Stance categories and example items.*

| Stance categories | Example items |
|---|---|
| **Modals and semi-modals** | |
| *Possibility, permission, ability* | can, could, may, might |
| *Necessity, obligation* | should, must, better, have to |
| *Prediction, volition* | would, will, shall, be going to |
| **Adverbials** | |
| *Communication* | confidentially, frankly, generally, honestly |
| *Certainty* | actually, always, certainly, definitely, indeed |
| *Likelihood* | apparently, perhaps, possibly, probably |
| *Attitudinal* | amazingly, curiously, disturbingly, hopefully |
| **Verb-controlled *that*-complement clauses** | |
| *Communication: argue* | argue, claim, maintain, insist |
| *Communication: declare* | declare, mention, say, report |
| *Communication: suggest* | advise, hint, imply, suggest, urge |
| *Certainty* | affirm, certify, conclude, confirm, prove |
| *Likelihood* | appear, assume, doubt, guess, hypothesize |
| *Attitudinal* | accept, admit, fear, hope, mind |
| **Noun-controlled *that*-complement clauses** | |
| *Certainty* | conclusion, conviction, knowledge, statement |
| *Likelihood* | assumption, belief, expectation, hypothesis |
| *Attitudinal* | fear, hope, thought |
| **Adjective-controlled *that*-complement clauses** | |
| *Certainty* | certain, clear, evident, observable, sure, true |
| *Likelihood* | likely, probable |

that could then be hand-checked for accuracy. For modals and adverbials, KWIC entries are printed based on string matches. For *that*-complement clauses, all occurrences of uncapitalized *that* were identified as potential stance features.[4] All occurrences of potential *that*-complement clauses were hand-checked, as well as occurrences of 'better' to ensure that 'better' functioned as a semi-modal and not as an adjective. Each potential complement clause was evaluated, and the KWIC file was updated to reflect the accurate

[4] For this analysis, we excluded capitalized 'That'. However, some of the occurrences of capitalized 'That' are stance complement clauses, and this is one area for further research. In addition, because the analysis is based on untagged texts, we do not analyse complement clauses in which the complementizer *that* has been omitted.

controlling word and stance category. The third and final stage of our iterative process occurred while coding the KWIC file. This stage involved identifying stance words controlling complement clauses not already in our lists and placing them within the grammatical and semantic categories if they indeed indicated the author's stance. The final step in the analysis was to write a second computer program to parse the KWIC file, creating counts for each lexical item and each grammatical and semantic category, normalizing those counts to 1,000 words.

## 12.5 Findings

In this section, we present our quantitative and qualitative results of the stance analysis in three text categories from the *PT* and the five non-*PT* categories of medical writing in *EMEMT.* Several interesting trends emerge. First, while there is no overall difference between *PT* categories and other text categories in the combined use of stance, there is variation within the three *PT* categories. As can be seen in Figure 12.1, letters contain the highest frequency of stance markers (c. twenty-three stance markers per 1,000 words). Reports, treatises on specific topics, regimens and surgical and anatomical treatises demonstrate similar rates of stance-marker use (c. twenty markers per 1,000 words). Book reviews and recipes contain the fewest stance markers of all categories (c. fifteen per 1,000 words in each).

Second, and perhaps most interesting, *that*-complement clauses controlled by stance verbs, nouns and adjectives are much more prevalent in the three *PT* categories than in other text categories. This suggests that the use of *that*-complement clauses is an innovation tied to the new purposes of the *PT* and reflects the use of more explicit evaluation in medical prose. This finding will be discussed in more detail below.

In addition to the two major findings summarized above, Figure 12.1 also reveals that modal verbs are the most frequently occurring stance structure across all text categories. In the three categories from the *PT*, *that*-complement clauses are slightly more frequent than stance adverbials, while rates for *that*-clauses and adverbials are more balanced in the remaining five text categories. In the next sections, we examine each stance feature in more detail.

### *12.5.1 The use of modals*

Across all text categories, modal verbs are the most frequently occurring stance markers, with an overall frequency of c. twelve to fifteen modals per 1,000 words (with the exception of book reviews, which contain only six to seven modals per 1,000 words). Figure 12.2 shows the distribution of

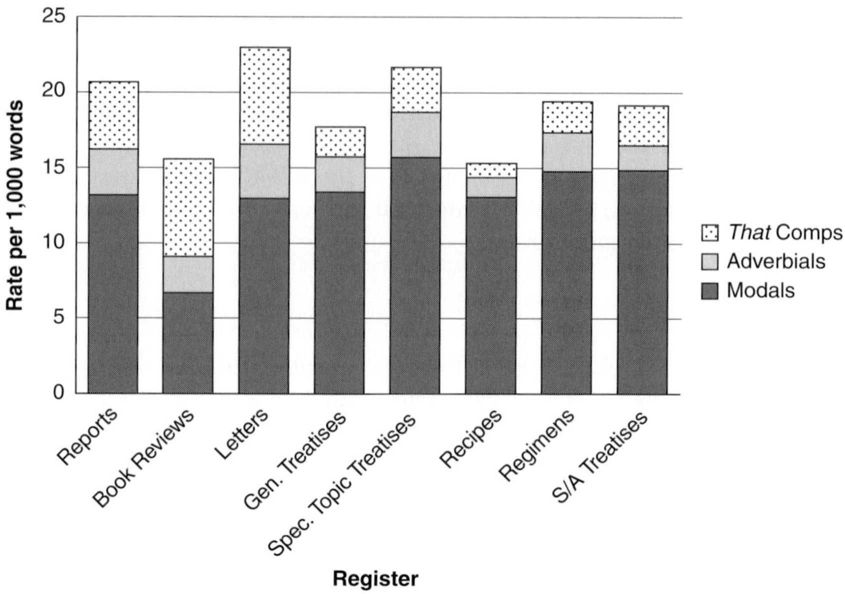


Figure 12.1 Distribution of grammatical structures.

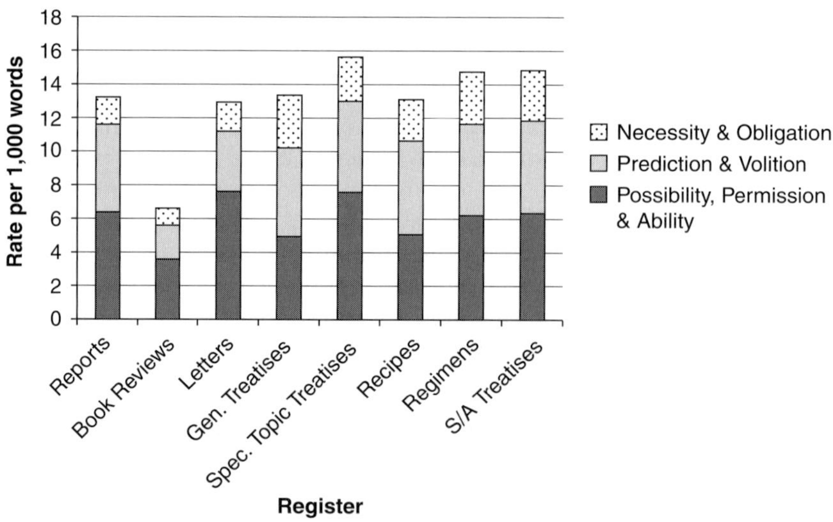


Figure 12.2 Distribution of modals.

the three modal types across categories. Except for in recipes and general treatises, possibility, permission and ability modals are the most frequent. Prediction and volition modals are second-most frequent, and necessity and obligation modals are the least frequent.

Within possibility, permission and ability modals, 'may' is the most frequent and occurs across all text categories, accounting for 55 per cent of all possibility, permission and ability modals. 'May' occurs less frequently in book reviews than other categories; however, it is still the most frequent modal used in that category (with a rate of 1.9 per 1,000 words). In these historical texts, 'may' occurs in several semantic contexts. First, 'may' can indicate a meaning of possibility, as in Example 3. Although traditionally thought to be expressed by 'can', the meaning of ability is also found with 'may' (Example 4).

(3) From hence **may** appear the danger of using Mercury in humane Bodies, so as that it **may** get into the Mass of Blood, especially into the Lungs (*EMEMT*; *PT*, 16, 1687–8: 486–8, report)
(4) All things being thus prepard, tie the Dogs on their sides towards one another so conveniently, that the Quill **may** go into each other (*EMEMT*; *PT*, 1, 1666: 353–8, report)

A third use of 'may' corresponds to the author's need not to impose thoughts or actions on the audience, in which an author uses 'may' to soften the assumption that the reader will agree with an interpretation or will follow an indirect directive. In Example 5, the writer directs the reader to attend to points he will soon summarize. In Example 6, the author uses 'may' to introduce an interpretation or claim.

(5) To represent distinctly, what he undertakes to make out in this Tract, we **may** take notice of these particulars: (*EMEMT*; *PT*, 2, 1667: 534–5, book review)
(6) The Analogy I have already mentioned, which we **may** rationally suppose between the manner of the propagation of Plants and Animals, does likewise make this probable. (*EMEMT*; *PT*, 16, 1687–8: 474–83, letter)

'Can' is less frequent (accounting for 25 per cent of all permission, possibility and ability modals) than 'may' but is still fairly stable across categories. 'Can' is used primarily to express ability, as in Example 7.

(7) A Muscle is an Instrument of voluntary motion, without which no part of the Body **can** move it self, it consists of fibrous flesh to make up its body, of Nerves (*EMEMT*; Culpeper 1651, specific treatises)

The prediction and volition modal 'will' is also frequent across categories, accounting for 45 per cent of all prediction and volition modals. 'Will' is particularly high in recipes and comparatively low in book reviews and letters. 'Will' is used most commonly to indicate future happenings or events (Example 8); however, a less frequent use also appears: a way of organizing discourse (Example 9).

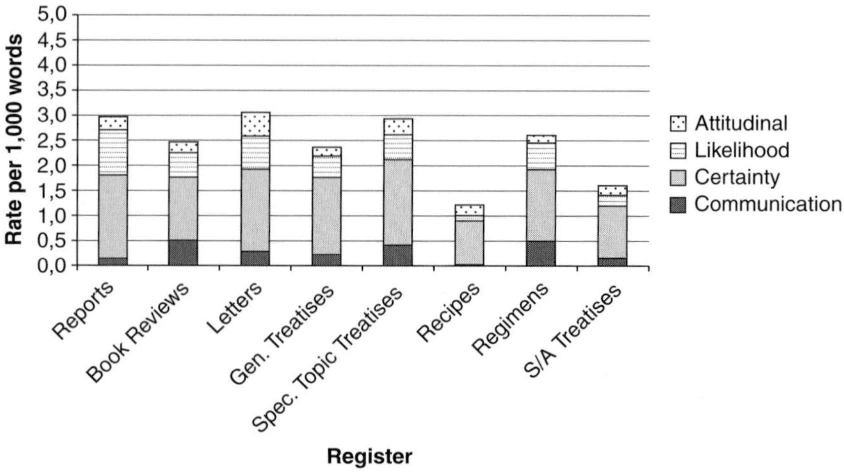


Figure 12.3 Distribution of stance adverbials.

(8) I confess this Difficulty is to me and the Gentlemen who have seen them dissected, a Mystery, which these Anatomists and their Approvers **will** discover to us when they shall think fit (*PT*, 27, 1710: 170–85, report)

(9) thus farre I have shewed you how the Pestilence happeneth, and how to prevent it; Now I **will** shew you briefly the simptomes and signes of it, and proceed to the cure. (*EMEMT*; Elkes 1651, recipes)

### *12.5.2 The use of stance adverbials*

Stance adverbials are relatively rare, used between one and three times per 1,000 words across categories (Figure 12.3). Recipes use the fewest stance adverbials, followed by surgical and anatomical treatises. Certainty adverbials are used more than any other stance adverbial class across all categories, followed by likelihood adverbials, while attitudinal and communication adverbials are less frequent.

As the most frequently occurring stance adverbials, certainty adverbials demonstrate that the author is confident in the accuracy of his statements, as in Examples 10 through 14 below. The two most common certainty adverbials, 'never' and 'always', signify an absolute certainty as to the frequency of occurrence of some phenomena (Examples 11 and 12).

(10) You have **doubtless** heard of a Mad-man, that hath been lately cured and restored to his Wits (*EMEMT*; *PT*, 2, 1667–8: 617–23, letter)

(11) but the Fever it self must **always** be cur'd with the Cortex (*EMEMT*; *PT*, 17, 1693: 717–28, book review)

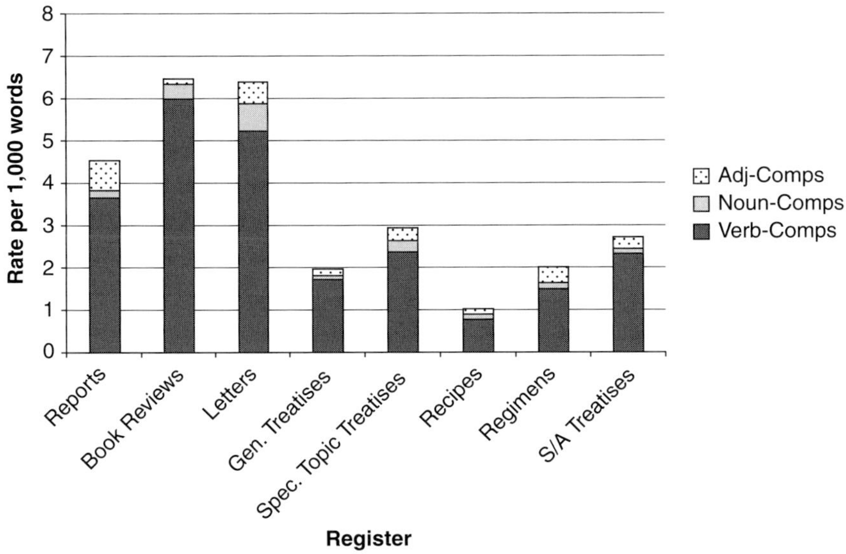


Figure 12.4 *That*-complement clause types.

(12) Of both which we cannot omit to give the Reader the substance in English, as follows, Having often observed in Anatomical Dissections of Men as well as Brutes, that the Optick Nerve does **never** answer just to the Middle of the bottom of the Eye (*EMEMT*; *PT*, 3, 1668: 668–71, report)

Hyland (1998: 353) claims that markers of certainty (what he calls 'boosters') can serve to position a claim or statement as 'consensually given' information, and this interpretation seems to hold true for many of the certainty adverbials here. In Examples 13 and 14, the use of 'of course' and 'surely' gives a sense that the audience will readily accept the statement to come without questioning the validity of the statement.

(13) And as they cannot be suppos'd to occasion such Sensations, without assigning 'em an influence upon our Organs and Liquors; so **of course**, they must needs be useful in Physick. (*EMEMT*; Tauvry 1700, specific treatises)

(14) **Surely**, all ingenius men will acknowledge, that the certain way of decidiug such Controversies as these, is a Publick Record, either written or printed, declaring the time and place of an Invention first proposed, the contrivance of the Method, to practise it, and the instances of the success in the Execution. (*EMEMT*; *PT*, 2, 1667: 517–25, report)

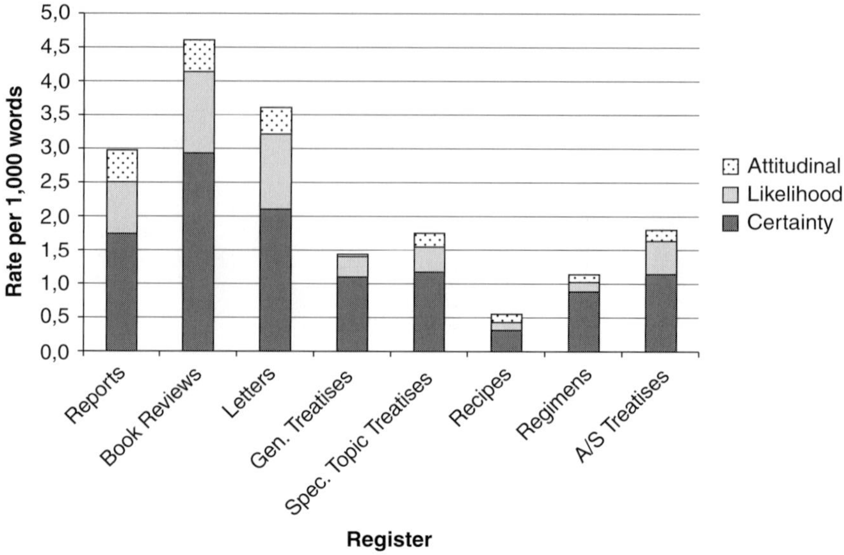


Figure 12.5 Non-communication verb-controlled *that*-complement clauses.

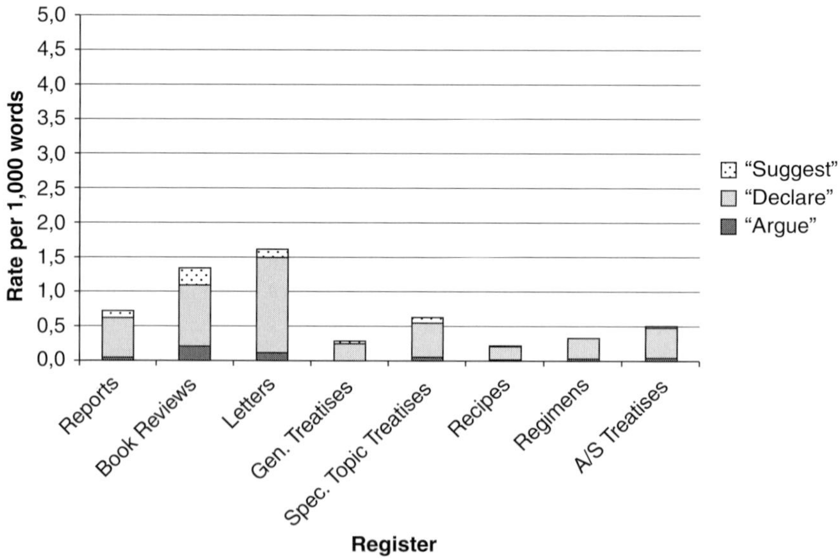


Figure 12.6 Communication verb-controlled *that*-complement clauses.

### *12.5.3 That-complement clauses*

*That*-complement clauses are more frequent in the three *PT* categories than in all others (see Figure 12.4). Book reviews, which to this point have demonstrated much lower rates of stance markers than other *PT* categories and non-*PT* text categories, exhibit the highest rate of occurrence for complement clauses. Across all categories, verb-controlled complement clauses are the most frequent.

Figures 12.5 and 12.6 display the distribution of non-communication verbs and communication verbs respectively. Non-communication stance verbs controlling *that*-clauses make up 75 per cent of all verb-controlled *that*-clauses in this corpus. Stance verbs expressing certainty are the most frequent, followed by those indicating some level of doubt or likelihood. Attitudinal verbs are the least frequent type in these non-communication verbs. All three semantic classes of non-communication stance verbs have a much higher rate of occurrence in the three *PT* categories than the remaining five text categories.

The most common stance verb found in this corpus is 'observe', a certainty verb. 'Observe' is used in two main ways. First, 'observe' is used frequently in the book-review category as a means of reporting what the author of the book being reviewed found in his investigations or wrote about in the book (see Example 15). In fact, book reviews contain the highest frequency of the verb 'observe'. However, 'observe' is also used by writers to report their own experiments and findings, often using the first person (Example 16). The relative high frequency of this verb reflects the value system of the scientific community, which placed an emphasis on observable phenomena and observation as the key to scientific enquiry. The value of observation is reflected in Example 17 below, where the writer offers up his observation 'for proof hereof'. Other certainty verbs that occurred across categories were 'affirm', 'conclude', 'find', 'know', 'prove', 'show' and 'understand'.

(15) He proceeds next to the manner of preparing Vegetables, **observing**, that in them lies hid a very subtil and pure aethereal, and a fixed substance, the cherisher and supporter (*EMEMT*; *PT*, 7, 1672: 5023–4, book review)

(16) When the Skin with the other Integuments were taken off, I **observed** that part of the Omentum had thrust itself thro the Annular Holes of the Abdominal Muscles on the Left Side (*EMEMT*; *PT*, 27, 1710: 32–5, report)

(17) For proof hereof, I **observd**, that Men would lie all night, and sleep on the Sands without hurt. (*EMEMT*; *PT*, 3, 1668: 699–709, report)

Contrasted with other stance verbs controlling *that*-complement clauses, communication stance verbs are comparatively rare, occurring less than twice per 1,000 words. The three *PT* categories have the highest rates of occurrence, with a steady increase in frequency of use from reports to book reviews to letters. Furthermore, across all categories, 'declare' communication verbs are the most frequent, with the second-most frequent stance verb being a declare-type verb: 'say'. 'Add' and 'tell' are the only other two declare-type verbs that occur regularly. In contrast, 'suggest' and 'argue' verbs are nearly absent in these texts.

In book reviews, the communication verbs are used to summarize and report the contents of the reviewed book and occur primarily with third-person subjects, as in Example 18. In all other categories, third-person subjects are also quite common in discussing what others have said prior to the current investigation (Example 19). This finding demonstrates the authors' concern with situating their own research or thoughts with what has been related before. This at times takes the form of an extraposed complement clause, illustrated in Example 20.

(18) *The Author of this Book* **declareth**, that his design in composing it was to shew, that in a Muscle neither the Parts of it can be distinctly named, nor its Motion duly considered (*EMEMT*; *PT*, 2, 1667–8: 627–8, book review)

(19) Of the number of these seems to be that *French Virtuoso, Gasper de Gurye de Montpoly, who in a late Letter of his to Monsieur Bourdelot*, **declares** to the World, that this is a very Ingenious Invention, and such an one, as may prove very useful; but withall, that, in his opinion, it is to be used with much caution (*EMEMT*; *PT*, 2, 1667: 517–25, report)

(20) *IT* **has been said** before, that from the Basis of the Heart of the Land Tortoise of America, there goes out four great Arteries. (*EMEMT*; *PT*, 27, 1710: 170–85, report)

Approximately 20 per cent of the communication verb-controlled complement clauses have first-person subjects, where the author of the text places himself in the discourse for two main reasons. First, the author may use the communication verb as a discourse organizer, as in Example 21. Second, the author may use this structure to interact with readers (Example 22).

(21) We come now unto the Parts contain'd within the Thorax, but before we speak of them, *I* **must tell** you that I took notice of something, I account admirable, and that was the unusual situation of the Diaphragm (*EMEMT*; *PT*, 18, 1693–4: 15–20, report)

(22) To your Quaere, Whether the said Ferment-vessels discharge as last all their Ferment into the Ductus Thoracicus, thence to be carry'd directly to the Heart, there to increase and to ferment the Blood, or whether they communicate their Ferment to other parts also? *I* **answer**, that most of the Juyce of the Milky vessels is discharged between the Tunicles of the Veines, Arteries, Lymphaticks (*EMEMT*; *PT*, 3, 1668: 791–2, letter)

### 12.5.4 *Stance adjective- and noun-controlled* that-*complement clauses*

*That*-complement clauses controlled by stance adjectives and nouns appear less than one time per 1,000 words (Figures 12.7 and 12.8). When authors employ them, they tend to use them to express certainty, likelihood and attitudes fairly evenly.

Fifty-six stance adjectives controlling *that*-complement clauses occurred in the corpus, and these were placed in the semantic framework of attitudinal (Example 23), certainty (Example 24) and likelihood (Example 25) stance markers. Some adjectives (like in Example 26) expressed evaluation rather than an affective state (e.g., 'fitting', 'remarkable', 'strange'), and these were included in the attitudinal category.

(23) **It is really admirable** that so small a part as this, should so wonderfully dilate and expand its Tunicles (*EMEMT*; *PT*, 18, 1693–4: 15–20, report)
(24) Thirdly, **It is certain** that a Comatose Disease proceeds from a Tumor that oppresses the Brain by its weight. (*EMEMT*; Pechey 1695, general treatises)
(25) The sudden appearance and displaying of all the Parts after Incubation makes it **probable**, that they are not then actually formed out of a Fluid (*EMEMT*; *PT*, 16, 1687–8: 474–83, letter)
(26) To me it was not necessary, but I conceive it **convenient**, that Velvet or some gentle Leather should be fastned to the Tabulous part next the eyes, to shadow them from (*EMEMT*; *PT*, 3, 1668: 727–31, letter)

Most stance adjectives occurred only a few times in the corpus, and few occurred in multiple categories. Adjectives that were more frequent and appeared across categories included the certainty adjectives 'certain', 'clear', 'evident', 'impossible', 'observable', 'sure', 'true' and the likelihood adjectives 'likely' and 'probable'. As reflected in the four examples above, most adjective-headed complement clauses are extraposed. Biber (2006) claims that although extraposed constructions show no overt marking of attribution, they are typically interpreted to reflect the author's stance.

Like stance adjectives, few stance nouns controlling *that*-complement clauses occurred frequently and across text categories. A few that did were 'observation', 'opinion', 'proof' and 'reason'. Many of the nouns are nominalizations that correspond to verbs also used to construct stance (e.g., 'argument', 'assertion', 'demonstration' and 'observation').

## 12.6 Characterizing stance use in Early Modern English medical texts

The detailed analysis of grammatical and semantic categories of overt stance markers and their distributions in the three *PT* categories and five non-*PT*

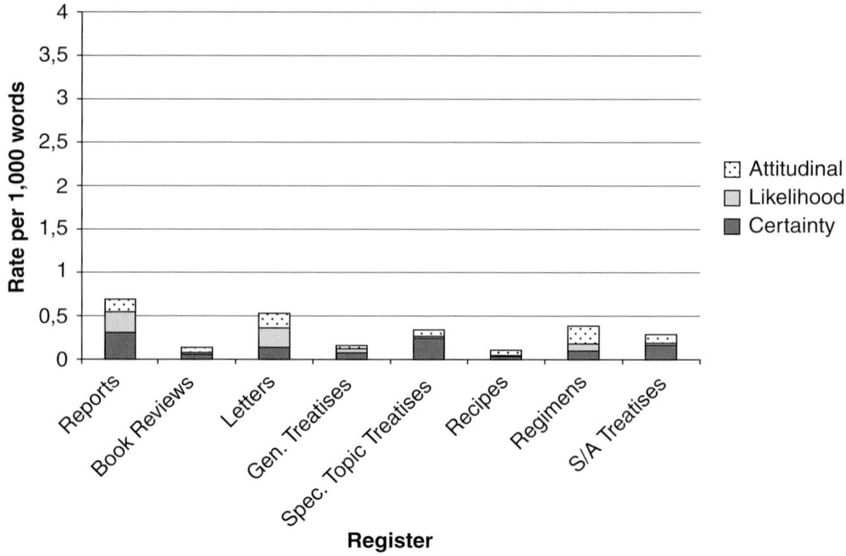


Figure 12.7 Adjective-controlled *that*-complement clauses.

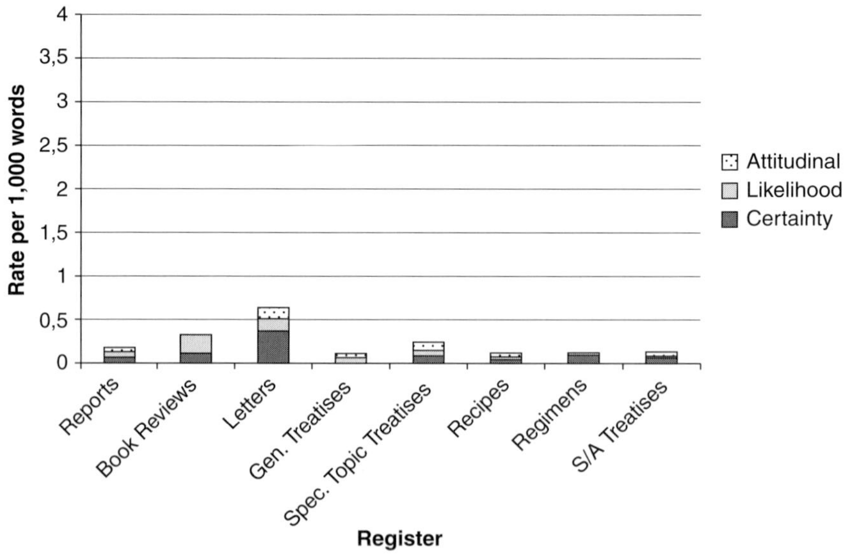


Figure 12.8 Noun-controlled *that*-complement clauses.

categories of medical prose from *EMEMT* has revealed two general findings. First, our analysis has revealed that general variation occurs across the many types of medical prose in circulation in the mid seventeenth century to the early eighteenth century. While these different types of texts are indeed similar in many ways, they also vary with regard to several stance features. Three interesting specific patterns emerge:

1. *PT* book reviews and traditional recipes contain the fewest lexico-grammatical markers of stance, while *PT* letters contain the most.
2. Across all categories, modality is the most frequent stance marker, with possibility, permission and ability modals being the most common, followed by prediction and volition modals.
3. Overall, the expression of epistemic certainty is more prevalent than other semantic stance meanings.

The most interesting general finding relates to the ways in which the *PT* is innovative when compared to the five traditional types of medical writing. That is, the various types of treatises, recipes and regimens in *EMEMT* represent the status quo of medical writing in this period, having been well established and in circulation historically. In contrast, publications from the *PT* were a new type of medical prose, associated with shifts in communicative purpose, target audience and discourse context. With these changes came innovations in the linguistic expression of knowledge. In the *PT* categories, the following innovations are particularly noteworthy (also illustrated in Table 12.3 below):

1. The three text categories from the *PT* (reports, book reviews and letters) exhibit a much higher use of verb + *that*-clause constructions than other categories of medical prose, particularly in the expression of epistemic stance.
2. The *PT* categories contain more communication stance markers, especially through the use of communication verbs controlling *that*-complement clauses.

Table 12.3 illustrates these two major findings with regard to the patterns within verb complement clauses. Taking the *PT* to represent virtual historical change (as these three text categories did not exist in earlier periods), we can see that the use of linguistic features to express epistemic stance (indicating the degree of certainty or doubt) began to develop in the early years of the *PT*, demonstrated by the much higher use of certainty and likelihood verb complement clauses.

The innovative use of verb-controlled *that*-complement clauses in the *PT* categories may reflect the primary purpose of *PT* publications to communicate research findings and procedures, as well as the importance of integrating and building upon prior discourse and research findings (a practice which has continued to be important in modern-day prose). While many

Table 12.3 *Stance patterns in the use of verb-controlled* that-*complement clauses.*

| | Reports | Book reviews | Letters | General treatises | Specific treatises | Recipes | Regimens | Surgical treatises |
|---|---|---|---|---|---|---|---|---|
| Communication: 'declare' | ■ | ■■ | ■■■ | □ | □ | □ | □ | □ |
| Communication: 'argue' | □ | □ | □ | □ | □ | □ | □ | □ |
| Communication: 'suggest' | □ | □ | □ | □ | □ | □ | □ | □ |
| Certainty | ■■■■ | ■■■■■■ | ■■■■ | ■■ | ■■ | □ | ■■ | ■■ |
| Likelihood | ■ | ■■ | ■■ | □ | □ | □ | □ | ■ |
| Attitudinal | ■ | ■ | □ | □ | □ | □ | □ | □ |

□ occurrences fewer than 0.5 times per 1,000 words.
■ occurrences about 0.5 times per 1,000 words.

of these complement clauses have first-person subjects, there are even more clauses with third-person subjects. As discussed above, *PT* authors used those constructions to bring other scholars' claims, findings and observations into their own discourse.

Epistemic stance indicating both certainty and likelihood is especially prevalent in the *PT* categories. Certainty markers are more common than likelihood, and the most commonly occurring epistemic stance verbs fall within two types of verbs: those that communicate and interpret research findings and observations (e.g., 'observe', 'find', 'show', 'conclude', 'prove') and those that indicate mental processes (e.g., 'believe', 'know'). However, the first type, in which observations are described and interpreted, are the most common. In Examples 27–9 below, the results of research are imparted. This use of verb + *that*-clause occurs across categories and includes both first-person and third-person subjects.

(27) I **observd**, that the Sea, which was Azure, and transparent in Sunshiny dayes, was black and dark-colourd (*EMEMT*; *PT*, 3, 1668: 699–709, report)
(28) One Dr Astendoff **found**, that the colour of the Salt, drawn from the Kings-and Hot-bath, was yellow (*EMEMT*; *PT*, 4, 1669: 977–82, letter)
(29) for by drawing to and fro the Medulla spinalis, we **found**, that a part of that also did not shine ill (*EMEMT*; *PT*, 7, 1672: 5108–16, letter)

The second use of certainty verbs is to relate research findings to implications. Unlike the verbs used to report findings, which occurred across text categories, verbs such as 'show' and 'prove' occur much more frequently in book reviews, where the author first summarizes the research findings and then indicates the meaning of those findings. Although this use also appears in reports and letters as in Example 30 below, it is much more prevalent in book reviews (see Example 31).

(30) If in falling they are handled and slightly pressed, there will stick a little skin to the finger, which **shews** that 'tis not seed, nor any thing like it (*EMEMT*; *PT*, 7, 1672: 4018–26, report)
(31) Then he **proves** by many cogent Arguments, that all universal Diseases, whether primarily such, do immediately arise from the Spirits (*EMEMT*; *PT*, 17, 1693: 717–28, book review)

In *PT* book reviews, stance is not generally as common as in other categories of medical prose, using approximately fifteeen overt markers of stance per 1,000 words (see Figure 12.1). However, these reviews are innovative in that they commonly use verb complement clauses to express stance. Book reviews also especially utilize modal verbs to indicate stance. If simple summary was the primary communicative purpose of book reviews, we would expect a high frequency of communication verbs. In fact, all *PT* text categories exhibit a higher use of communication stance markers than non-*PT* categories. While communication verbs (particularly the rather neutral declare verbs) are more frequent in book reviews than in the non-*PT* categories, they are actually more common in the *PT* category of letters.

Rather, book-review authors use frequent certainty verbs, particularly 'observe', to describe the contents of a reviewed item, focusing on the actions and findings of the author (in contrast to the author's ideas or theories). Example 32 below illustrates a book-review passage with a high use of certainty verbs followed by *that*-complement clauses.

(32) To resolve both which our Author, having disproved the Filtration of the liquor, held by Curvey and Everhard out of the Chorion into the Amnion, and **evinced**, [that the liquor in the Allantoides, interjected between these two is Urinous,] he **concludes**, [that the alimentary Juyce passes through the Umbilical Vessels by a proper Artery, depositing it in those Membranes we speak of, and reserving it there for the use of the Foetus.] Concerning the Humors, he **affirms**, [that all of them in all Animals are Nutritive, except that in the Allantoides.] He **observes** also, [that most of Oviparous Fishes have Eggs or Spawn,] as to sense of one only colour, and but one humor; yet [that the Spawn of a Skate hath a White and a Yolk.] (*EMEMT*; *PT*, 2, 1667: 506–12, book review)

Gotti (Chapter 11, this volume) and Atkinson (1996) point out the highly dialogic nature of publications in the *PT*. Letters can be particularly dialogic because they can provide a venue for directly addressing a peer or a previous critique. This dialogic nature seems to correspond with higher rates of stance use in letters, particularly modal verbs expressing possibility, permission and ability, communication verbs and certainty verbs. In Examples 33 and 34, we see the use of communication verbs to summarize previous communications on the topic, indicating an ongoing dialogue and orienting the reader to the discussion. In addition to communication verbs, the examples illustrate the use of certainty adverbials, communication adverbials, modals, and non-communication verbs.

(33) In a Letter to Mr. Oldenburg, in the Year, 1674. I **mentioned** [that I could not otherwise **perceive** but [that the Scarf-insensible-skin consisted of small round Scales] and **declared** my Sense of the Skins fabrick thus, [That continually as it was worn away on the outside, it was supplied from beneath], and in several Observations since I have found nothing new; for viewing them **always** by a common Microscope they shewed as at H, Fig.4, which Scales I **judged** of that Minuteness, [that a Sand ***might*** cover two hundred or more of them]; but viewing them with a better Microscope, I find they are not formed by … (*EMEMT*; *PT*, 17, 1693: 646–9, letter)

(34) I *shall* begin with **telling** you, [that in a Conversation last Winter, where I had the good fortune to make one of the number, the discourse was of an Opinion of M, Dela Chambre], who, to **prove** [that the Spirits are animated], alledges, among other arguments, their Aptness to discern; by which he **supposes**, [that in the heat of their anger they gather the Poison from the several parts of the blood, and therewith convey themselves to the teeth of the irritated animal, from whence they are afterwards transfused into the wound by biting.] This conceit was by some of the Company received with much applause, because they knew, how difficult a thing it was, to come to an explanation of that poison, which M. Dela Chambre makes mention of in general, That the spirits proceed from the Blood of the irritated animal. (*EMEMT*; *PT*, 7, 1672: 5060–7, letter)

Gotti (Chapter 11, this volume) and Atkinson (1996) emphasize three characteristics of publications in early volumes of the *PT* that can readily be seen through the category's use of stance markers:

1. the place of the researcher as integral to the text and the science reported on, i.e. the researcher as a participant in the research activities;
2. the need to accurately portray the research activities carried out and to state conclusions with appropriate levels of certainty or uncertainty;
3. the adherence to politeness norms within the discourse community.

Considering Examples 35 and 36 below, we can see the authors' attention to these characteristics. In Example 35, the attitudinal verb 'desire' brings the author's own attitudes and wishes into the discourse, while the possibility modal 'may' lessens the force of the author's sort of directive to the audience to consider (and implicitly agree with) the observations he will offer up in the following sections. In Example 36, the high use of modals (particularly possibility modals) is apparent.

(35) To confirm and illustrate all which, I **desire**, [that the following familiar Observations *may* be Considered]: (*EMEMT*; *PT*, 1, 1666: 316–20, report)

(36) This Experiment, as it hath raised Disputes among the Curious both here and abroad; so it hath put some of them upon considering such ways, and given such cautions, as may render the use of it safe and beneficial. Of the number of these seems to be that French Virtuoso, Gasper de Gurye de Montpoly, who in a late Letter of his to Monsieur Bourdelot, **declares** to the World, [that this is a very Ingenious Invention], and such an one, as *may* prove very useful; but withall, that, in his opinion, it is to be used with much caution, as not being like to be practiced innoxiously, if imprudent men do mannage it, and the concourse of two differing sorts of Blood requiring

> many tryals, and a careful observation of many circumstances, to give assurance. He **supposes**, [that the Blood of every Animal is endowed with its peculiar Temper, and contains in the Aggregate of its parts, different natures, principles, figures, and even a different Center.] Whence he **concludes**, [that two Substances thus differing, and containing plenty of Spirits, are not reducible to one and the same Center, nor to one and the same Body without Fermentation]; and [that this Operation ***may*** prove of danger to him, that ***shall*** have admitted into his Veins a strange Blood (wont to be free in its native Vessels) without passing through those degrees, that ***must*** give it Impressions sutable to the temper and functions of the Vitals of the Recipient] (*EMEMT*; *PT*, 2, 1667: 517–25, report)

This example illustrates the high use of communication and non-communication verbs, in addition to demonstrating how modal verbs are used to balance commitment with possibility, thus enabling the author to follow the norms of the scientific community.

## 12.7 Concluding remarks

This study has sought to uncover patterns of variation across three categories within the *PT* as compared with the other five categories of Early Modern English medical prose in *EMEMT*. The analysis has revealed that authors of these texts use stance adverbials, modal and semi-modal verbs and *that*-complement clauses to indicate their evaluations, attitudes and level of commitment towards the information and claims they present. In addition, the use of these features varies systematically across all types of medical prose.

More specifically, the three types of publications from the *PT* exhibit variation both in contrast to the non-*PT* categories and within the three *PT* categories. The higher use of verb + *that*-clause in the *PT* categories reflects the new communicative purpose of the *PT* to summarize and to disseminate research findings and observations (rather than to provide instruction) and to build a dialogic relationship among those interested in medical topics. Within the *PT* categories, book reviews in particular exhibit a high use of this innovation, which contrasts with their low use of other stance markers. This finding is related to the purpose of the book reviews in offering a summary of a medical book.

While this chapter investigated three major grammatical structures as markers of stance (modal verbs, stance adverbials and *that*-complement clauses headed by stance nouns, verbs and adjectives), future research should also consider other features that signal an author's stance. For example, a commonly investigated stance structure such as *to*-complement clauses should also be investigated in order to gain a fuller picture of stance use in these medical texts. Furthermore, future research focusing on aspects of language use not previously investigated under the 'stance' label may lead to a more robust description of stance. For instance, two features we noted as possibly indicating stance throughout our analysis include the use of emphatic 'do' (Example 37) and concessive clauses (Examples 38–9).

(37) Continuation of the Discourse concerning Vitriol, begun in Numb. 103. shewing, That Vitriol is usually produced by Sulphur, acting on, and concoagulating with, a Metal; and then making out, that Allom is likewise the Result of the said Sulphur; as also evincing, that Vitriol, Sulphur, and Allom, **do agree** in the Saline Principle; (*EMEMT*; *PT*, 9, 1674: 66–73, report)

(38) I also observd many long and very clear Particles; the longest of which, **as far as I could judge**, was about the Diameter of a Hair of ones Head (*EMEMT*; *PT*, 27, 1710: 529–34, letter)

(39) A description is also made of the Urachus, found in all Viviparous Creatures, **though by many Writers denied to be in Man**, who notwithstanding hath need, as well as other such Animals, somewhere to lodge his Urine. (*EMEMT*; *PT*, 4, 1669: 1018–19, book review)

While such features are not overt in expressing a particular stance, they do seem attitudinal, and, thus, a description of their use could provide an important additional perspective on the ways in which authors situate their ideas within discourse.

# Appendix A: Raw data tables corresponding to Figures 4.3–4.14

Table A1 *Raw frequencies of modal auxiliaries and their type by category (see Figure 4.3).*

| | *Category* | | | | | |
|---|---|---|---|---|---|---|
| Type | General | Specialized | Recipes | Regimens | Surgical | *PT* |
| Deontic | 30 | 38 | 16 | 36 | 57 | 3 |
| Epistemic | 24 | 50 | 18 | 25 | 22 | 6 |
| None | 144 | 506 | 262 | 234 | 255 | 133 |

Table A2 *Raw frequencies of modal auxiliaries and their type on the timeline (see Figure 4.4).*

| | *Time period* | | | |
|---|---|---|---|---|
| Type | 1500–50 | 1550–1600 | 1600–50 | 1650–1700 |
| Deontic | 50 | 53 | 21 | 53 |
| Epistemic | 27 | 38 | 37 | 54 |
| None | 89 | 179 | 155 | 333 |

Table A3 *Trends in the use of pronominal subjects in the categories (see Figure 4.5).*

| | | *Category* | | | | | |
|---|---|---|---|---|---|---|---|
| Gram. Subject | Polarity | General | Specialized | Recipes | Regimens | Surgical | *PT* |
| First-person plural | negative | 1 | 8 | 7 | 0 | 2 | 1 |
| | positive | 6 | 34 | 14 | 7 | 6 | 6 |
| First-person singular | negative | 6 | 28 | 18 | 4 | 13 | 10 |
| | positive | 10 | 77 | 37 | 19 | 15 | 23 |
| Second-person singular | negative | 2 | 6 | 0 | 3 | 4 | 1 |
| | positive | 35 | 72 | 27 | 34 | 57 | 10 |

Table A3 (*cont.*)

| Gram. Subject | Polarity | *Category* General | Specialized | Recipes | Regimens | Surgical | *PT* |
|---|---|---|---|---|---|---|---|
| Third-person plural | negative | 4 | 10 | 7 | 4 | 1 | 3 |
| | positive | 6 | 16 | 9 | 8 | 11 | 2 |
| Third-person singular | negative | 7 | 6 | 2 | 2 | 2 | 2 |
| | positive | 17 | 32 | 9 | 20 | 22 | 11 |

Table A4 *Polarity in relation to category (see Figure 4.6).*

| Polarity | *Category* General | Specialized | Recipes | Regimens | Surgical | *PT* |
|---|---|---|---|---|---|---|
| Positive | 177 | 521 | 237 | 288 | 307 | 107 |
| Negative | 30 | 108 | 64 | 25 | 49 | 33 |

Table A5 *Polarity in relation to timeline (Figure 4.7).*

| Polarity | *Time period* 1500–50 | 1550–1600 | 1600–50 | 1650–1700 |
|---|---|---|---|---|
| Positive | 288 | 469 | 293 | 587 |
| Negative | 23 | 74 | 59 | 153 |

Table A6 *Changes in the knower class on the timeline (see Figure 4.8).*

| Knower | *Time period* 1500–50 | 1550–1600 | 1600–50 | 1650–1700 |
|---|---|---|---|---|
| Divine | 2 | 2 | 2 | 6 |
| Authority | 5 | 10 | 7 | 17 |
| Author | 8 | 64 | 83 | 152 |
| Medical community | 40 | 91 | 46 | 186 |
| Reader | 195 | 218 | 111 | 209 |
| All/lay | 50 | 71 | 40 | 108 |

Table A7 *Knower classes of third-person-singular subjects in relation to category (see Figure 4.9).*

| | Category | | | | | |
|---|---|---|---|---|---|---|
| Knower | General | Specialized | Recipes | Regimens | Surgical | *PT* |
| Divine | 1 | 0 | 0 | 0 | 0 | 0 |
| Authority | 1 | 10 | 2 | 2 | 1 | 2 |
| Medical community | 60 | 7 | 2 | 9 | 4 | 11 |
| Reader | 10 | 2 | 1 | 6 | 13 | 0 |
| All/lay | 3 | 16 | 5 | 5 | 2 | 0 |

Table A8 *Knower classes of third-person plural subjects in relation to category (see Figure 4.10).*

| | Category | | | | | |
|---|---|---|---|---|---|---|
| Knower | General | Specialized | Recipes | Regimens | Surgical | *PT* |
| Authority | 1 | 0 | 0 | 2 | 0 | 0 |
| Medical community | 3 | 9 | 11 | 1 | 7 | 4 |
| Reader | 0 | 1 | 0 | 0 | 1 | 0 |
| All/lay | 2 | 9 | 3 | 9 | 1 | 1 |

Table A9 *Topoi in relation to timeline (see Figure 4.11).*

| | Time period | | | |
|---|---|---|---|---|
| Topos | 1500–50 | 1550–1600 | 1600–50 | 1650–1700 |
| Assertive | 98 | 223 | 165 | 481 |
| Practical | 205 | 234 | 108 | 206 |
| Epistemic | 5 | 10 | 5 | 11 |

Table A10 *Sub-topoi of assertive knowledge (see Figure 4.12).*

| | Century | |
|---|---|---|
| Sub-topos | Sixteenth | Seventeenth |
| Assertive | 222 | 353 |
| Declarative | 61 | 217 |
| Negative attribution | 38 | 76 |

Table A11 *Sub-topoi of practical knowledge (see Figure 4.13).*

| | Century | |
|---|---|---|
| Sub-topos | Sixteenth | Seventeenth |
| Practical | 235 | 238 |
| Didactic | 204 | 113 |

Table A12 *Topoi of knowledge in relation to category (see Figure 4.14).*

| | Category | | | | | |
|---|---|---|---|---|---|---|
| Sub-topos | General | Specialized | Recipes | Regimens | Surgical | *PT* |
| Assertive | 77 | 354 | 190 | 109 | 116 | 121 |
| Practical | 103 | 231 | 221 | 163 | 178 | 14 |
| Epistemic | 8 | 9 | 3 | 6 | 5 | 0 |

# Appendix B: Raw data tables corresponding to Figures 8.1–8.4

Table B1 *Raw and normalized frequencies of all overt references to the reader in the texts (see Figure 8.1).*

| Text | Total word count | Raw frequency | Normalized to 1,000 words |
|---|---|---|---|
| Miles: *Countrymans Friend* | 7,148 | 175 | 24.48 |
| Winter: *Pretious Treasury* | 5,089 | 107 | 21.03 |
| Elkes: *Approved Medicines* | 8,683 | 125 | 14.40 |
| Woolley: *Compleat Servant-Maid* | 4,419 | 55 | 12.45 |
| Hawes: *Poore-Mans Plaster-Box* | 10,842 | 116 | 10.70 |
| Salmon: *Pharmacopœia Bateana* | 9,755 | 74 | 7.59 |
| Wood: *Alphabetical Book* | 10,694 | 81 | 7.57 |
| Charas: *Royal Pharmacopœa* | 9,732 | 58 | 5.96 |
| Culpeper: *London Dispensatory* | 11,235 | 60 | 5.34 |

Table B2 *Raw and normalized frequencies of references to reader as patient, with percentage of all reader references in each text (see Figure 8.2).*

| Text | Total word count | Raw frequency | Normalized to 1,000 words | Percentage |
|---|---|---|---|---|
| Miles: *Countrymans Friend* | 7,148 | 89 | 12.45 | 50.9 |
| Winter: *Pretious Treasury* | 5,089 | 55 | 10.81 | 51.4 |
| Elkes: *Approved Medicines* | 8,683 | 41 | 4.72 | 32.8 |
| Woolley: *Compleat Servant-Maid* | 4,419 | 19 | 4.30 | 34.6 |
| Hawes: *Poore-Mans plaster-Box* | 10,842 | 36 | 3.32 | 31.0 |
| Salmon: *Pharmacopœia Bateana* | 9,755 | 0 | 0 | 0 |
| Wood: *Alphabetical Book* | 10,694 | 39 | 3.65 | 48.2 |
| Charas: *Royal Pharmacopœa* | 9,732 | 0 | 0 | 0 |
| Culpeper: *London Dispensatory* | 11,235 | 0 | 0 | 0 |

Table B3 *Raw and normalized frequencies of references to the patient in the second and third person, with percentage of all patient references in each text (see Figure 8.3).*

| Text | Total word count | Second person | | | Third person | | |
|---|---|---|---|---|---|---|---|
| | | *Raw* | *Norm.* | % | *Raw* | *Norm.* | % |
| Miles: *Countrymans Friend* | 7,148 | 89 | 12.45 | 51.7 | 83 | 11.61 | 48.3 |
| Hawes: *Poore-Mans Plaster-Box* | 10,842 | 36 | 3.32 | 16.7 | 180 | 16.6 | 83.3 |
| Winter: *Pretious Treasury* | 5,089 | 55 | 10.81 | 60.4 | 36 | 7.07 | 39.6 |
| Elkes: *Approved Medicines* | 8,683 | 41 | 4.72 | 27.5 | 108 | 12.44 | 72.5 |
| Woolley: *Compleat servant-maid* | 4,419 | 19 | 4.30 | 44.2 | 24 | 5.43 | 55.8 |
| Wood: *Alphabetical Book* | 10,694 | 39 | 3.65 | 43.8 | 50 | 4.68 | 56.2 |
| Culpeper: *London Dispensatory* | 11,235 | 0 | 0 | 0 | 66 | 5.87 | 100 |
| Salmon: *Pharmacopœia Bateana* | 9,755 | 0 | 0 | 0 | 48 | 4.92 | 100 |
| Charas: *Royal Pharmacopœa* | 9,732 | 0 | 0 | 0 | 31 | 3.19 | 100 |

Table B4 *Raw and normalized frequencies of classical terminology by category (see Figure 8.4).*

| Text | Total word count | Set expressions | | Technical terms | | Spontaneous language | |
|---|---|---|---|---|---|---|---|
| | | *Raw* | *Normalized* | *Raw* | *Normalized* | *Raw* | *Normalized* |
| Woolley: *Compleat Servant-Maid* | 4,419 | 1 | 0.23 | 15 | 3.39 | 0 | 0 |
| Hawes: *Poore-Mans Plaster-Box* | 10,842 | 2 | 0.18 | 41 | 3.78 | 0 | 0 |
| Winter: *Pretious Treasury* | 5,089 | 2 | 0.39 | 33 | 6.48 | 6 | 1.18 |
| Miles: *Countrymans Friend* | 7,148 | 76 | 10.63 | 28 | 3.92 | 0 | 0 |
| Elkes: *Approved Medicines* | 8,683 | 43 | 4.95 | 108 | 12.44 | 8 | 0.92 |
| Wood: *Alphabetical Book* | 10,694 | 180 | 16.83 | 166 | 15.52 | 5 | 0.47 |
| Culpeper: *London Dispensatory* | 11,235 | 8 | 0.71 | 340 | 30.26 | 27 | 2.4 |
| Salmon: *Pharmacopœia Bateana* | 9,755 | 87 | 8.92 | 257 | 26.35 | 2 | 0.21 |
| Charas: *Royal Pharmacopœa* | 9,732 | 53 | 5.45 | 246 | 25.28 | 267 | 27.44 |

# Appendix C: Stance markers used in the analysis in Chapter 12

Table C1 *Forms used in the analysis of stance.*

| Stance category | Forms |
|---|---|
| ***Modals and semi-modals*** | |
| Possibility, permission, ability | can, cannot, could, may, might |
| Necessity, obligation | should, shouldn't, must, better, have to |
| Prediction, volition | would, wouldn't, will, won't, shall, be going to |
| ***Adverbials*** | |
| Communication (show point of view, manner of speaking, source of information) | confidentially, figuratively speaking, frankly speaking, generally, honestly, in general, mainly, reportedly, strictly, technically speaking, truthfully |
| Attitudinal (show speaker's attitude; must be able to state the attitude) | admirably, agreeably, amazingly, astonishingly, confidently, confusedly, conveniently, curiously, desperately, disturbingly, even worse, faithfully, fortunately, gladly, grievously, happily, hopefully, humbly, importantly, indifferently, intolerably, ironically, regrettably, remarkably, rightly, sadly, sensibly, surprisingly, unbelievably, unfortunately, unhappily, willingly, wisely |
| Certainty (express certainty) | absolutely, actually, alwaies, always, certainly, clearly, definitely, doubtless, for certain, for certan, in fact, indeed, inevitably, never, no doubt, obviously, of course, really, surely, undoubtedly, universally, without doubt |
| Likelihood (show some degree of certainty (but not certainty); express doubt) | apparently, doubtfully, evidently, improbably, kind of, largely, maybe, most cases, most instances, perhaps, possibly, predictably, probably, roughly, seemingly, sort of, usually |
| ***Verb-controlled* that*-complement clauses*** [a] | |
| Communication: suggest | advise, alledge, hint, imply, insinuate, intimate, persuade, recommend, request, suggest, urge |
| Communication: declare | add, advertise, assert, answer, bear in hand, call to mind, confess, declare, depose, emphasize, import, inform, mention, present, publish, put in mind, relate, remark, remind, reply, report, represent, say, set down, take notice, tell, write |
| Communication: argue | argue, aver, avouch, claim, command, commit, contend, insist, maintain, profess, promise, propose, swear |

Table C1 (*cont.*)

| Stance category | Forms |
|---|---|
| Attitudinal | accept, admire, admit, admonish, agree, allow, anticipate, approve, assent, beware, blame, bragg, boast, complain, concede, cry, deny, desire, dream, ensure, exhort, expect, fancy, fear, feel, forget, forsee, guarantee, hope, marvel, mind, object, prefer, pretend, protest, reflect, rejoice, require, resolve, suffice, threaten, trust, wish, wonder, worry |
| Certainty | acknowledge, affirm, apprehend, ascertain, assure, calculate, certify, check, come to pass, conclude, confirm, construe, convince, decide, decree, deem, demonstrate, determine, discern, discover, evidence, evince, experience, find, follow, happen, know, learn, manifest, mean, note, notice, observe, own, prove, realize, recall, recognize, recollect, record, remember, see, show, signify, submit, testify, understand |
| Likelihood | appear, assume, believe, bet, conceive, conjecture, consider, deduce, deduct, detect, doubt, estimate, figure, gather, guess, hypothesize, imagine, indicate, infer, intend, judge, perceive, postulate, predict, presume, presuppose, reckon, seem, sense, speculate, suppose, suspect, think, wager |
| *Adjective-controlled* **that**-*complement clauses* | |
| Attitudinal, evaluative[b] | absurd, acceptable, adamant, admirable, advisable, afraid, agitated, agreable, agreeable, alarmed, amazed, amazing, amused, angry, annoyed, annoying, anomalous, appropriate, astonishd, astonished, astonishing, aware, awful, bad, careful, carefull, cheerful, conceivable, concernd, concerned, concerning, concern'd, confusd, confused, contemptible, critical, crucial, curious, degraded, dejected, deplorable, depressed, deprest, deserving, desirable, desired, disagreeable, disappointed, disappointing, discontented, discouraging, displeased, dissatisfied, distressed, disturbd, disturbed, dreadful, embarrassing, encouraged, envious, essential, excellent, excessive, exciting, expected, extraordinary, fabulous, fair, favourable, fearful, feasible, fit, fitting, fortunate, frightened, frightening, frighten'd, fundamental, funny, glad, good, grateful, gratifying, great, grievous, happy, honored, honourable, hopeful, horrible, hurt, ideal, imaginable, imperative, important, importuning, incidental, inconceivable, incredible, incredulous, indisputable, interesting, ironic, irritated, irritating, jealous, livid, lucky, mad, natural, neat, necessary, nervous, nice, noble, notable, noteworthy, noticeable, notorious, obligatory, odd, odde, offended, okay, outrageous, paradoxical, |

Table C1 (*cont.*)

| Stance category | Forms |
|---|---|
| | peculiar, peculier, perfect, pertinent, pissed, pleasant, pleasd, pleased, pleas'd, preferable, prejudicial, pressing, proper, proud, reasonable, reassured, recommendable, redundant, relievd, relieved, remarkable, remarquable, ridiculous, right, rotten, rough, sad, satisfactory, satisfied, satisfyd, sensible, shocked, shocking, silly, sorry, speculative, strang, strange, stupid, sufferable, sufficient, suitable, super, sure, surprised, surprising, surpris'd, surprizd, surprizing, sutable, sweet, terrible, thankful, tolerable, touched, tragic, troubled, troublesome, typical, unacceptable, unaware, uncertain, uncomfortable, uncommon, unconceivable, understandable, uneasy, unfair, unfortunate, unhappy, unlucky, unpleasing, unreasonable, unthinkable, untypical, unusual, upsetting, usual, vehement, vital, wild, willing, wonderful, wonderfull, wondrous, worried |
| Certainty | accepted, apparent, certain, certan, clear, cleer, common, confident, convincd, convinced, convincing, correct, evident, false, impossible, inevitable, observable, obvious, palpable, plain, positive, provd, proved, right, sure, true, undeniable, undoubted, visible, well known |
| Likelihood | doubtful, dubious, improbable, likely, plausible, possible, probable, unlikely |
| *Noun-controlled* that-*complement clauses* | |
| Attitudinal | admonition, amusement, complaint, concession, disparagement, fear, ground, grounds, hope, hopes, lamentation, objection, reason, reasons, view, thought, thougt, wonder |
| Certainty | account, argument, assertion, conclusion, conviction, demonstration, discovery, doctrine, doubt, evidence, fact, knowledge, mandate, maxim, observation, principle, proof, realization, result, rule, statement, truth |
| Likelihood | assumption, belief, claim, contention, expectation, feeling, hypothesis, idea, implication, impression, indication, inference, notion, opinion, perception, possibility, presumption, probability, rumor, sense, sign, suggestion, suspicion, thesis |

*Notes:* [a] This list includes the base form of the verbs. Other verb forms (e.g., for third person, past tense, etc.) and their variant spellings were also included for these verbs.
[b] The adjectives listed here were included in the analysis as potential stance features. We have labelled them *attitudinal* or *evaluative* here, although their stance meanings were not always clear-cut. However, the most frequently occurring adjectives controlling *that*-clauses (listed in Table 12.2) fit clearly within their semantic categories.

# Appendix D: Preliminary list of texts in the corpus of *Early Modern English Medical Texts* (*EMEMT*)

## CATEGORY 1: GENERAL TREATISES AND TEXTBOOKS

| | | |
|---|---|---|
| 1545 | Langton, Christopher | *Introduction into Phisycke* |
| 1547 | Langton, Christopher | *Uery Brefe Treatise* |
| 1554 | Anonymous | *Prognosticacion* |
| 1574 | Jones, John | *Galens Bookes of Elementes* |
| 1582 | Batman, Stephen | *Batman vppon Bartholome* |
| 1586 | Galen | *Methodus Medendi* |
| 1606 | Fage, John | *Speculum Aegrotorum* |
| 1609 | Pomarius, Petrus | *Enchiridion Medicum* |
| 1632 | Bruele, Walter | *Praxis Medicinae* |
| 1648 | Brugis, Thomas | *Marrow of Physicke* |
| 1651 | Biggs, Noah | *Mataeotechnia Medicinae* |
| 1652 | Culpeper, Nicholas | *Galens Art of Physick* |
| 1652 | Fioravanti, Leonardo | *Discourse of the Secrets* |
| 1671 | Archer, John | *Every Man his own Doctor* |
| 1679 | Hall, John | *Select Observations* |
| 1680 | Couch, Robert | *Praxis Catholica* |
| 1694 | Chamberlen, Hugh | *Practice of Physick* |
| 1695 | Pechey, John | *Store-House of Physical Practice* |
| 1695 | Sydenham, Thomas | *Compleat Method of Curing* |
| 1697 | Durant, John | *Art and Nature* |
| 1700 | Harvey, Gideon | *The Vanities of Philosophy and Physick* |

## CATEGORY 2: TREATISES ON SPECIFIC TOPICS

*Category 2a: Texts on specific diseases*

| | | |
|---|---|---|
| 1552 | Caius, John | *Against Sweatyng Sicknesse* |
| 1566 | Jones, John | *Dial for all Agves* |
| 1586 | Bright, Timothy | *Treatise of Melancholy* |
| 1596 | Clowes, William | *Lves Venerea* |
| 1598 | Wateson, George | *Cvres of the Diseased* |
| 1599 | Laurentius, Andreas | *Preservation of Sight* |
| 1602 | Clowes, William | *Cure of Struma* |
| 1616 | Bailey, Walter | *Preservation of Eie-Sight* |
| 1621 | Burton, Robert | *Anatomy of Melancholy* |

| | | |
|---|---|---|
| 1633 | Holland, Philemon | *Gutta Podagrica* |
| 1662 | Sennert, Daniel | *Sixth Book of Practical Physick* |
| 1665 | Drage, William | *Daimonomageia* |
| 1666 | Harvey, Gideon | *Morbus Anglicus* |
| 1670 | Harvey, Gideon | *Little Venus Unmask'd* |
| 1685 | Lamport, John | *Small-Pox* |
| 1697 | Cockburn, W. | *Continuation of the Account of Distempers* |

*Category 2b: Texts on specific methods of diagnosis or treatment*

| | | |
|---|---|---|
| 1525 | Anonymous | *Seynge of Uryns* |
| 1547 | Recorde, Robert | *Vrinal of Physick* |
| 1556 | Cocles, Bartholomeus | *Epitomye of Phisiognomie* |
| 1562 | Turner, William | *Booke of Bathes* |
| 1596 | Hester, John | *Key of Philosophie* |
| 1601 | Harward, Simon | *Phlebotomy* |
| 1631 | Simotta, George | *Planetary Houres* |
| 1637 | Brian, Thomas | *Pisse-Prophet* |
| 1640 | Bartlet, John | *Warming Stone* |
| 1658 | Culpeper, Nicholas | *Semeiotica Uranica* |
| 1659 | Culpeper, Nicholas | *School of Physick, Astrology* |
| 1659 | Culpeper, Nicholas | *School of Physick, Lapidary* |
| 1659 | Culpeper, Nicholas | *School of Physick, Urinal* |
| 1671 | Blagrave, Joseph | *Astrological Practice of Physick* |
| 1675 | Cock, Thomas | *Miscelanea Medica* |
| 1696 | Maynwaringe, Everard | *True Purgation* |
| 1698 | Colbatch, John, Sir | *Physico-Medical Essay Concerning Alkaly and Acid* |
| 1699 | Brown, Andrew | *Epilogue to Five Papers* |
| 1700 | Tauvry, Daniel | *Treatise of Medicines* |

*Category 2c: Texts on specific therapeutic substances*

| | | |
|---|---|---|
| 1550 | Bacon, Roger | *Waters Artyfycialles* |
| 1574 | Baker, George | *Oleum Magistrale* |
| 1584 | Chaloner, Thomas | *Vertue of Nitre* |
| 1585 | Bailey, Walter | *Mithridatium* |
| 1588 | Bailey, Walter | *Three Kindes of Peppers* |
| 1602 | Philaretes | *Work for Chimny-Sweepers* |
| 1602 | Russel, Thomas | *Diacatholicon Avrevm* |
| 1611 | Gardiner, Edmund | *The Triall of Tobacco* |
| 1615 | T., C. | *How to Plant Tobacco* |
| 1631 | Jorden, Edward | *Natvrall Bathes* |
| 1632 | Rowzee, Lodwick | *Queenes Welles* |
| 1664 | Lockyer, Lionel | *Advertisement Concerning Pills* |
| 1673 | Daffy, Anthony | *Elixir Salutis* |
| 1674 | Nendick, Humphrey | *Popular Pill* |
| 1682 | Talbor, Robert, Sir | *English Remedy* |
| 1693 | Packe, Christopher | *Mineralogia* |
| 1700 | Daffy, Anthony | *Directions for Taking Elixir Salutis* |

*Category 2d: Texts on midwifery and children's diseases*

| | | |
|---|---|---|
| 1540 | Roesslin, Eucharius | *Byrth of Mankynde* |
| 1546 | Phayer, Thomas | *Boke of Chyldren* |
| 1603 | Jorden, Edward | *Suffocation of the Mother* |
| 1612 | Guillemeau, Jacques | *Child-Birth* |
| 1612 | Guillemeau, Jacques | *Nvrsing of Children* |
| 1636 | Sadler, John | *Sick Womans Looking-Glasse* |
| 1651 | Culpeper, Nicholas | *Directory for Midwives* |
| 1653 | Pemell, Robert | *De Morbis Puerorum* |
| 1671 | Sharp, Jane | *Midwives Book* |
| 1684 | Anonymous | *Aristoteles Master-Piece* |

*Category 2e: Texts on plague*

| | | |
|---|---|---|
| 1578 | Brasbridge, Thomas | *Poore Mans Iewel* |
| 1603 | Balmford, James | *Plagves Infection* |
| 1603 | Lodge, Thomas | *Treatise of the Plague* |
| 1636 | Bradwell, Stephen | *Physick for the Plagve* |
| 1636 | Royal College of Physicians | *Certain Necessary Directions* |
| 1665 | Wharton, Thomas | *Directions for the Plague* |
| 1691 | Willis, Thomas | *Plain and Easie Method* |

## CATEGORY 3: RECIPE COLLECTIONS AND *MATERIA MEDICA*

| | | |
|---|---|---|
| 1525 | Anonymous | *Newe Mater* |
| 1526 | Anonymous | *Grete Herball* |
| 1526 | Anonymous | *Treasure of Pore Men* |
| 1528 | Anonymous | *Lytell Boke of the .xxiiii. Stones* |
| 1548 | Anonymous | *Ten Recipes by Henry VIII* |
| 1548 | Turner, William | *Names of Herbes* |
| 1552 | Anonymous | *Antidotharius* |
| 1561 | Braunschweig, Hieronymus | *Homish Apothecarye* |
| 1562 | Ruscelli, Girolamo | *Secretes of Alexis of Piemovnt* |
| 1563 | Gale, Thomas | *Antidotarie* |
| 1570 | Feckenham, John | *Booke of Sovereigne Medicines* |
| 1573 | Partridge, John | *Tresurie of Commodious Conceits* |
| 1580 | Bright, Timothy | *Sufficiencie of English Medicines* |
| 1580 | Monardes, Nicolás | *Ioyfvll Newes* |
| 1595 | Partridge, John | *Widdowes Treasure* |
| 1596 | Clowes, William | *Booke of Obseruations* |
| 1596 | Dawson, Thomas | *Good Huswifes Iewell* |
| 1598 | Langham, William | *Garden of Health* |
| 1602 | Plat, Hugh | *Delightes for Ladies* |
| 1617 | Anonymous | *Secrets of Albertus Magnus* |
| 1633 | Gerard, John | *Generall Historie of Plantes* |
| 1634 | Hawes, Richard | *Poore-Mans Plaster-Box* |
| 1639 | Wood, Owen | *Alphabetical Book* |
| 1649 | Culpeper, Nicholas | *London Dispensatory* |

| | | |
|---|---|---|
| 1649 | Rondelet, Guillaume | *Countrey-Man's Apothecary* |
| 1649 | Winter, Salvator and Dickinson, Francisco | *Pretious Treasury* |
| 1651 | Elkes, Richard | *Approved Medicines* |
| 1652 | Culpeper, Nicholas | *English Physician* |
| 1653 | Grey, Elizabeth | *Choice Manual* |
| 1655 | Paracelsus | *Supreme Mysteries of Nature* |
| 1658 | Porta, Giambattista della | *Natural Magick* |
| 1659 | Parmer, Archdale | *Recipe Book* |
| 1662 | Miles, Abraham | *Countrymans Friend* |
| 1665 | D., T. | *Food and Physick* |
| 1673 | Woolley, Hannah | *Gentlewomans Companion* |
| 1677 | Woolley, Hannah | *Compleat Servant-Maid* |
| 1678 | Charas, Moyse | *Royal Pharmacopoea* |
| 1679 | M., W. | *Queens Closet Opened* |
| 1694 | Pechey, John | *Herbal of Physical plants* |
| 1700 | Salmon, William | *Pharmacopoeia Bateana* |
| 1700 | Salmon, William | *Phylaxa Medicinae* |
| 1700 | Woolley, Hannah | *Supplement to the Compleat Servant Maid* |

## CATEGORY 4: REGIMENS AND HEALTH GUIDES

| | | |
|---|---|---|
| 1506 | Anonymous | *Kalendar of Shepherdes* |
| 1506 | Lydgate, John | *Gouernall of Helthe* |
| 1528 | Copland, Robert | *Secrete of Secretes* |
| 1528 | Mediolano, Joannes de | *Regimen Sanitatis Salerni* |
| 1539 | Moulton, Thomas | *Myrrour or Glasse of Helth* |
| 1540 | Anonymous | *Compost of Ptholomeus* |
| 1550 | Boorde, Andrew | *Boke for to Lerne a Man* |
| 1541 | Elyot, Thomas, Sir | *Castel of Helth* |
| 1542 | Boorde, Andrew | *Dyetary of Helth* |
| 1547 | Boorde, Andrew | *Breuiary of Helthe* |
| 1559 | Gesner, Conrad | *Treasure of Evonymus* |
| 1565 | Moore, Philip | *Hope of Health* |
| 1574 | Gratarolo, Guglielmo | *Health of Magistrates and Studentes* |
| 1581 | Mulcaster, Richard | *Training vp of Children* |
| 1588 | Cogan, Thomas | *Haven of Health* |
| 1595 | Bullein, William | *Gouernement of Health* |
| 1604 | Manning, James | *Complexions Castle* |
| 1607 | Mediolano, Joannes de | *School of Salerne* |
| 1620 | Venner, Tobias | *Via Recta ad Vitam Longam* |
| 1625 | Bacon, Francis | *Of Regiment of Health* |
| 1631 | Ghesel, John | *Rule of Health* |
| 1633 | Hart, James | *Klinike* |
| 1638 | Bacon, Francis | *Historie of Life and Death* |
| 1656 | D., D. | *Skilful Physician* |
| 1676 | Cock, Thomas | *Kitchin-Physick* |
| 1683 | Maynwaringe, Everard | *Method and Means* |
| 1696 | Tryon, Thomas | *Miscellania, Tract 2* |

## CATEGORY 5: SURGICAL AND ANATOMICAL TREATISES

| | | |
|---|---|---|
| 1525 | Braunschweig, Hieronymus | *Handy Warke of Surgeri* |
| 1543 | Vigo, Johannes de | *Most Excellent Workes of Chirurgerye* |
| 1553 | Geminus, Thomas | *Compendiosa Totius Anatomie Delineatio* |
| 1562 | Bullein, William | *Bulleins Bulwarke* |
| 1563 | Gale, Thomas | *Enchiridion of Chirurgerie* |
| 1563 | Gale, Thomas | *Institution of a Chirurgian* |
| 1563 | Gale, Thomas | *Treatise of Wounds* |
| 1575 | Banister, John | *Treatise of Chyrurgerie* |
| 1577 | Vicary, Thomas | *Anatomie of Mans Body* |
| 1578 | Banister, John | *Historie of Man* |
| 1579 | Chauliac, Guy de | *Guydos Questions* |
| 1597 | Guillemeau, Jacques | *Frenche Chirurgerye* |
| 1612 | Lowe, Peter | *Whole Art of Chyrurgerie* |
| 1615 | Crooke, Helkiah | *Mikrokosmografia* |
| 1617 | Woodall, John | *Svrgions Mate* |
| 1630 | Bonham, Thomas | *Chyrvrgians Closet* |
| 1634 | Paré, Ambroise | *Workes of Ambrose Parey* |
| 1650 | Read, Alexander | *Workes of that Famous Physitian* |
| 1651 | Brugis, Thomas | *Vade Mecum* |
| 1652 | Fioravanti, Leonardo | *Treatise of Chirurgery* |
| 1652 | Ross, Alexander | *Arcana Microcosmi* |
| 1653 | Harvey, William | *Anatomical Exercises* |
| 1654 | Turner, Robert | *Mikrokosmos* |
| 1676 | Wiseman, Richard | *Of Wounds* |
| 1686 | Hildanus, Gulielmus Fabritius | *Cista Militaris* |
| 1686 | Minderer, Raymund | *Medicina Militaris* |
| 1687 | Barbette, Paul | *Thesaurus Chirurgiae* |
| 1689 | Prat, Ellis | *Vade Mecum* |
| 1693 | Cooke, James | *Marrow of Chirurgery* |
| 1696 | Tryon, Thomas | *Miscellania, Tract 1* |
| 1698 | Colbatch, John | *Novum Lumen Chirurgicum* |

## CATEGORY 6: *PHILOSOPHICAL TRANSACTIONS*

| | |
|---|---|
| 1665–6 | *Philosophical Transactions 1* |
| 1667–8 | *Philosophical Transactions 2* |
| 1668 | *Philosophical Transactions 3* |
| 1669–70 | *Philosophical Transactions 4* |
| 1672 | *Philosophical Transactions 7* |
| 1674 | *Philosophical Transactions 9* |
| 1686–91 | *Philosophical Transactions 16* |
| 1693–4 | *Philosophical Transactions 17* |
| 1693–4 | *Philosophical Transactions 18* |

## APPENDIX: MEDICINE IN SOCIETY

| | | |
|---|---|---|
| 1537 | Erasmus, Desiderius | *Declamatio in Lavdem Nobilissimae Artis Medicinae* |
| 1564 | Bullein, William | *Dialogve Against Feuer Pestilence* |
| 1566 | Securis, John | *Detection of Daily Enormities* |
| 1569 | Agrippa, Heinrich Cornelius | *Vanitie and Vncertaintie* |
| 1576 | Elizabeth I, Queen | *Orders by her Maiestie* |
| 1580 | Mexía, Pedro | *Pleasaunt Dialogue* |
| 1591 | Du Chesne, Joseph | *Breefe Avnswere* |
| 1595 | Middleton, Thomas | *Cornucopiae* |
| 1604 | Dekker, Thomas | *Meeting of Gallants* |
| 1605 | Bacon, Francis | *Aduancement of Learning* |
| 1616 | Cotta, John | *Triall of Witch-Craft* |
| 1625 | Spenser, Benjamin | *Vox Civitatis* |
| 1633 | Fletcher, Phineas | *Purple Island* |
| 1649 | Chamberlaine, Joseph | *Prognostication* |
| 1649 | Dade, William | *Prognostication* |
| 1649 | Swallow, John | *Almanack* |
| 1649 | White, John | *Prognostication for 1649* |
| 1652 | B., J. | *Faire in Spittle Fields* |
| 1653 | Bacon, Francis | *History of Winds* |
| 1655 | Boyle, Robert | *Philaretvs to Empyricus* |
| 1655 | Hartlib, Samuel | *Chymical Addresses* |
| 1655 | Starkey, George | *George Riplye's Epistle* |
| 1655 | Anonymous | *Vrim and Thummim* |
| 1660 | L'Estrange, Roger, Sir | *Physician Cure Thy Self* |
| 1670 | Goddard, Jonathan | *Unhappy Condition of Physick* |
| 1672 | Josselyn, John | *New-Englands Rarities* |
| 1688 | Pond, Edward | *Almanack* |
| 1689 | Coley, Henry | *Merlinus Anglicus Junior* |
| 1692 | Saunders, Richard | *Apollo Anglicanus* |
| 1694 | Gadbury, John | *Ephemeris* |
| 1698 | Emes, Thomas | *Dialogue Between Alkali and Acid* |
| 1700 | Anonymous | *Letter Concerning Acid and Alkali* |

# Bibliography

## PRIMARY SOURCES

### Texts in the corpus of *Early Modern English Medical Texts* (*EMEMT*) preliminary version


*The Antidotharius* (1530).

*Aristoteles Master-Piece* (1684). *Aristoteles Master-Piece or the Secrets of Generation Displayed in all the Parts thereof* ... London: J. How.

Bailey, Walter (1588) *A Short Discourse of the Three Kindes of Peppers in Common Use, and Certaine Special Medicines Made of the Same, Tending to the Preseruation of health,* [London?: Eliot's Court Press?] Facsimile edition 1972: The English Experience No. 425, Amsterdam and New York: Theatrum Orbis Terrarum and Da Capo Press.

Banister, John (1575) *A Needefvll, New, and Necessarie Treatise of Chyrurgerie, Briefly Comprehending the Generall and Particuler Curation of Vlcers, Drawen Foorth of Sundrie Worthy Wryters, but especially of Antonius Calmeteus Vergesatus, and Ioannes Tagaltius, by Iohn Banister Gent. Practiser in Physicke and Chyrurgerie. Hereunto is Annexed Certaine Experimentes of mine Ovvne Inuention, Truely Tried, and Daily of me Practised*, London: Thomas Marshe. Facsimile edition 1971: The English Experience No. 350, Amsterdam and New York: Theatrum Orbis Terrarum and Da Capo Press.

Biggs, Noah (1651) *Mataeotechnia Medicinae Praxeos. The Vanity of the Craft of Physick. Or, a New Dispensatory*, London: Giles Calvert.

Blagrave, Joseph (1671) *Blagrave's Astrological Practice of Physick Discovering, the True Way to Cure all Kinds of Diseases and Infirmities which are Naturally Incident to the Body of Man* ... London: S. G. and B. G. for Obad. Blagrav.

Bonham, Thomas (1630) *The Chyrvrgians Closet: Or, an Antidotarie Chyrurgicall* ... London: George Miller for Edvvard Brevvster. Facsimile edition 1968: The English Experience No. 31, Amsterdam and New York: Theatrum Orbis Terrarum and Da Capo Press.

Boorde, Andrew (1547) *The Breuiary of Helthe, for all Maner of Syckenesses and Diseases the Whiche may be in Man, or Woman doth Folowe. Expressynge the Obscure Termes of Greke, Araby, Latyn, and Barbary. in to Englysh Concerning Phisicke and Chierurgye Compyled by Andrewe Boord of Phisicke Doctour an Englysh Man*, London: Wyllyam Myddelton. Facsimile edition 1971: The English Experience No. 362, Amsterdam and New York: Theatrum Orbis Terrarum and Da Capo Press.

Bradwell, Stephen (1636) *Physick for the Sicknesse, Commonly Called the Plagve. With all the Particular Signes and Symptoms, Whereof the Most are too Ignorant. Collected, out of the Choycest Authors, and Confirmed with Good Experience; for the Benefit and Preservation of all, both Rich and Poore*, London: Beniamin Fisher. Facsimile edition 1977: The English Experience No. 852, Amsterdam and Norwood: Theatrum Orbis Terrarum and Walter J. Johnson.

Brasbridge, Thomas (1578) *The Poore Mans Ievvel, that is to say, a Treatise of the Pestilence. Unto the Which is Annexed a Declaration of the Vertues of the Hearbs Carduus Benedictus, and Angelica: which are very Medicinable, both Against the Plague, and also Against Many other Diseases. Gathered out of the Bookes of Diuers Learned Physitians*, London: George Byshop.

Braunschweig, Hieronymus (1525) *The Noble Experyence of the Vertuous Handy Warke of Surgeri*, London: Petrus Treueris. Facsimile edition 1973: The English Experience No. 531, Amsterdam and New York: Theatrum Orbis Terrarum and Da Capo Press.

(1561) *A Most Excellent and Perfecte Homish Apothecarye or Homely Physick Booke / for all the Grefes and Diseases of the Bodye. Translated out the Allmaine Speche into English by Ihon Hollybush*, Collen: [The heirs of] Arnold Birckman. Facsimile edition 1968: The English Experience No. 43, Amsterdam and New York: Theatrum Orbis Terrarum and Da Capo Press.

Bright, Timothy (1580) *A Treatise: Wherein is Declared the Sufficiencie of English Medicines, for Cure of all Diseases, Cured with Medicine*, London: Henrie Middleton for Thomas Man. Facsimile edition 1977: The English Experience No. 854, Amsterdam and Norwood, NJ: Theatrum Orbis Terrarum and Walter J. Johnson.

(1586) *A Treatise of Melancholy. Containing the Causes thereof, and Reasons of the Straunge Effects it Worketh in our Minds and Bodies:* … London: Iohn VVindet.

Brown, Andrew (1699) *The Epilogue to the Five Papers Lately Past Betwixt the Two Physicians Dr. O. and Dr. E. Containing Some Remarks, Pleasant and Profitable, Concerning that Debate, and the Usefulness of Vomiting and Purging in Fevers*, Edinburgh: John Reid.

Brugis, Thomas (1648) *The Marrow of Physicke. Or a Learned Discourse of the Severall Parts of Mans Body* … London: T. H. and M. H.

Bullein, William (1562) *Bulleins Bulwarke of Defe~ce Againste all Sicknes, Sornes, and Woundes, that dooe Daily Assaulte Mankinde, whiche Bulwarke is Kepte with Hillarius the Gardiner, Health the Phisician, with their Chyrurgian, to Helpe the Wounded Soldiors* … London: Ihon Kyngston. Facsimile edition 1971: The English Experience No. 350, Amsterdam and New York: Theatrum Orbis Terrarum and Da Capo Press.

Caius, John (1552) *A Boke, or Counseill Against the Disease Commonly Called the Sweate, or Sweatyng sicknesse made by Jhon Caius Doctour in Phisicke. Uery Necessary for Everye Personne and Much Requisite to be had in the Handes of Al Sortes, for their Better Instruction, Preparation and Defence, Against the Soubdein Comyng, and Fearful Assaultyng of the Same Disease*, London: Richard Grafton.

Charas, Moyse (1678) *The Royal Pharmacopœa, Galenical and Chymical, According to the Practice of the Most Eminent and Learned Physitians of France, and Publish'd with their Several Approbations* … London: John Starkey.

de Chauliac, Guy (1579) *Gvydos Questions, Newly Corrected. Wherevnto is Added the Thirde and Fourth Booke of Galen, with a Treatise for the Helps of all the Outward Parts of Mans Body. And also an Excellent Antidotary Containing Diuers Receipts, as well of Auncient as Latter Wryters: Faythfully Corrected by Men Skilfull in the Sayd Arte* … London: Thomas East. Facsimile edition 1968: The English Experience, No. 35, Amsterdam and New York: Theatrum Orbis Terrarum and Da Capo Press.

Clowes, William (1596a) *A Briefe and Necessary Treatise, Tovching the Cvre of the Disease now vsvally called lves Venerea, by Vnctions and other Approoued Waies of Curing: Newly Corrected and Augmented in the Yeere of our Lord 1596 by William Clowes one of hir Maiesties Chirurgions*, London: Edm. Bollifant for Thomas Dawson.

(1596b) *A Profitable and Necessarie Booke of Obseruations, for all those that are Burned with the Flame of Gun Powder, &c. and also for Curing of Wounds made with Musket and Caliuer Shot, and other Weapons of War Commonly vsed at this Day both by Sea and Land, as heerafter shall be Declared:* … London: Edm. Bollifant for Thomas Dawson.

(1602) *A Right Frvtefvll and Approoved Treatise, for the Artificiall Cure of that Malady called in Latin Struma, and in English, the Euill, Cured by Kinges and Queenes of England. Very Necessary for all Young Practizers of Chyrurgery*, London: Edward Allde. Facsimile edition 1970: The English Experience No. 238, Amsterdam and New York: Theatrum Orbis Terrarum and Da Capo Press.

Colbatch, John, Sir (1698) *Novum Lumen Chirurgicum: Or, a New Light of Chirurgery wherein is Discover'd a much more Safe and Speedy Way of Curing Wounds than has heretofore bin usually Practis'd. Illustrated with Several Experiments made in Flanders in the Year 1694*, London: J. D. for D. Brown.

Cooke, James (1693) *Mellificium Chirurgiæ: Or, the Marrow of Chirurgery. With the Anatomy of Human Bodies according to the Most Modern Anatomists; illustrated with many Anatomical Observations. Institutions of Physick, with Hippocrates's Aphorisms largely Commented Upon. The Marrow of Physick, Shewing the Causes, Signs and Cures of Most Diseases Incident to Human Bodies. Choice Experienced Receits for the Cure of Several Distempers*, London: W. M.

Culpeper, Nicholas (1649) *A Physicall Directory or a Translation of the London Dispensatory made by the Colledge of Physicians in London. Being that Book by which all Apothicaries are Strictly Commanded to make all their Physick with Many Hundred Additions which the Reader may find in Every Page Marked with this Letter A* … London: Peter Cole.

(1651) *A Directory for Midwives: Or, a Guide for Women, in their Conception, Bearing, and Suckling their Children* … London: Peter Cole.

(1652a) *Galens Art of Physick: Wherein is Laid Down, 1. A Description of Bodies, Healthful, Unhealthful, and Neutral. 2. Signs of Good and Bad Constitutions. 3. Signs of the Brain, Heart, Liver, Testicles being too Hot, Cold, Dry, Moist: Signs of the Temperature, Lungues, Stomach, &c. Being too Hot and Dry, Hot and Moist, Cold and Dry, Cold and Moist. 4. Sign and Causes of Sickness. With many other Excellent Things, the Particular of which the Table of Chapters will Specifie. Translated into English, and Largely Commented on; Together with Convenient Medicines for all Particular Distempers of the Parts, a Description of the Complexions, their Conditions, and what Diet and Exercise is Fittest for them*, London: Peter Cole.

(1652b) *The English Physitian: or an Astrologo-Physical Discourse of the Vulgar Herbs of this Nation – Being a Compleat Method of Physick, whereby a Man may Preserve his Body in Health; or Cure Himself, being Sick, for Three Pence Charge, with Such Things Only as Grows in England, they Being Most Fit for English Bodies*, London: Peter Cole.

(1659) *Culpeper's School of Physick. Or The Experimental Practice of the Whole Art*, London: N. Brook.

Daffy, Anthony (1673) *Elixir Salutis: The Choice Drink of Health or, Health-Bringing Drink* … London: Printed with Allowance for the Author, by W. G.

Dawson, Thomas (1596) *The Good Husvvifes Iewell. VVherein is to be Found Most Excellend and Rare Deuises for Conceites in Cookery, found out by the Practise of Thomas Dawson* … London: [E. Allde] for Edward White.

Elkes, Richard (1651) *Approved Medicines of Little Cost, to Preserve Health and also to Cure those that are Sick. Provided for the Souldiers Knap-sack, and the Country Mans Closet*, London: Robert Ibbitson.

Feckenham, John (1990) *'This Booke of Sovereigne Medicines' … : An Edition of Folger Ms. V.B.129 (ca. 1570)*, ed. Elizabeth Rawson Macgill, Ann Arbor, Mich.: University of Michigan. First published 1570.

Fioravanti, Leonardo (1652a) *Three Exact Pieces of Leonard Phioravant Knight, and Doctor in Physick, viz. his Rationall Secrets, and Chirurgery, Reviewed and Revived, Together with a Book of Excellent Experiments and Secrets, Collected out of the Practises of Severall Expert Men in Both Faculties* … London: G. Dawson.

(1652b) *A Treatise of Chirurgery: Published wih Many Excellent Experiments and Secrets*, London: G. Dawson.

Gale, Thomas (1563a) *An Antidotarie Conteyning Hidde and Secrete Medicines Simple and Compounde: As also all Suche as are Required in Chirurgerie*, London: Rouland Hall, for Thomas Gale.

(1563b) *An Excellent Treatise of VVounds Made VVith Gonneshot, in which is Confuted Bothe the Grose Errour of Ierome Brunswicke, Iohn Uigo, Alfonse Ferrius, and Others: in that they make the Wounde Venemous, whiche Commeth Through the Common Pouder and Shotte: And also there is Set Out a Perfect and Trew Methode of Curyng these Woundes. Newly Compiled and Published by Thomas Gale Maister in Chirurgerie*, London: Rouland Hall.

(1563c) *An Institution of a Chirurgian, Conteynynge the Sure Groundes and Principles of Chirurgerie Most Necessarie and Mete for all those that will Attaine the Arte Perfectly: For whose Cause it is Compiled by Thomas Gale, Maister in Chirurgerie*, London: Rouland Hall, for Thomas Gale.

Gesner, Conrad (1559) *The Treasure of Evonymvs, Conteyninge the VVonderfull Hid Secretes of Nature, Touchinge the Most Apte Formes to Prepare and Destyl Medicines, for the Conseruation of Helth:* … London: Iohn Daie. Facsimile edition 1969: The English Experience No. 97, Amsterdam and New York: Theatrum Orbis Terrarum and Da Capo Press.

Ghesel, John (1631) *The Rvle of Health. Wherein are Contained Divers Instructions for the Preservation of the Life of Man*, Oxford: J. Lichfield. Facsimile edition 1932: *A Facsimile of The Rule of Health by John Ghesel, as Printed by John Lichfield, at Oxford, in the Year 1631*, with an introduction by H. T. Price, Michigan Facsimile Series, No. 1, Ann Arbor, Mich.: Edwards Brothers.

Grey, Elizabeth (1653) *A Choice Manval of Rare and Select Secrets in Physick and Chyrurgery; Collected and Practised by the Right Honourable, the Countesse of Kent Late Deceased. As also Most Exquisite Ways of Preserving, Conserving, Candying, &c*, London: R. Norton.

Hall, John (1679) *Select Observations on English Bodies of Eminent Persons in Desperate Diseases. First Written in Latin by Mr. John Hall, Physician: After Englished by James Cook, Author of the Marrow of Chirurgery. To which is now added, an Hundred like Counsels and Advices, for Several Honourable Persons: By the Same Author* ... London: J. D. for Benjamin Shirley.

Hart, James (1633) *Klinike, or the Diet of the Diseased. Divided into Three Bookes. VVherein is Set Downe at Length the Whole Matter and Nature of Diet for those in Health, but Especially for the Sicke; the Aire, and other Elements; Meat and Drinke, with Divers other Things; Various Controversies Concerning this Subject are Discussed: Besides Many Pleasant Practicall and Historicall Relations, both of the Authours Owne and other Mens, &c* ... London: John Beale for Robert Allot.

Hartlib, Samuel (1655) *Chymical, Medicinal, and Chyrurgical Addresses: Made to Samuel Hartlib, Esquire* ... London: G. Dawson for Giles Calvert.

Harvey, Gideon (1700) *The Vanities of Philosophy and Physick: Together with Directions and Medicines Easily Prepared by any of the Least Skill, whereby to Preserve Health, and Prolong Life, as well in those that Live Regularly, as others that Live Irregularly* ... London: W. Turner.

Harvey, William (1653) *The Anatomical Exercises of Dr. William Harvey Professor of Physick, and Physician to the Kings Majesty, Concerning the Motion of the Heart and Blood. With the Preface of Zachariah Wood Physician of Roterdam. To which is added Dr. James De Back his Discourse of the Heart, Physician in Ordinary to the Town of Roterdam*, London: Francis Leach for Richard Lowndes.

Harward, Simon (1601) *Harwards Phlebotomy: Or, a Treatise of Letting of Bloud, Fitly Seruing, as well for an Aduertisement and Remembrance to Well Minded Chirurgians, as also to giue a Caueat Generally to all Men to Beware of the Manifold Dangers, which may Ensue vpon Rash and Vnaduised Letting of Bloud. Comprehended in Two Bookes: Written by Simon Harvvard*, London: F. Kingston for Simon Waterson. Facsimile edition 1973: The English Experience No. 526, Amsterdam and New York: Theatrum Orbis Terrarum and Da Capo Press.

Hawes, Richard (1634) *The Poore-Mans Plaster-Box Furnished with Diverse Excellent Remedies for Sudden Mischances, and Usuall Infirmities, which Happen to Men, Women, and Children in this Age* ... London: Tho. Cotes for Francis Grove. Facsimile edition 1974: The English Experience No. 664, Amsterdam and Norwood, New Jersey: Theatrum Orbis Terrarum and Walter J. Johnson.

Holland, Philemon (1633) *Gutta Podagrica: A Treatise of the Govt. The Severall Sorts thereof. VVhat Diet is Good for such as are Troubled Therewith. And some Approved Medicines and Remedies for the Same*, London: Thomas Harper.

Jones, John (1566) *A Dial for all Agves; Conteininge the Names in Greeke, Latten, and Englyshe, with the Diuersities of them, Symple and Compounde, Proper and Accident, Definitions, Deuisions, Causes, and Signes, Comenly Hetherto Knowen: Uery Profitable for Al Men, Compendiously Compiled (and Confirmed as may Appeare out of the Auctors Following by Iohn Iones Phisitio~*. London: VVilliam Seres.

Jorden, Edward (1603) *A Briefe Discovrse of a Disease called the Suffocation of the Mother. Written Vppon Occasion which hath beene of late taken thereby, to*

*Suspect Possession of an Euill Spirit, or some such like Supernaturall Power …* London: Iohn Windet.

(1631) *Discovrse of Natvrall Bathes, and Minerall Waters. Wherein first the Originall of Fountaines in Generall is Declared. Then the Nature and Differences of Minerals, with examples of Particular Bathes from most of them. Next the Generation of Minerals in the Earth, …* London: Thomas Harper.

*Kalendar of Shepherdes* (1506) *Here Begynneth the Kalender of Shepherdes*, London: Rycharde Pynson. Facsimile edition 1892: *The Kalendar of Shepherdes: the Edition of Paris 1503 in Photographic Facsimile and a Faithful Reprint of R. Pynson's Edition of London 1506*, ed. Oskar H. Sommer, London: Kegan Paul.

Lamport, John (1685) *A Direct Method of Ordering and Curing People of that Loathsome Disease, the Small-Pox; Teaching the Common Sort of People (to whom the Care of the Sick is for the Most Part Committed) how to go Thorow their Business, with Much More Safety, Ease, Speed, and Certainty than hath been hitherto Commonly Known …* London: J. Gain for the author.

Langton, Christopher (1545) *An Introduction into Phisycke, wyth an Vniuersal Dyet, Gathered by Christofer Langton*, London: Edwarde Whytchurche. Facsimile edition 1970: The English Experience No. 281, Amsterdam and New York: Theatrum Orbis Terrarum and Da Capo Press.

(1547) *A Uery Brefe Treatise, Ordrely Declaring the Pricipal Partes of Phisick, that is to Saye: Thynges Natural. Thynges not Naturall. Thynges Agaynst Nature. Gathered, and Sette Forth by Christopher Langton*, London: Edvvard VVhitchurche.

*Letter Concerning Acid and Alkali* (1700) *A Letter to a Physician Concerning Acid and Alkali. Being an Answer to a Late Piece, Intituled, A Dialogue between Alkali and Acid*, London: Andrew Bell.

Lockyer, Lionel (1664). *An Advertisement, Concerning those most Excellent Pills called Pillulæ Radijs Solis Extractæ …* London: s.n.

Lodge, Thomas (1603) *A Treatise of the Plague: Containing the Nature, Signes, and Accidents of the Same, with the Certaine and Absolute Cure of the Feuers, Botches and Carbuncles that Raigne in these Times: …* London: [Thomas Creede and Valentine Simmes] for Edward White and N[icholas] L[ing]. Facsimile edition 1979: The English Experience No. 938, Amsterdam and Norwood, NJ: Theatrum Orbis Terrarum and Walter J. Johnson.

*Lytell Boke of the .xxiiii. Stones* (1528) *Here Begynneth a Lytell Boke of the .xxiiii. Stones Pryncipalles / that Profyteth Most to Mans body as y=e= day & the Nyght Hath .xxiiii. Houres / so be there .xxiiii. Stones Pryncipall*, London: R. Pynson.

M., W. (1679) *The Queens Closet Opened Incomparable Secrets in Physick, Chyrurgery, Preserving and Candying, &c. which were Presented unto the Queen: By the Most Experienced Persons of the Times, many wherof were had in Esteem when she Pleased to Descend to Private Recreations*, London: Obadiah Blagrave.

Miles, Abraham (1662) *The Countrymans Friend, and no Circumventing Mountebanck but a Rare Method of Chyrurgery and Physick, Teaching the Country People Excellent Cures, the like was Never Laid Open in any Age Before. Besides here are Four Arts, Three of them Concerning Horses, and the Fourth an Art to keep a Field of Corn from any Manner of Fowles, that Devour Grain, this Art is only by

*Anointing a Few Crow Feathers, for neither Pidgeon, Sparrow, Rook nor Crow will Endure the Field where they Stick*, London: E. Andrews.

Moore, Philip (1565) *The Hope of Health, wherein is Conteined a Goodlie Regiment of Life: As Medicine, Good Diet, and the Goodly Vertues of Sondrie Herbes, doen by Philip Moore*, London: Ihon Kingston.

Moulton, Thomas (1539) *This is the Myrrour or Glasse of Helth Necessary and Nedefull for Euery Person to Loke in, that wil Kepe their Bodye from the Syckenesse of the Pestilence, and it Sheweth how the Planettes do Raygne in Euery Houre of the Daye and Nyghte, with the Natures and Exposicio~s of the xii Sygnes, Deuyded by the .xii. Monethes of the Yeare, and Shewed the Remedies for Many Dyuers Infirmities and Dyseases that Hurteth the Bodye of Manne*, London: Robert Wyer.

Nendick, Humphrey (1674) *A Compendium of the Vertues, Operations, and use of that Applauded Antipancronicon called Nendicks Popular Pill* ... London: s.n.

Packe, Christopher (1693) *Mineralogia: Or, an Account of the Preparation, Manifold Vertues and uses of a Mineral Salt, both in Physick and Chyrurgery*; ... London: D. Newman.

Palmer, Archdale (1659) 'The Recipe Book', facsimile edition of the manuscript in Uden, Grant (ed.), *The Recipe Book 1659–1672 of Archdale Palmer, Gent. Lord of the Manor of Wanlip in the County of Leicestershire*, Wymondham: Sycamore, pp. 156–231.

Paracelsus (1655) *Of the Supreme Mysteries of Nature. Of the Spirits of the Planets. Occult Philosophy. The Magical, Sympathetical, and Antipathetical Cure of Wounds and Diseases. The Mysteries of the Twelve Signs of the Zodiack*, London: J. C. for N. Brook and J. Harison.

Paré, Ambroise (1634) *The Workes of that Famous Chirurgion Ambrose Parey*, London: Th. Cotes and R. Young.

Partridge, John (1573) *The Treasurie of Commodious Conceits, & Hidden Secrets. And may be called, the Huswiues Closet, of Healthfull Prouision. Mete and Necessarie for the Profitable vse of all Estates both Men and Women: And also Pleasaunt for Recreation, with a Necessary Table of all Things herein Contayned. Gathered Out of Sundrye Experiments Lately Practised by Men of Great Knowledge. By I. Par.*, London: Richarde Iones.

(1595) *The Widdowes Treasure. Plentifully Furnished with Sundry Precious and Approued Secrets in Phisicke and Chirurgery, for the Health and Pleasure of Mankinde. Heereunto are Adioyned, Sundry Prittie Practises and Conclusions of Cookerie, with many Profitable and Wholsome Medicines, for Sundrie Diseases in Cattell*, London: I. Roberts for Edward VVhite.

Pechey, John (1695) *The Store-House of Physical Practice: Being a General Treatise of the Causes and Signs of all Diseases Afflicting Human Bodies. Together with the Shortest, Plainest and Safest Way of Curing them, by Method, Medicine and Diet. To which is added, for the Benefit of Young Practisers, Several Choice Forms of Medicines used by the London Physicians*, London: Henry Bonwicke.

Pemell, Robert (1653) *De Morbis Puerorum, or, a Treatise of the Diseases of Children; with their Causes, Signs, Prognosticks, and Cures, for the Benefit of Such as do not Understand the Latine Tongue, and Very Useful for all such as are House-Keepers, and have Children. With the Contents of the Several Chapters, as also an Alphabetical Table of all the Diseases Mentioned Herein*, London: J. Legatt for Philemon Stephens.

Philaretes (1602) *VVork for Chimny-Sweepers: Or a Warning for Tabacconists* ... 1st edn, London: T. Este [and Thomas Creede], for Thomas Bushell.

*Philosophical Transactions* 1–18, 1665–94 [various articles]. Reprint: New York: Johnson Reprint Corporation and Kraus Reprint Corporation, 1963.

Plat, Hugh (1602) *Delightes for Ladies, to Adorne their Persons, Tables, Closets and Distillatories. With Beauties, Banquets, Perfumes and Waters. Reade, Practise, and Censure*, London: Peter Short.

Pomarius, Petrus (1609) *Enchiridion Medicum: Containing, an Epitome of the Whole Covrse of Physicke:* ... London: Henry Ballard for George Potter.

Porta, Giambattista della (1658) *Natural Magick by John Baptista Porta, a Neapolitane: In Twenty Books: ... Wherein are Set Forth all the Riches and Delights of the Natural Sciences*, London: Thomas Young and Samuel Speed.

Prat, Ellis (1689) *Vade Mecum: Or, a Companion for a Chirurgion. Fitted for Sea, or Land; Peace, or War. Shewing the use of his Instruments, and Virtues of Medicines Simple and Compound most in use, and how to make them up after the Best Method* ... London: T. Sawbridge.

*Prognosticacion* (1554) *Prognosticacion Drawen Out of the Bookes of Ipocras, Auicen, and other Notable Auctours of Physycke, Shewynge the Daunger of Dyuers Syckenesses, that is to say, whether Peryll of Death be in them or not, the Pleasure of Almyghtye God Reserued*, London: Robert Wyer.

Recorde, Robert (1547) *The Urinal of Physick. Composed by Mayster Robert Recorde: Doctor of Physicke*, London: Reynolde Wolfe.

Ruscelli, Girolamo (1562) *The Secretes of the Reverende Maister Alexis of Piemovnt. Containing Excellente Remedies Against Diuers Diseases, Woundes, and other Accidents, with the Manner to make Distillations, Parfumes, Confitures, Diynges, Colours, Fusions and Meltynges* ... London: Rouland Hall for Nycolas England.

Russel, Thomas (1602) *Diacatholicon Avrevm: Or a Generall Powder of Gold, Purging all Offensiue Humours in Mans Bodie: Good in Generall for all Diseases, where there Needeth any Purgation:* ... London: [S. Stafford] for Iohn Flasket.

Sadler, John (1636) *The Sicke VVomans Private Looking-Glasse Wherein Methodically are Handled all Uterine Affects, or Diseases Arising from the Wombe; Enabling Women to Informe the Physician about the Cause of their Griefe*, London: Anne Griffin for Philemon Stephens and Christopher Meridith. Facsimile edition 1977: The English Experience No. 891, Amsterdam and Norwood, NJ: Theatrum Orbis Terrarum and Walter J. Johnson.

Salmon, William (1700a) *Pharmacopœia Bateana: Or Bate's Dispensatory. Translated from the Last Edition of the Latin Copy, Published by Mr. James Shipton. Containing his Choice and Select Recipe's, their Names, Compositions, Preparations, Vertues, Uses, and Doses, as they are Applicable to the Whole Practice of Physick and Chirurgery ... The Second Edition, with Emendations, and Enlarged with Several Extraordinary Preparations not in the Former Impression, and above a Thousand Other Additions Interspersed Thro' the Body of the Work*, London: S. Smith and B. Walford.

(1700b) *Phylaxa Medicinae. The Cabinet of Physick Containing, a Set of the Best Medical Preparations now used in the Art of Physick, as they are Prepared, and Daily Prescribed in the Continual Practise of the Author hereof, William Salmon, M.D. Living in the Great House, Near Black-Fryers Stairs, London*, London: I. Dawks.

Sennert, Daniel (1662) *The Sixth Book of Practical Physick. Of Occult or Hidden Diseases; in Nine Parts* … London: Peter Cole.

*Seynge of Uryns* (1525) *Here Begynneth the Seynge of Uryns / of all the Colours that Uryns be of / with Medycynes Annexed to Euery Uryne / & Euery Uryne his Urynall / not Imprynted in Englysshe before this Tyme / Moche Profytable for Euery Man to Knowe*, London: [J. Rastell for] Rycharde Bancke.

Sharp, Jane (1671) *The Midwives Book; or, The Whole Art of Midwifry Discovered: Directing Childbearing Women how to Behave Themselves in their Conception, Breeding, Bearing, and Nursing of Children* … London: Simon Miller.

Starkey, George (1655) 'Sir George Riplye's Epistle to King Edward Unfolded', in Samuel Hartlib, *Chymical, Medicinal, and Chyrurgical Addresses: Made to Samuel Hartlib, Esquire* … London: G. Dawson for Giles Calvert, pp. 19–47.

Tauvry, Daniel (1700) *A Treatise of Medicines Containing an Account of their Chymical Principles, the Experiments made upon 'em, their Various Preparations, their Vertues, and the Modern way of using them* … London: Richard Wellington, Arthur Bettesworth, and Bernard Lintott.

*Ten Recipes by Henry VIII* (1548) 'Ten Recipes by Henry VIII and his Physicians, Dr. Augustyne, Dr. Butts, and Dr. Cromer', in *The Anatomie of the Bodie of Man, by T. Vicary … The Edition of 1548 … With a Life of Vicary, Notes on Surgeons in England, Bartholomew's Hospital, and London, in Tudor Times, an Appendix of Documents, and Illustrations*, ed. F. J. Furnivall and P. Furnivall, EETS Extra 53, London: Oxford University Press, pp. 220–30.

*Treasure of Pore Men* (1526) *Here Begynneth a Newe Boke of Medecynes Intytulyd or callyd the Treasure of Pore Men / whiche sheweth many Dyuerse Good Medecines for Dyuerse Certayn Dysseases as in the Table of this Present Boke more Playnly shall Appere*, London: [J. Rastell for] Rycherd Bankes.

Turner, William (1562) *A Booke of the Natures and Properties as well of the Bathes in England as of Other Bathes in Germany and Italy / Very Necessary for all Seik Persones that can not be Healed without the Helpe of Natural Bathes / Gathered by William Turner Doctor of Physik*, Collen: Arnold Birckman.

Vicary, Thomas (1577) *A Profitable Treatise of the Anatomie of Mans Body* … London: Henry Bamforde.

de Vigo, Johannes (1543) *The Most Excellent Workes of Chirurgerye, Made and Set Forth by Maister John Vigon, Heed Chirurgie[n] of our Tyme in Italie, Translated into English. Whereunto is added an Exposition of Straunge Termes [and] Vnknowen Symples, Belongyng to the Arte.* [London?]: Edwarde Whytchurch. Facsimile edition 1968: The English Experience No. 67, Amsterdam and New York: Theatrum Orbis Terrarum and Da Capo Press.

Winter, Salvator and Dickinson, Francisco (1649) *A Pretious Treasury: Or a New Dispensatory. Contayning 70. Approved Physicall Rare Receits. Most Necessary and Needfull for all sorts of People to have in their Families. Collected out of the Most Approved Authors, Both in Physick and Chyrurgery: By Salvator Winter, and Signieur Francisco Dickinson, Expert Operators. In Two Bookes*, London: Richard Harper.

Wiseman, Richard (1676) 'A treatise of wounds', in Richard Wiseman, *Severall Chirurgicall Treatises*, London: E. Flesher and J. Macock, for R. Royston

… and B. Took, pp. 337–403. Facsimile edition 1977: *Of Wounds, of Gun-Shot Wounds, of Fractures and Luxations by Richard Wiseman, a Facsimile, of Books V, VI and VII from 'Severall Chirurgical Treatises'*, ed. J. Kirkup, Bath: Kingsmead Press.

Wood, Owen (1639) *An Alphabetical Book of Physicall Secrets, for all those Diseases that are most Predominant and Dangerous (Curable by Art) in the Body of Man* … London: Walter Edmonds.

Woolley, Hannah (1670) *The Queen-Like Closet; or, Rich Cabinet: Stored with all Manner of Rare Receipts for Preserving, Candying & Cookery. Very Pleasant and Beneficial to all Ingenious Persons of the Female Sex*, London: R. Lowndes.

(1677) *The Compleat Servant-Maid; or, the Young Maidens Tutor. Directing them how they may Fit, and Qualifie Themselves for any of these Employments*, London: T. Passinger.

(1700) *A Supplement to the Compleat Servant Maid; Containing the Choicest Receipts and Rarest Secrets in Physick and Chirurgery. Fitted to the Capacity of the Meanest Housekeeper, and if put into Practice may Prevent the Frequent Expences, and Charges which most Families are at upon Doctory and Chirurgery*, London: Eben Tracy.

## Other primary sources

Anonymous (1670–80) *Elixir Magnum Vitæ: or, The Great Elixir of Life*, [London: s.n.].

(1680) *The so much Fam'd Tablets*, [London: s.n.].

Brugis, Thomas (1689) *Vade Mecum: Or, a Companion for a Chirurgion*, 7th edn, London: Printed for B. T. and T. S. and sold by Fr. Hubbert, next the Crown Tavern in Duck-lane.

Bullein, William (1888) *A Dialogue Against the Feuer Pestilence: From the Edition of 1578, Collated with the Earlier Editions of 1564 and 1573*, eds. Mark W. Bullen and A. H. Bullen. EETS Extra 52, London: Oxford University Press.

Burton, T. L. (ed.) (1998) *Sidrak and Bokkus: A Parallel-Text Edition from Bodleian Library, MS Laud Misc. 559 and British Library, MS Lansdowne 793*. EETS O.S. 312, Oxford: Oxford University Press.

Cawdrey, Robert (1604) *A Table Alphabetical*, London: Printed by I. R[oberts] for Edmund Weauer.

Colbatch, John, Sir (1696) *Physico-Medical Essay Concerning Alkaly and Acid* … London: printed for Dan. Browne at the Black Swan without Temple-Bar.

(1698) *The Doctrine of Acids in the Cure of Diseases farther asserted* … London: printed for Dan. Brown at the Black Swan and Bible without Temple-Bar; and Abel Roper at the Black-Boy in Fleet-street.

(1700) *A Letter to a Physician Concerning Acid and Alkali. Being an Answer to a Late Piece, Intituled, A Dialogue Between Alkali and Acid, Written by a Gentleman*, London: Printed for Andrew Bell.

Dekker, Thomas (1609) *The Guls Horne-booke*. Imprinted at London: [by Nicholas Okes] for R. S[ergier?]. Published 1904, ed. R. B. McKerrow, London: De la More Press.

Emes, Thomas (1698) *A Dialogue between Alkali and Acid Containing Divers Philosophical and Medicinal Consideration* … London: Printed for R. Cumberland … and Tho. Speed.

(1700) *A Letter to a Gentleman Concerning Alkali and Acid. Being an Answer to a Late Piece, Intituled, A Letter to a Physician Concerning Acid and Alkali* … London: Printed for Tho. Speed.

Fletcher, R. (1677) *The Vertues of that Well Known and Often-Experienced Medicine Fletchers Powder*, London: Printed by Thomas James for the Author with Allowance.

Hinde, Thomas (1673) *Under God, Humbly Desiring His Blessing to this Famous and Wonderful Never-Failing Cordial Drink of the World* … London: Printed for the Author, with Allowance.

Jonson, Ben (1601) *Everyman Out of His Humour*, London: Printed for William Holme. Published 1954 in *Ben Jonson*, ed. C. H. Herford and Percy Simpson, vol. III, Oxford: Clarendon Press.

Locke, John (1690) *An Essay Concerning Human Understanding*, London: Printed by Eliz. Holt for Thomas Basset. Published 1997, ed. Roger B. Jones, Research Centre for Humanities Computing. Available online at http://humanum.arts.cuhk.edu.hk/Philosophy/Locke/echu (accessed 9 May 2009).

Lomax, Nathaniel (1680?) *Delaun reviv'd, viz. A Plain and Short Discourse of that Famous Doctor's Pills, their Use and Virtues* … [London: s.n.].

Marbecke, Roger (1602) *A Defence of Tabacco. VVith a Friendly Answer to the Late Printed Booke called Worke for Chimny-Sweepers, &c*, London: Printed by Richard Field for Thomas Man. STC (2nd edn) 6468.

Markham, Gervase (1615) *Countrey Contentments or the English Huswife, Containing the Inward and Outward Vertues which ought to be in a Compleate Woman, by her skill in Physicke, Surgerie* … London: J. Beale for R. Jackson.

(Maynwaringe, Everard) (1684) *The Catholic Medicine, and Soverain Healer* … London: Printed by J. Gain; for R. Horn, T. Bassett and C. Blount.

*Philosophical Transactions* 27, 1710 (various articles).

Poynter, F. N. L. and Bishop, W. J. (eds.) (1951) *A Seventeenth Century Doctor and his Patients: John Symcotts, 1592?–1662*, Streatley: Bedfordshire Historical Record Society.

Simpson, William (1669) *Hydrologia Chymica* … London: Printed by W. G. for Richard Chiswel.

Turner, William (1551) *A new Herball, wherin are Conteyned the Names of Herbes in Greke, Latin, Englysh, Duch & Frenche, and in the Potecaries and Herbaries Latin, with the Properties Degrees and Naturall Places of the same, Gathered and Made by Wylliam Turner, Phisicion vnto the Duke of Somersettes Grace*, London: Steven Mierdman.

Wedel, Georg (1685) *An Introduction to the Whole Practice of Physick*, London: printed for William Thackery at the Angel, and Thomas Yeate at the Bell in Duck-lane.

Winter, Salvatore (1664) *Directions for the use of my Elixir, my Philosophical Petza or Plaister, my Balsom, and also my Purging Drink*, [London: s.n.].

Witherden, Thomas (1679) *Elixir Salutis or the Great Preservative of Health called by some the Never-Failing Cordial of the World* … [London: s.n.].

Woodward, Daniel (1690?) *Amicus Naturæ. An Advertisement of the Virtues of Woodward's Cordial Pills, and Elixir Salutis* … [London: s.n.].

## SECONDARY SOURCES


Aijmer, Karin (1997) '*I Think*: An English Modal Particle', in Toril Swan and Olaf Jansen Westvik (eds.), *Modality in Germanic Languages: Historical and Comparative Perspectives*, Berlin and New York: Mouton De Gruyter, pp. 1–48.

Allen, Bryce, Qin, Jian and Lancaster, F. W. (1994) 'Persuasive Communities: A Longitudinal Analysis of References in the *Philosophical Transactions* of the Royal Society, 1665–1990', *Social Studies of Science*, 24 (2): 279–310.

Alonso Almeida, Francisco and Cabrera-Abreu, Mercedes (2002) 'The Formulation of Promise in Medieval English Medical Recipes: A Relevance-Theoretic Approach', *Neophilologus*, 86 (1): 137–54.

Aristotle (1928) *Topics*, trans. W. A. Pickard-Cambridge, Oxford: Clarendon Press.

(1924) *Metaphysics*, trans. W. D. Ross, Oxford: Oxford University Press. Available online at http://classics.mit.edu/Aristotle/metaphysics.html (accessed 24 August 2010).

Atkinson, Dwight (1992) 'The Evolution of Medical Research Writing from 1735 to 1985: The Case of the *Edinburgh Medical Journal*', *Applied Linguistics*, 13 (4): 337–74.

(1996) 'The *Philosophical Transactions* of the Royal Society of London, 1675–1975: A Sociohistorical Discourse Analysis', *Language in Society*, 25 (3): 333–71.

(1999) *Scientific Discourse in Sociohistorical Context: The* Philosophical Transactions *of the Royal Society of London, 1675–1975*, Mahwah, NJ: Lawrence Erlbaum.

auf dem Keller, Caren (2004) *Textual Structures in Eighteenth-Century Newspaper Advertising*, Aachen: Shaker Verlag.

Bach, Ulrich (1997) *Englische Flugtexte im 17. Jahrhundert: Historisch-pragmatische Untersuchungen zur frühen Massenkommukation*, Heidelberg: C. Winter.

Barber, Charles (1976) *Early Modern English*, London: Deutsch.

Barnes, Eugene B. (1947) 'The International Exchange of Knowledge in Western Europe, 1680–89', Ph.D. thesis, Graduate Library School, University of Chicago.

Bates, Don (1995a) 'Scholarly Ways of Knowing: An Introduction', in Don Bates (ed.), *Knowledge and the Scholarly Medical Traditions*, Cambridge: Cambridge University Press, pp. 1–22.

(ed.) (1995b) *Knowledge and the Scholarly Medical Traditions*, Cambridge: Cambridge University Press.

Bazerman, Charles (1988) *Shaping Written Knowledge: The Genre and Activity of the Experimental Article in Science*, Madison, Wisc.: The University of Wisconsin Press.

Bennett, H. S. (1969) *English Books & Readers, 1475 to 1557: Being a Study in the History of the Book Trade from Caxton to the Incorporation of the Stationers' Company*, 2nd edn, Cambridge: Cambridge University Press.

Bensly, Edward (1904) 'King's "Classical and Foreign Quotations,"' *Notes and Queries*, 10 (41): 281. Available online at http://nq.oxfordjournals.org/cgi/issue_pdf/frontmatter_pdf/s10-II/41.pdf (accessed 15 December 2009).

Bevan, Michael (2004) 'Emes, Thomas (*d.* 1707)', in Lawrence Goldman (ed.), *Oxford Dictionary of National Biography*, Oxford: Oxford University Press.

Available online at http://www.oxforddnb.com/view/article/8789 (accessed 7 December 2009).

Bhatt, R. M. (2008) 'In Other Words: Language Mixing, Identity Representations, and *Third Space*', *Journal of Sociolinguistics*, 12 (2): 177–200.

Biber, Douglas (1988) *Variation across Speech and Writing*, Cambridge: Cambridge University Press.

(1993) 'Representativeness in Corpus Design', *Literary and Linguistic Computing*, 8 (4): 243–57.

(2004a) 'Historical Patterns for the Grammatical Marking of Stance: A Cross-Register Comparison', *Journal of Historical Pragmatics*, 5 (1): 107–36.

(2004b) 'Modal Use across Registers and Time', in Anne Curzan and Kimberly Emmons (eds.), *Studies in the History of the English Language II: Unfolding Conventions*, Berlin: Mouton De Gruyter, pp. 189–216.

(2006) 'Stance in Spoken and Written University Registers', *Journal of English for Academic Purposes*, 5 (2): 97–116.

Biber, Douglas, Conrad, Susan and Reppen, Randi (1998) *Corpus Linguistics: Investigating Language Structure and Use*, Cambridge: Cambridge University Press.

Biber, Douglas and Finegan, Edward (1988) 'Adverbial Stance Types in English', *Discourse Processes*, 11 (1): 1–34.

(1989) 'Styles of Stance in English: Lexical and Grammatical Marking of Evidentiality and Affect', *Text*, 9 (1): 93–124.

Biber, Douglas, Johansson, Stig, Leech, Geoffrey, Conrad, Susan and Finegan, Edward (1999) *Longman Grammar of Spoken and Written English*, London: Longman.

Blair, Ann (2008) 'Student Manuscripts and the Textbook', in Emidio Campi, Simone De Angelis, Anja-Silvia Goeing and Anthony Grafton (eds.), *Scholarly Knowledge: Textbooks in Early Modern Europe*, Geneva: Droz, pp. 39–73.

Blommaert, Jan (2005) *Discourse: A Critical Introduction*, Cambridge: Cambridge University Press.

Brayman Hackel, Heidi (2004) 'Rhetorics and Practices of Illiteracy or the Marketing of Illiteracy', in Ian Frederick Moulton (ed.), *Reading and Literacy in the Middle Ages and Renaissance*, Turnhout: Brepols, pp. 169–83.

(2005) *Reading Material in Early Modern England: Print, Gender, and Literacy*, Cambridge: Cambridge University Press.

Bühler, Curt F. (1961) 'A Middle English Medical Manuscript from Norwich', in Macedward Leach (ed.), *Studies in Medieval Literature in Honor of Professor Albert Croll Baugh*, Philadelphia, Pa.: University of Pennsylvania Press, pp. 285–98.

Bullock, Barbara E. and Toribio, Almeida Jacqueline (eds.) (2009) *The Cambridge Handbook of Linguistic Code-Switching*, Cambridge: Cambridge University Press.

Burke, Peter (1978) *Popular Culture in Early Modern Europe*, London: Temple Smith.

Burrow, J. A. (1986) *The Ages of Man: A Study in Medieval Writing and Thought*, Oxford: Clarendon.

Butchvarov, Panayot (1970) *The Concept of Knowledge*, Evanston, Ill.: Northwestern University Press.

Bylebyl, Jerome J. (1985) 'Disputation and Description in the Renaissance Pulse Controversy', in A. Wear, R. K. French and I. M. Lonie (eds.), *The Medical Renaissance of the Sixteenth Century*, Cambridge: Cambridge University Press, pp. 223–45.

Callahan, Laura (2004) *Spanish/English Codeswitching in a Written Corpus*, Amsterdam and Philadelphia, Pa.: John Benjamins.

Cameron, M. L. (1993) *Anglo-Saxon Medicine*, Cambridge: Cambridge University Press.

Capp, Bernard (1979) *Astrology and the Popular Press: English Almanacs, 1500–1800*, London and Boston, Mass.: Faber and Faber.

Chafe, Wallace (1986) 'Evidentiality in English Conversation and Academic Writing', in Wallace Chafe and Johanna Nichols (eds.), *Evidentiality: The Linguistic Coding of Epistemology*, Norwood, NJ: Ablex, pp. 261–72.

Chafe, Wallace and Nichols, Johanna (eds.) (1986) *Evidentiality: The Linguistic Coding of Epistemology*, Norwood, NJ: Ablex.

Charles, Maggie (2003) '"This Mystery ...": A Corpus-Based Study of the Use of Nouns to Construct Stance in Theses from Two Contrasting Disciplines', *Journal of English for Academic Purposes*, 2 (4): 313–26.

(2006) 'The Construction of Stance in Reporting Clauses: A Cross-Disciplinary Study of Theses', *Applied Linguistics*, 27 (3): 492–518.

Chartier, Roger (1988) *Cultural History: Between Practices and Representations*, Cambridge: Polity Press.

(1995) *Forms and Meanings: Texts, Performances and Audiences from Codex to Computer*, Philadelphia, Pa.: University of Pennsylvania Press.

Claridge, Claudia (2001) 'Structuring Text: Discourse Deixis in Early Modern English Texts', *Journal of English Linguistics*, 29 (1): 55–71.

Cody, Lisa Forman (ed.) (2002) *Writings on Medicine*, Aldershot: Ashgate.

Colman, Eric (1999) 'The First English Medical Journal: *Medicina Curiosa*', *Lancet*, 354 (9175): 324–6.

Considine, John (2004) 'Wolley, Hannah (*b.* 1622?, *d.* in or after 1674)', in Lawrence Goldman (ed.), *Oxford Dictionary of National Biography*, Oxford: Oxford University Press. Available online at http://www.oxforddnb.com/view/article/29957 (accessed 17 August 2009).

Cook, Harold J. (1986) *The Decline of the Old Medical Regime in Stuart London*, Ithaca, NY: Cornell University Press.

(2004) 'Colbatch, Sir John (*bap.* 1666?, *d.* 1729)', in Lawrence Goldman (ed.), *Oxford Dictionary of National Biography*, Oxford: Oxford University Press. Available online at http://www.oxforddnb.com/view/article/5833 (accessed 7 December 2009).

Coste, Joel (2008) 'Le Médecine pratique et ses genres littéraires en France à l'époque moderne', *Medic@*, available online at http://www.bium.univ-paris5.fr/histmed/medica/medpratique.htm (accessed 18 August 2009).

Crawford, Patricia (1984) 'Printed Advertisements for Women Medical Practitioners in London, 1670–1710', *Bulletin, Society for the Social History of Medicine*, 35: 66–70.

Crespo, Begoña and Moskowich, Isabel (2006) 'Latin Forms in Vernacular Scientific Writing: Code-Switching or Borrowing?', in R. W. McConchie, Olga Timofeeva, Heli Tissari and Tanja Säily (eds.), *Selected Proceedings of the*

*2005 Symposium on New Approaches in English Historical Lexis (HEL-LEX)*, Somerville, Mass.: Proceedings Project, pp. 51–9.
Cressy, David (1980) *Literacy and the Social Order: Reading and Writing in Tudor and Stuart England*, Cambridge: Cambridge University Press.
(2003) *Society and Culture in Early Modern England*, Aldershot: Ashgate.
Crisciani, Chiara (1990) 'History, Novelty, and Progress in Scholastic Medicine', *Osiris*, 2nd Series, 6: 118–39.
Crombie, A. C. (1994) *Styles of Scientific Thinking in the European Tradition: The History of Argument and Explanation, Especially in the Mathematical and Biomedical Sciences and Arts*, 3 vols., London: Duckworth.
(1995) 'Commitments and Styles of European Scientific Thinking', *History of Science*, 33: 225–38.
Cunningham, Andrew (1989) 'Thomas Sydenham: Epidemics, Experiments, and the "Good Old Cause,"' in Roger French and Andrew Wear (eds.), *The Medical Revolution of the Seventeenth Century*, Cambridge: Cambridge University Press, pp. 164–91.
Curth, Louise Hill (2002) 'The Commercialisation of Medicine in the Popular Press: English Almanacs 1640–1700', *The Seventeenth Century*, 17 (1): 48–69.
(2006) 'Medical Advertising in the Popular Press: Almanacs and the Growth of Proprietary Medicines', in Louise Hill Curth (ed.), *From Physick to Pharmacology: Five Hundred Years of British Drug Retailing*, Aldershot: Ashgate, pp. 29–48.
(2007) *English Almanacs, Astrology and Popular Medicine, 1550–1700*, Manchester: Manchester University Press.
Daston, Lorraine (1998) 'The Language of Strange Facts in Early Modern Science', in Timothy Lenoir (ed.), *Inscribing Science: Scientific Texts and the Materiality of Communication*, Palo Alto: Stanford University Press, pp. 20–38.
Debus, Allen G. (1987) *Chemistry, Alchemy, and the New Philosophy* 1550–1700, London: Variorum Reprints.
(2002) *The French Paracelsians: The Chemical Challenge to Medical and Scientific Tradition in Early Modern France*, Cambridge: Cambridge University Press.
Engelhardt, H. Tristram, Jr. and Caplan, Arthur L. (1987a) 'Patterns of Controversy and Closure: The Interplay of Knowledge, Values, and Political Forces', in H. Tristram Engelhardt and Arthur L. Caplan (eds.), *Scientific Controversies: Case Studies in the Resolution and Closure of Disputes in Science and Technology*, Cambridge: Cambridge University Press, pp. 1–23.
(eds.) (1987b) *Scientific Controversies: Case Studies in the Resolution and Closure of Disputes in Science and Technology*, Cambridge: Cambridge University Press.
*English Short-Title Catalogue*, London: British Library. Online at http://estc.bl.uk (accessed 24 November 2009).
Fahnestock, Jeanne and Secor, Marie (1988) 'The Stases in Scientific and Literary Argument', *Written Communication*, 5 (4): 427–43.
(1991) 'The Rhetoric of Literary Criticism', in Charles Bazerman and James Paradis (eds.), *Textual Dynamics of the Professions: Historical and Contemporary Studies in Writing in Professional Communities*, Madison, Wisc.: University of Wisconsin Press, pp. 77–96.

Fanego, Teresa, Méndez-Naya, Belén and Seoane, Elena (eds.) (2002) *Sounds, Words, Texts and Change: Selected Papers from 11 ICEHL, Santiago de Compostela, 7–11 September 2000*, Amsterdam and Philadelphia, Pa.: John Benjamins.
Feather, John (1994) *Publishing, Piracy, and Politics: An Historical Study of Copyright in Britain*, London: Mansell.
Fishman, J. A. (1979) 'The Relationship between Micro- and Macro-Sociolinguistics in the Study of who Speaks what Language to Whom and When', in J. B. Pride and Janet Holmes (eds.), *Sociolinguistics: Selected Readings*, Harmondsworth: Penguin, pp. 15–32.
Fissell, Mary E. (2007) 'The Marketplace of Print', in Mark S. R. Jenner and Patrick Wallis (eds.), *Medicine and the Market in England and Its Colonies, c. 1450–c. 1850*, Basingstoke and New York: Palgrave Macmillan, pp. 108–32.
Ford, Wyn (1993) 'The Problem of Literacy in Early Modern England', *History*, 78 (252): 22–37.
Fox, Adam (2000) *Oral and Literate Culture in England, 1500–1700*, Oxford: Clarendon Press.
Frank, Robert G., Jr. (1980) *Harvey and the Oxford Physiologists: A Study of Scientific Ideas*, Berkeley, Calif.: University of California Press.
French, Roger (1994) *William Harvey's Natural Philosophy*, Cambridge: Cambridge University Press.
(2002) *Ancients and Moderns in the Medical Sciences: From Hippocrates to Harvey*, Aldershot: Ashgate.
(2003) *Medicine before Science: The Rational and Learned Doctor from the Middle Ages to the Enlightenment*, Cambridge: Cambridge University Press.
French, Roger and Wear, Andrew (eds.) (1989) *The Medical Revolution of the Seventeenth Century*, Cambridge: Cambridge University Press.
Fries, Udo (1997) 'Electuarium Mirabile: Praise in 18th-Century Medical Advertisements', in Jan Aarts, Inge De Mönnink and Herman Wekker (eds.), *Studies in English Language and Teaching: in Honour of Flor Aarts*, Amsterdam: Rodopi, pp. 57–73.
Fritz, Gerd (2003) 'Dialogical Structures in 17th Century Controversies', in M. Bondi and S. Stati (eds.), *Dialogue Analysis, 2000*, Tübingen: Niemeyer, pp. 199–208.
(2005) 'First Person Singular in 17th Century Controversies', in Pierluigi Barrotta and Marcelo Dascal (eds.), *Controversies and Subjectivity*, Amsterdam and Philadelphia, Pa.: John Benjamins, pp. 235–50.
(2010) 'Controversies', in Andreas H. Jucker and Irma Taavitsainen (eds.), *Historical Pragmatics*, Berlin and New York: De Gruyter Mouton, pp. 451–81.
Furdell, Elizabeth Lane (2002) *Publishing and Medicine in Early Modern England*, Rochester, NY and Woodbridge: University of Rochester Press and Boydell & Brewer.
(2005) *Textual Healing: Essays on Medieval and Early Modern Medicine*, Leiden and Boston, Mass.: Brill Academic Publishers.
(2008) 'Bate, George (1608–1668)', in Lawrence Goldman (ed.), *Oxford Dictionary of National Biography*, Oxford: Oxford University Press. Available online at http://www.oxforddnb.com/view/article/1661 (accessed 18 August 2009).

Garrison, Fielding H. (1934) 'The Medical and Scientific Periodicals of the 17th and 18th Centuries', *Bulletin of the Institute of the History of Medicine*, 2 (5): 285–343.

Genette, Gérard (1997) *Paratexts: Thresholds of Interpretation*, trans. J. E. Lewin, Cambridge: Cambridge University Press.

Gentilcore, David (2006) *Medical Charlatanism in Early Modern Italy*, Oxford: Oxford University Press.

George, Philip (1952) 'The Scientific Movement and the Development of Chemistry in England, as Seen in the Papers Published in the *Philosophical Transactions* from 1664/5 until 1750', *Annals of Science*, 8: 302–22.

Getz, Faye Marie (1990) 'Charity, Translation, and the Language of Medical Learning in Medieval England', *Bulletin of the History of Medicine*, 64 (1): 1–17.

(1998) *Medicine in the English Middle Ages*, Princeton, NJ: Princeton University Press.

Gieszinger, Sabine (2000) 'Two Hundred Years of Advertising in *The Times*: The Development of Text Type Markers', in Friedrich Ungerer (ed.), *English Media Texts Past and Present*, Amsterdam and Philadelphia, Pa.: John Benjamins, pp. 85–110.

Gil, Fernando (1985) 'Science and Controversy', in Marcelo Dascal (ed.), *Dialogue: An Interdisciplinary Approach*, Amsterdam and Philadelphia, Pa.: John Benjamins, pp. 353–65.

Glaisyer, Natasha and Pennell, Sara (2003) 'Introduction', in Natasha Glaisyer and Sara Pennell (eds.), *Didactic Literature in England 1500–1800: Expertise Constructed*, Aldershot: Ashgate, pp. 1–18.

Gloning, Thomas (1999) 'The Pragmatic Form of Religious Controversies around 1600: A Case Study in the Osiander vs. Scherer and Rosenbusch Controversy', in Andreas H. Jucker, Gerd Fritz and Franz Lebsanft (eds.), *Historical Dialogue Analysis*, Amsterdam and Philadelphia, Pa.: John Benjamins, pp. 81–110.

Gorham, Geoffrey (1994) 'Mind–Body Dualism and the Harvey-Descartes Controversy', *Journal of the History of Ideas*, 55 (2): 211–34.

Görlach, Manfred (2002) 'A Linguistic History of Advertising, 1700–1890', in Teresa Fanego, Belén Méndez-Naya and Elena Seoane (eds.), *Sounds, Words, Texts and Change: Selected Papers from 11 ICEHL, Santiago de Compostela, 7–11 September 2000*, Amsterdam and Philadelphia, Pa.: John Benjamins, pp. 83–104.

Gotti, Maurizio (2001) 'The Experimental Essay in Early Modern English', *European Journal of English Studies*, 5 (2): 221–39.

(2005) 'Advertising Discourse in Eighteenth-Century English Newspapers', in Janne Skaffari, Matti Peikola, Ruth Carroll, Risto Hiltunen and Brita Wårvik (eds.), *Opening Windows on Texts and Discourses of the Past*, Amsterdam and Philadelphia, Pa.: John Benjamins, pp. 23–38.

(2006a) 'Communal Correspondence in Early Modern English: The *Philosophical Transactions* Network', in Marina Dossena and Susan M. Fitzmaurice (eds.), *Business and Official Correspondence: Historical Investigations*, Bern: Peter Lang, pp. 17–46.

(2006b) 'Disseminating Early Modern Science: Specialized News Discourse in the *Philosophical Transactions*', in Nicholas Brownlees (ed.), *News Discourse in Early Modern Britain*, Bern: Peter Lang, pp. 41–70.

(2008) *Investigating Specialized Discourse*, 2nd edn, Bern: Peter Lang.

(in press) 'Managing Disputes with Civility: Language and Politeness in 17th-Century Argumentative Discourse', in Ulrich Busse and Axel Hübler (eds.), *From the Metacommunicative Lexicon to Historical Pragmatics*, Amsterdam: John Benjamins.

Grafton, Anthony, Shelford, April and Siraisi, Nancy (1992) *New Worlds, Ancient Texts: The Power of Tradition and the Shock of Discovery*, Cambridge, Mass. and London: The Belknap Press of Harvard University Press.

Greenhill, W. A. (2004) 'Marbeck, Roger (1536–1605)', rev. Sarah Bakewell, in Lawrence Goldman (ed.), *Oxford Dictionary of National Biography*, Oxford: Oxford University Press. Available online at http://www.oxforddnb.com/view/article/18027 (accessed 7 December 2009).

Gross, Alan G., Harmon, Joseph E. and Reidy, Michael S. (2000) 'Argument and 17th-Century Science: A Rhetorical Analysis with Sociological Implications', *Social Studies of Science*, 30 (3): 371–96.

(2002) *Communicating Science: The Scientific Article from the 17th Century to the Present*, Oxford: Oxford University Press.

Grund, Peter (2003) 'The Golden Formulas: Genre Conventions of Alchemical Recipes in the Middle English Period', *Neuphilologische Mitteilungen*, 104 (4): 455–75.

Gumperz, John J. (1982) *Discourse Strategies*, Cambridge: Cambridge University Press.

Hall, Marie Boas (1991) *Promoting Experimental Learning: Experiment and the Royal Society, 1660–1727*, Cambridge: Cambridge University Press.

(2004) 'Henry Oldenburg (c. 1619–1677)', in Lawrence Goldman (ed.), *Oxford Dictionary of National Biography*, Oxford: Oxford University Press. Available online at http://www.oxforddnb.com/view/article/20676 (accessed 7 October 2009).

Halliday, M. A. K. and Hasan, Ruqaiya (1976) *Cohesion in English*, London: Longman.

Harkness, Deborah E. (2007) *The Jewel House: Elizabethan London and the Scientific Revolution*, New Haven, Conn.: Yale University Press.

Harley, David (1993) 'The Beginnings of the Tobacco Controversy: Puritanism, James I, and the Royal Physicians', *Bulletin of the History of Medicine*, 67 (1): 28–50.

Harris, Tim (1995) 'Problematising Popular Culture', in Tim Harris (ed.), *Popular Culture in England, c. 1500–1850*, Basingstoke and London: Macmillan, pp. 1–27.

Harrison, Peter (2001) 'Curiosity, Forbidden Knowledge, and the Reformation of Natural Philosophy in Early Modern England', *Isis*, 92 (2): 265–90.

Hartley, Harold (ed.) (1960) *The Royal Society: Its Origins and Founders*, London: The Royal Society.

Haycock, David Boyd and Wallis, Patrick (eds.) (2005) *Quackery and Commerce in Seventeenth-Century London: The Proprietary Medicine Business of Anthony Daffy*, London: The Wellcome Trust Centre for the History of Medicine at UCL.

Heilbron, J. L. (1983) *Physics at the Royal Society during Newton's Presidency*, Los Angeles, Calif.: William Andrews Clark Memorial Library.

Heller, Monica (ed.) (1988) *Codeswitching: Anthropological and Sociolinguistic Perspectives*, Berlin: Mouton De Gruyter.

Hickey, Raymond (2003) *Corpus Presenter: Software for Language Analysis*, Amsterdam: John Benjamins.

Hiltunen, Turo and Tyrkkö, Jukka (2009) ''Tis Well Known to Barbers and Laundresses: Overt References to Knowledge in English Medical Writing from the Middle Ages to the Present Day', in Antoinette Renouf and Andrew Kehoe (eds.), *Corpus Linguistics: Refinements and Reassessments*, Amsterdam and New York: Rodopi, pp. 67–86.

Hoey, Michael (2005) *Lexical Priming: A New Theory of Words and Language*, London and New York: Routledge.

Hull, Suzanne W. (1996) *Women According to Men: The World of Tudor-Stuart Women*, Walnut Creek, Calif.: Altamira Press.

Hunston, Susan (1994) 'Evaluation and Organization in a Sample of Written Academic Discourse', in Malcolm Coulthard (ed.), *Advances in Written Text Analysis*, London: Routledge, pp. 191–218.

Hunston, Susan and Thompson, Geoff (eds.) (2000) *Evaluation in Text: Authorial Stance and the Construction of Discourse*, Oxford: Oxford University Press.

Hunt, Tony (1990) *Popular Medicine in Thirteenth-Century England: Introduction and Texts*, Cambridge: Brewer.

(2000) 'Code-Switching in Medical Texts', in D. A. Trotter (ed.), *Multilingualism in Later Medieval Britain*, Cambridge: D. S. Brewer, pp. 131–47.

(2010) 'The Old French Translations in the Wellcome Library for the History and Understanding of Medicine MS 546', in Anneli Aejmelaeus and Päivi Pahta (eds.), *Translation, Interpretation and Meaning*, Helsinki: Helsinki Collegium for Advanced Studies. Available online at http://www.helsinki.fi/collegium/e-series.

Hunt, Tony and Benskin, Michael (eds.) (2001) *Three Receptaria from Medieval England: The Languages of Medicine in the Fourteenth Century*, Oxford: The Society for the Study of Medieval Languages and Literature.

Hunter, Lynette (1997) 'Women and Domestic Medicine: Lady Experimenters, 1570–1620', in Lynette Hunter and Sarah Hutton (eds.), *Women, Science and Medicine, 1500–1700: Mothers and Sisters of the Royal Society*, Stroud: Sutton Publishing, pp. 89–107.

(2002) 'Books for Daily Life: Household, Husbandry, Behaviour', in John Barnard and D. F. McKenzie (eds.), *The Cambridge History of the Book in Britain*, vol. IV: *1557–1695*, Cambridge: Cambridge University Press, pp. 514–32.

Hunter, Michael (1981) *Science and Society in Restoration England*, Cambridge: Cambridge University Press.

(1989) *Establishing the New Science: The Experience of the Early Royal Society*, Woodbridge: Boydell Press.

Hyland, Ken (1996) 'Writing Without Conviction? Hedging in Science Research Articles', *Applied Linguistics*, 17 (4): 433–54.

(1998) 'Boosting, Hedging and the Negotiation of Academic Knowledge', *Text*, 18 (3): 349–82.

(1999) 'Talking to Students: Metadiscourse in Introductory Coursebooks', *English for Specific Purposes*, 18 (1): 3–26.

(2000) *Disciplinary Discourses: Social Interactions in Academic Writing*, Harlow: Pearson Education.

(2001) 'Bringing in the Reader: Addressee Features in Academic Articles', *Written Communication*, 18 (4): 549–74.

(2002) 'Authority and Invisibility: Authorial Identity in Academic Writing', *Journal of Pragmatics*, 34 (8): 1091–112.

(2005) 'Stance and Engagement: A Model of Interaction in Academic Discourse', *Discourse Studies*, 7 (2): 173–92.

Hyland, Ken and Tse, Polly (2005) 'Evaluative *That* Constructions: Signalling Stance in Research Abstracts', *Functions of Language*, 12 (1): 39–63.

Hymes, Dell (1974) *Foundations in Sociolinguistics: An Ethnographic Approach*, Philadelphia, Pa.: University of Pennsylvania Press.

Isaac, Peter (1998) 'Pills and Print', in Robin Myers and Michael Harris (eds.), *Medicine, Mortality, and the Book Trade*, Folkestone and New Castle, Del.: St Paul's Bibliographies and Oak Knoll Press, pp. 25–47.

Jardine, Lisa (1999) *Ingenious Pursuits: Building the Scientific Revolution*, London: Little, Brown.

Jenner, Mark S. R. and Wallis, Patrick (eds.) (2007) *Medicine and the Market in England and Its Colonies, c. 1450–c. 1850*, Basingstoke and New York: Palgrave Macmillan.

Jones, Claire (1998) 'Formula and Formulation: "Efficacy Phrases" in Medieval English Medical Manuscripts', *Neuphilologische Mitteilungen*, 99 (2): 199–209.

Jones, Peter Murray (1995) 'Reading Medicine in Tudor Cambridge', in Vivian Nutton and Roy Porter (eds.), *The History of Medical Education in Britain*, Amsterdam and Atlanta, Ga.: Rodopi, pp. 153–83.

(1996) 'Book Ownership and the Lay Culture of Medicine in Tudor England', in Hilary Marland and Margaret Pelling (eds.), *The Task of Healing: Medicine, Religion and Gender in England and the Netherlands, 1450–1800*, Rotterdam: Erasmus Publishing, pp. 49–68.

(2000) 'Medical Libraries and Medical Latin 1400–1700', in Wouter Bracke and Herwig Deumens (eds.), *Medical Latin from the Late Middle Ages to the Eighteenth Century*, Brussels: Koninklijke Academie Voor Geneeskunde Van Belgie, pp. 115–35.

(2006) 'Medical Libraries', in Elisabeth Leedham-Green and Teresa Webber (eds.), *The Cambridge History of Libraries in Britain and Ireland*, vol. 1: *To 1640*, Cambridge: Cambridge University Press, pp. 461–71.

(2008) 'Witnesses to Medieval Medical Practice in the Harley Collection', *Electronic British Library Journal*. Available online at http://www.bl.uk/eblj/2008articles/article8.html (accessed 16 December 2009).

Jucker, Andreas H., Fritz, Gerd and Lebsanft, Franz (eds.) (1999) *Historical Dialogue Analysis*, Amsterdam and Philadelphia, Pa.: John Benjamins.

Jucker, Andreas H., Schreier, Daniel and Hundt, Marianne (eds.) (2009) *Corpora: Pragmatics and Discourse: Papers from the 29th International Conference on English Language Research on Computerized Corpora (ICAME 29)*, Amsterdam and New York: Rodopi.

Jucker, Andreas H. and Taavitsainen, Irma (eds.) (2010) *Historical Pragmatics*, Berlin and New York: De Gruyter Mouton.

Kassell, Lauren (2005) *Medicine and Magic in Elizabethan London: Simon Forman, Astrologer, Alchemist, and Physician*, Oxford: Clarendon Press.

Katritzky, M. A. (2007) *Women, Medicine and Theatre, 1550–1750: Literary Mountebanks and Performing Quacks*, Aldershot: Ashgate.

Kay, Christian (1994) 'Word Lists for a Changing World', in Werner Hüllen (ed.), *The World in a List of Words*, Tubingen: M. Niemeyer, pp. 67–75.

Klein, Lawrence (1994) '"Politeness" as Linguistic Ideology in Late Seventeenth- and Eighteenth-Century England', in Dieter Stein and Ingrid Tieken-Boon Van Ostade (eds.), *Towards a Standard English, 1600–1800*, Berlin: Mouton De Gruyter, pp. 31–50.

Koecher, Paul H. (1950) 'The Idea of God in Elizabethan Medicine', *Journal of the History of Ideas*, 11 (1): 3–29.

Koivisto-Alanko, Päivi (2000) *Abstract Words and Abstract Worlds: Directionality and Prototypical Structure in the Semantic Change in English Nouns of Cognition*, Helsinki: Société Néophilologique.

Kronick, David A. (1976) *A History of Scientific and Technical Periodicals: The Origins and Development of the Scientific and Technical Press, 1665–1790*, 2nd edn, Metuchen, NJ: The Scarecrow Press.

(1988) 'Anonymity and Identity: Editorial Policy in the Early Scientific Journal', *Library Quarterly*, 58 (3): 221–37.

Kurzon, Dennis (1985) 'Signposts for the Reader: A Corpus-Based Study of Text Deixis', *Text*, 5 (3): 187–200.

Kytö, Merja (1996) *Manual to the Diachronic Part of the Helsinki Corpus of English Texts: Coding Conventions and Source Texts*, 3rd edn, Helsinki: Department of English, University of Helsinki. Available online at http://helmer.aksis.uib.no/icame/hc/index.htm (accessed 21 December 2009).

Lancashire, Ian (2002) '"Dumb Significants" and Early Modern English Definition', in Jens Brockmeier, Min Wang and David R. Olson (eds.), *Literacy, Narrative and Culture*, Richmond: Curzon, pp. 131–54.

Landau, Sidney (2001) *Dictionaries: The Art and Craft of Lexicography*, 2nd edn, Cambridge: Cambridge University Press.

Lee, David (1992) *Competing Discourses: Perspective and Ideology in Language*, London and New York: Longman.

Leech, Geoffrey (2007) 'New Resources or Just Better Old Ones? The Holy Grail of Representativeness', in Marianne Hundt, Nadja Nesselhauf and Carolin Biewer (eds.), *Corpus Linguistics and the Web*, Amsterdam and New York: Rodopi, pp. 133–49.

LeFanu, W. R. (1984) *British Periodicals of Medicine: A Chronological List 1640–1899*, rev. edn, ed. Jean Loudon, Oxford: University of Oxford and Wellcome Unit for the History of Medicine.

Leong, Elaine (2008) 'Making Medicines in the Early Modern Household', *Bulletin of the History of Medicine*, 82 (1): 145–68.

Leong, Elaine and Pennell, Sara (2007) 'Recipe Collections and the Currency of Medical Knowledge in the Early Modern "Medical Marketplace"', in Mark S. R. Jenner and Patrick Wallis (eds.), *Medicine and the Market in England and Its Colonies, c. 1450–c. 1850*, Basingstoke and New York: Palgrave Macmillan, pp. 133–52.

Lindemann, Stephanie and Mauranen, Anna (2001) '"It's Just Real Messy": The Occurrence and Function of *Just* in a Corpus of Academic Speech', *English for Specific Purposes*, 20 (Supplement 1): 459–75.

Locke, John (1997) *An Essay Concerning Human Understanding*, ed. Roger B. Jones. First published 1690. Available online at the Research Centre for Humanities Computing, http://humanum.arts.cuhk.edu.hk/Philosophy/Locke/echu (accessed 9 May 2009).

Lyons, John (1968) *Introduction to Theoretical Linguistics*, Cambridge: Cambridge University Press.

Maclean, Ian (1980) *The Renaissance Notion of Woman: A Study in the Fortunes of Scholasticism and Medical Science in European Intellectual Life*, Cambridge: Cambridge University Press.

McCarl, M. R. (1996) 'Publishing the Works of Nicholas Culpeper, Astrological Herbalist and Translator of Latin Medical Works in Seventeenth-Century London', *Canadian Bulletin of Medical History/Bulletin Canadien d'Histoire de la Médecine*, 13 (2): 225–76.

McConchie, R. W. (1997) *Lexicography and Physicke: The Record of Sixteenth-Century English Medical Terminology*, Oxford: Clarendon Press.

(2002) 'Doctors and Dictionaries in Sixteenth-Century England', in Jacek Fisiak (ed.), *Studies in English Historical Linguistics and Philology: A Festschrift for Akio Oizumi*, Frankfurt: Peter Lang, pp. 267–92.

McDermott, Anne (2002) 'Early Dictionaries of English and Historical Corpora: In Search of Hard Words', in Javier E. Díaz Vera (ed.), *A Changing World of Words: Studies in English Historical Lexicography, Lexicology and Semantics*, Amsterdam and New York: Rodopi, pp. 197–226.

McEnery, Tony, Xiao, Richard and Tono, Yukio (2006) *Corpus-Based Language Studies: An Advanced Resource Book*, London and New York: Routledge.

McKitterick, David (2003) *Print, Manuscript and the Search for Order, 1450–1830*, Cambridge: Cambridge University Press.

McVaugh, M. (1997) 'Bedside Manners in the Middle Ages', *Bulletin of the History of Medicine*, 71 (2): 201–23.

Mäkinen, Martti (2002) 'On Interaction in Herbals from Middle English to Early Modern English', *Journal of Historical Pragmatics*, 3 (2): 229–51.

(2004) 'Herbal Recipes and Recipes in Herbals: Intertextuality in Early English Medical Writing', in Irma Taavitsainen and Päivi Pahta (eds.), *Medical and Scientific Writing in Late Medieval English*, Cambridge: Cambridge University Press, pp. 144–73.

(2006) 'Between Herbals et alia: Intertextuality in Medieval English Herbals', Ph.D. thesis, University of Helsinki. Available online at http://ethesis.helsinki.fi/julkaisut/hum/engla/vk/makinen (accessed 9 September 2009).

Matthews, Leslie G. (1964) 'Licensed Mountebanks in Britain', *Journal of the History of Medicine and Allied Sciences*, 19 (1): 30–45.

Mendelsohn, Everett (1987) 'The Political Anatomy of Controversy in Sciences', in H. Tristram Engelhardt and Arthur L. Caplan (eds.), *Scientific Controversies: Case Studies in the Resolution and Closure of Disputes in Science and Technology*, Cambridge: Cambridge University Press, pp. 93–124.

Meyer, Paul (1997) 'Hedging Strategies in Written Academic Discourse: Strengthening the Argument by Weakening the Claim', in Raija Markkanen and Hartmut Schröder (eds.), *Hedging and Discourse: Approaches to the Analysis of a Pragmatic Phenomenon in Academic Texts*, Berlin: Walter De Gruyter, pp. 21–41.

*Middle English Dictionary* (1952–2001) eds. Hans Kurath, Sherman M. Kuhn, John Reidy and Robert E. Lewis, Ann Arbor, Mich.: University of Michigan Press. Available online at http://quod.lib.umich.edu/m/med (accessed 25 August 2010).

Milroy, James (1992) *Linguistic Variation and Change: On the Historical Sociolinguistics of English*, Oxford: Blackwell.

Moss, Jean Dietz (1993) *Novelties in the Heavens: Rhetoric and Science in the Copernican Controversy*, Chicago, Ill.: The University of Chicago Press.

Mühlhäusler, Peter and Harré, Rom (1990) *Pronouns and People: The Linguistic Construction of Social and Personal Identity*, Oxford and Cambridge, Mass.: Basil Blackwell.

Nagy, Doreen Evenden (1988) *Popular Medicine in Seventeenth-Century England*, Madison, Wisc.: Bowling Green State University Popular Press.

Norri, Juhani (1992) *Names of Sicknesses in English, 1400–1550: An Exploration of the Lexical Field*, Helsinki: Academia Scientiarum Fennica.

(1998) *Names of Body Parts in English, 1400–1550*, Helsinki: Academia Scientiarum Fennica.

(2004) 'Entrances and Exits in English Medical Vocabulary, 1400–1550', in Irma Taavitsainen and Päivi Pahta (eds.), *Medical and Scientific Writing in Late Medieval English*, Cambridge: Cambridge University Press, pp. 100–43.

Nurmi, Arja (1999) *A Social History of Periphrastic DO*, Helsinki: Société Néophilologique.

Nurmi, Arja and Pahta, Päivi (2004) 'Social Stratification and Patterns of Code-Switching in Early English Letters', *Multilingua*, 23 (4): 417–56.

(2010) 'Preacher, Scholar, Brother, Friend: Social Roles and Code-Switching in the Writings of Thomas Twining', in Päivi Pahta, Minna Nevala, Arja Nurmi and Minna Palander-Collin (eds.), *Social Roles and Language Practices in Late Modern English*, Amsterdam and Philadelphia, Pa.: John Benjamins, pp. 135–62.

Orlin, Lena Cowen (1998) 'Gertrude's Closet', *Shakespeare-Jahrbuch*, 134: 44–67.

*Oxford English Dictionary* (1989–2009) online edn, Oxford University Press. http://dictionary.oed.com/.

Pahta, Päivi (2001) 'Creating a New Genre: Contextual Dimensions in the Production and Transmission of Early Scientific Writing', *European Journal of English Studies*, 5 (2): 205–20.

(2003) 'On Structures of Code-Switching in Medical Texts from Medieval England', *Neuphilologische Mitteilungen*, 104 (2): 197–210.

(2004a) 'Code-Switching in Medieval Medical Writing', in Irma Taavitsainen and Päivi Pahta (eds.), *Medical and Scientific Writing in Late Medieval English*, Cambridge: Cambridge University Press, pp. 73–99.

(2004b) '*So Seiþ* Idem Comentator: Code-Switching and Organization of Knowledge in John Trevisa's Translation of *De Proprietatibus Rerum*', in Alicia Rodríguez Álvarez and Francisco Alonso Almeida (eds.), *Voices on the Past: Studies in Old and Middle English Language and Literature*, A Coruña: Netbiblo, pp. 35–48.

(2007) 'Flowers, *Cum Multis Aliis Quae Nunc Praescribere Longum Est*: on Code-Switching in Early Modern English Medical Texts', in Ute Smit, Stefan Dollinger, Julia Hüttner, Gunther Kaltenböck and Ursula Lutzky (eds.), *Tracing English through Time: Explorations in Language Variation*, Vienna: Braumüller, pp. 259–72.

Pahta, Päivi and Nurmi, Arja (2006) 'Code-Switching in the Helsinki Corpus: A Thousand Years of Multilingual Practices', in Nikolaus Ritt, Herbert Schendl, Christiane Dalton-Puffer and Dieter Kastovsky (eds.), *Medieval English and Its Heritage: Structure, Meaning and Mechanisms of Change*, Frankfurt: Peter Lang, pp. 203–20.

(2009) 'Negotiating Interpersonal Identities in Writing: Code-Switching Practices in Charles Burney's Correspondence', in Arja Nurmi, Minna Nevala and Minna Palander-Collin (eds.), *The Language of Daily Life in England, 1450–1800*, Amsterdam and Philadelphia: John Benjamins, pp. 27–52.

Pahta, Päivi and Taavitsainen, Irma (2004) 'Vernacularisation of Scientific and Medical Writing in Its Sociohistorical Context', in Irma Taavitsainen and Päivi Pahta (eds.), *Medical and Scientific Writing in Late Medieval English*, Cambridge: Cambridge University Press, pp. 1–18.

Palander-Collin, Minna (1999) *Grammaticalization and Social Embedding: I THINK and METHINKS in Middle and Early Modern English*, Helsinki: Société Néophilologique.

(2009) 'Self-Reference and Mental Processes in Early English Personal Correspondence: A Corpus Approach to Changing Patterns of Interaction', in Andreas H. Jucker, Daniel Schreier and Marianne Hundt (eds.), *Corpora: Pragmatics and Discourse: Papers from the 29th International Conference on English Language Research on Computerized Corpora (ICAME 29)*, Amsterdam and New York: Rodopi, pp. 105–25.

Palmer, Frank R. (2001) *Mood and Modality*, 2nd edn, Cambridge: Cambridge University Press.

Parry, Richard (2007) 'Episteme and Techne', in Edward N. Zalta (ed.), *The Stanford Encyclopedia of Philosophy (Summer 2007 Edition)*, Palo Alto, Calif.: Metaphysics Research Lab, Center for the Study of Language and Information, Stanford University. Online at http://plato.stanford.edu/archives/sum2007/entries/episteme-techne (accessed 5 October 2009).

Pelling, Margaret (2003) *Medical Conflicts in Early Modern London: Patronage, Physicians, and Irregular Practitioners, 1550–1640*, Oxford: Oxford University Press.

Pelling, Margaret and Webster, Charles (1979) 'Medical Practitioners', in Charles Webster (ed.), *Health, Medicine and Mortality in the Sixteenth Century*, Cambridge: Cambridge University Press, pp. 165–237.

Pennell, Sara (2004a) 'Perfecting Practice? Women, Manuscript Recipes and Knowledge in Early Modern England', in Victoria E. Burke and Jonathan Gibson (eds.), *Early Modern Women's Manuscript Writing: Selected Papers from the Trinity/Trent Colloquium*, Aldershot: Ashgate, pp. 237–55.

(ed.) (2004b) *Women in Medicine: Remedy Books, 1533–1865*, Woodbridge, Conn.: Primary Source Microfilm.

Perelman, Chaïm and Olbrechts-Tyteca, L. (1971) *The New Rhetoric: A Treatise on Argumentation*, 2nd edn, Notre Dame, Ind.: University of Notre Dame Press.

Pollard, A. W., Redgrave, G. R., Jackson, W. A., Ferguson, F. S., Pantzer, Katharine F. and Rider, Philip R. (comps.) (1976–91) *A Short-Title Catalogue of Books*

*Printed in England, Scotland and Ireland and of English Books Printed Abroad, 1475–1640*, 2nd rev. edn, London: Bibliographical Society.
Porter, Roy (1989a) *Health for Sale: Quackery in England, 1660–1850*, Manchester and New York: Manchester University Press.
(1989b) 'The Early Royal Society and the Spread of Medical Knowledge', in Roger French and Andrew Wear (eds.), *The Medical Revolution of the Seventeenth Century*, Cambridge: Cambridge University Press, pp. 272–93.
(1996) 'Medical Science', in Roy Porter (ed.), *The Cambridge Illustrated History of Medicine*, Cambridge: Cambridge University Press, pp. 154–201.
(2000) *Quacks: Fakers and Charlatans in English Medicine*, Stroud: Tempus.
Poynter, F. N. L. (1953) 'A Seventeenth-Century Medical Controversy: Robert Witty Versus William Simpson', in E. A. Underwood (ed.), *Science, Medicine, and History: Essays on the Evolution of Scientific Thought and Medical Practice Written in Honour of Charles Singer*, vol. II, London: Oxford University Press, pp. 72–81.
Precht, Kristen (2003) 'Stance Moods in Spoken English: Evidentiality and Affect in British and American Conversation', *Text*, 23 (2): 239–57.
Rapp, Christof (2002) 'Aristotle's Rhetoric', in Edward N. Zalta (ed.), *The Stanford Encyclopedia of Philosophy (Summer 2002 Edition)*, Palo Alto, Calif.: Metaphysics Research Lab, Center for the Study of Language and Information, Stanford University. Available online at http://plato.stanford.edu/archives/sum2002/entries/aristotle-rhetoric (accessed 22 May 2006).
Ratia, Maura (2005) 'Personal Pronouns in Argumentation: An Early Tobacco Controversy', in Janne Skaffari, Matti Peikola, Ruth Carroll, Risto Hiltunen and Brita Wårvik (eds.), *Opening Windows on Texts and Discourses of the Past*, Amsterdam and Philadelphia, Pa.: John Benjamins, pp. 123–41.
(2006) '"*Con* and *Pro*": Early Modern Texts in Dialogue', in Irma Taavitsainen, Juhani Härmä and Jarmo Korhonen (eds.), *Dialogic Language Use/Dimensions du Dialogisme/Dialogischer Sprachgebrauch*, Helsinki: Société Néophilologique, pp. 87–106.
Raymond, Joad (2003) *Pamphlets and Pamphleteering in Early Modern Britain*, Cambridge: Cambridge University Press.
Read, Allen Walker (2003) 'The Beginnings of English Lexicography', *Dictionaries*, 24: 187–226.
Renouf, Antoinette and Kehoe, Andrew (eds.) (2009) *Corpus Linguistics: Refinements and Reassessments*, Amsterdam and New York: Rodopi.
Rissanen, Matti (1989) 'Three Problems Connected with the Use of Diachronic Corpora', *ICAME Journal*, 13: 16–19.
(1991) 'Spoken Language and the History of *Do*-Periphrasis', in Dieter Kastovsky (ed.), *Historical English Syntax*, Berlin and New York: Mouton De Gruyter, pp. 321–42.
(2006) 'Latin Influence on an Old English Idiom: "To Wit"', in John Walmsley (ed.), *Inside Old English: Essays in Honour of Bruce Mitchell*, Oxford: Blackwell, pp. 222–41.
(2008) 'Corpus Linguistics and Historical Linguistics', in Anke Lüdeling and Merja Kytö (eds.), *Corpus Linguistics: An International Handbook*, Berlin and New York: Walter De Gruyter, pp. 53–68.

Rissanen, Matti and Koivisto-Alanko, Päivi (2002) 'We Give You to Wit: Semantics and Grammaticalisation of the Verb Wit in the History of English', in Helena Raumolin-Brunberg, Minna Nevala, Arja Nurmi and Matti Rissanen (eds.), *Variation Past and Present: VARIENG Studies on English for Terttu Nevalainen*, Helsinki: Société Néophilologique, pp. 13–32.

Rissanen, Matti, Kytö, Merja and Palander-Collin, Minna (eds.) (1993) *Early English in the Computer Age: Explorations through the Helsinki Corpus*, Berlin and New York: Mouton De Gruyter.

Robinson, Richard (1954) *Definition*, Oxford: Clarendon Press.

Sampson, George (1970) *The Concise Cambridge History of English Literature*, 3rd edn, Cambridge: Cambridge University Press.

Sanderson, Jonathan (1999) 'Medical Secrets and the Book Trade: Ownership of the Copy of the College of Physicians' *Pharmacopoeia* (1618–50)', in Peter C. G. Isaac and Barry McKay (eds.), *The Human Face of the Book Trade: Print Culture and Its Creators*, Winchester: St Paul's Bibliographies, pp. 65–80.

Schendl, Herbert (2000) 'Linguistic Aspects of Code-Switching in Medieval English Texts', in D. A. Trotter (ed.), *Multilingualism in Later Medieval Britain*, Cambridge: D. S. Brewer, pp. 77–92.

(2002) 'Mixed Language Texts as Data and Evidence for English Historical Linguistics', in Donka Minkova and Robert P. Stockwell (eds.), *Studies in the History of the English Language: A Millennial Perspective*, Berlin and New York: Mouton De Gruyter, pp. 51–78.

Selosse, Philippe (2005) 'The Underlying Pattern of the Renaissance Botanical Genre *Pinax*', in Janne Skaffari, Matti Peikola, Ruth Carroll, Risto Hiltunen and Brita Wårvik (eds.), *Opening Windows on Texts and Discourses of the Past*, Amsterdam and Philadelphia, Pa.: John Benjamins, pp. 161–78.

Shapin, Steven (1984) 'Pump and Circumstance: Robert Boyle's Literary Technology', *Social Studies of Science*, 14 (4): 481–520.

(1994) *A Social History of Truth: Civility and Science in Seventeenth-Century England*, Chicago, Ill.: University of Chicago Press.

(1996) *The Scientific Revolution*, Chicago, Ill.: University of Chicago Press.

Shapiro, Barbara J. (2000) *A Culture of Fact: England, 1550–1720*, Ithaca, NY: Cornell University Press.

Sharpe, Kevin (2000) *Reading Revolutions: The Politics of Reading in Early Modern England*, New Haven, Conn.: Yale University Press.

Shepard, Leslie (1973) *The History of Street Literature*, Newton Abbot: David & Charles.

Sinclair, John (1991) *Corpus, Concordance, Collocation*, Oxford: Oxford University Press.

(2005) 'Corpus and Text: Basic Principles', in Martin Wynne (ed.), *Developing Linguistic Corpora: A Guide to Good Practice*, Oxford: Oxbow Books, pp. 1–16. Available online at http://ahds.ac.uk/linguistic-corpora (accessed 15 May 2009).

Siraisi, Nancy G. (1990) *Medieval and Early Renaissance Medicine: An Introduction to Knowledge and Practice*, Chicago, Ill.: University of Chicago Press.

Skaffari, Janne, Peikola, Matti, Carroll, Ruth, Hiltunen, Risto and Wårvik, Brita (eds.) (2005) *Opening Windows on Texts and Discourses of the Past*, Amsterdam and Philadelphia: John Benjamins.

Slack, Paul (1979) 'Mirrors of Health and Treasures of Poor Men: The Uses of the Vernacular Medical Literature of Tudor England', in Charles Webster (ed.), *Health, Medicine and Mortality in the Sixteenth Century*, Cambridge: Cambridge University Press, pp. 237–73.

Spencer, L. (1958) 'The Professional and Literary Connections of George Thomason', *The Library*, 5th Series, 13 (2): 102–18.

Spiller, Elizabeth (2004) *Science, Reading, and Renaissance Literature*, Cambridge: Cambridge University Press.

Stannard, Jerry (1982) 'Rezeptliteratur As Fachliteratur', in William Eamon (ed.), *Studies in Medieval Fachliteratur*, Brussels: Omirel, pp. 59–73.

Stine, Jennifer K. (1996) 'Opening Closets: The Discovery of Household Medicine in Early Modern England', unpublished Ph.D. thesis, Stanford University.

Studer, Patrick (2008) *Historical Corpus Stylistics: Media, Technology, and Change*, London: Continuum.

Styles, John (2000) 'Product Innovation in Early Modern London', *Past and Present*, 168: 124–69.

Swales, John (1990) *Genre Analysis: English in Academic and Research Settings*, Cambridge: Cambridge University Press.

Swales, John M. and Burke, Amy (2003) '"It's Really Fascinating Work": Differences in Evaluative Adjectives across Academic Registers', in Pepi Leistyna and Charles F. Meyer (eds.), *Corpus Analysis: Language Structure and Language Use*, Amsterdam: Rodopi, pp. 1–18.

Symons, John (2006) 'Scientific and Medical Libraries: The Rise of the Institution', in Giles Mandelbrote and K. A. Manley (eds.), *The Cambridge History of Libraries in Britain and Ireland, vol. II: 1640–1850*, Cambridge: Cambridge University Press, pp. 388–404.

Taavitsainen, Irma (1999) 'Dialogues in Late Medieval and Early Modern English Medical Writing', in Andreas H. Jucker, Gerd Fritz and Franz Lebsanft (eds.), *Historical Dialogue Analysis*, Amsterdam and Philadelphia, Pa.: John Benjamins, pp. 243–68.

(2001a) 'Changing Conventions of Writing: The Dynamics of Genres, Text Types, and Text Traditions', *European Journal of English Studies*, 5 (2): 139–50.

(2001b) 'Evidentiality and Scientific Thought-Styles: English Medical Writing in Late Middle English and Early Modern English', in Maurizio Gotti and Marina Dossena (eds.), *Modality in Specialized Texts: Selected Papers of the 1st CERLIS Conference*, Bern: Peter Lang, pp. 21–52.

(2001c) 'Middle English Recipes: Genre Characteristics, Text Type Features and Underlying Traditions of Writing', *Journal of Historical Pragmatics*, 2 (1): 85–113.

(2002) 'Historical Discourse Analysis: Scientific Language and Changing Thought-Styles', in Teresa Fanego, Belén Méndez-Naya and Elena Seoane (eds.), *Sounds, Words, Texts and Change: Selected Papers from 11 ICEHL, Santiago de Compostela, 7–11 September 2000*, Amsterdam and Philadelphia, Pa.: John Benjamins, pp. 201–26.

(2004) 'Transferring Classical Discourse Conventions into the Vernacular', in Irma Taavitsainen and Päivi Pahta (eds.), *Medical and Scientific Writing in Late Medieval English*, Cambridge: Cambridge University Press, pp. 37–72.

(2005) 'Genres and the Appropriation of Science: *Loci Communes* in English in the Late Medieval and Early Modern Period', in Janne Skaffari, Matti Peikola, Ruth Carroll, Risto Hiltunen and Brita Wårvik (eds.), *Opening Windows on Texts and Discourses of the Past*, Amsterdam and Philadelphia, Pa.: John Benjamins, pp. 179–96.

(2006) 'Key Word in Context: Semantic and Pragmatic Meaning of *Humour*', in Graham D. Caie, Carole Hough and Irené Wotherspoon (eds.), *The Power of Words: Essays in Lexicography, Lexicology and Semantics, in Honour of Christian J. Kay*, Amsterdam and New York: Rodopi, pp. 209–19.

(2009a) 'Authority and Instruction in Two Sixteenth-Century Medical Dialogues', in Matti Peikola, Janne Skaffari and Sanna-Kaisa Tanskanen (eds.), *Instructional Writing in English: Studies in Honour of Risto Hiltunen*, Amsterdam and Philadelphia, Pa.: John Benjamins, pp. 105–24.

(2009b) '"Joyful News Out of the Newfound World": Medical and Scientific News Reports in Early Modern England', in Andreas H. Jucker (ed.), *Early Modern English News Discourse: Newspapers, Pamphlets and Scientific News Discourse*, Amsterdam and Philadelphia: John Benjamins, pp. 189–204.

(2009c) 'The Pragmatics of Knowledge and Meaning: Corpus Linguistic Approaches to Changing Thought-Styles in Early Modern Medical Discourse', in Andreas H. Jucker, Daniel Schreier and Marianne Hundt (eds.), *Corpora: Pragmatics and Discourse: Papers from the 29th International Conference on English Language Research on Computerized Corpora (ICAME 29)*, Amsterdam and New York: Rodopi, pp. 37–62.

Taavitsainen, Irma and Fitzmaurice, Susan (2007) 'Historical Pragmatics: What It Is and How to Do It', in Susan Fitzmaurice and Irma Taavitsainen (eds.), *Methods in Historical Pragmatics*, Berlin and New York: Mouton De Gruyter, pp. 11–36.

Taavitsainen, Irma and Jucker, Andreas H. (2010) 'Trends and Developments in Historical Pragmatics', in Andreas H. Jucker and Irma Taavitsainen (eds.), *Historical Pragmatics*, Berlin and New York: De Gruyter Mouton, pp. 3–30.

Taavitsainen, Irma and Pahta, Päivi (1995) 'Scientific "Thought-Styles" in Discourse Structure: Changing Patterns in a Historical Perspective', in Brita Wårvik, Sanna-Kaisa Tanskanen and Risto Hiltunen (eds.), *Organization in Discourse: Proceedings from the Turku Conference*, Turku: University of Turku, pp. 519–29.

(1997a) 'The Corpus of Early English Medical Writing', *ICAME Journal*, 21: 71–8.

(1997b) 'The Corpus of Early English Medical Writing: Linguistic Variation and Prescriptive Collocations in Scholastic Style', in Terttu Nevalainen and Leena Kahlas-Tarkka (eds.), *To Explain the Present: Studies in the Changing English Language in Honour of Matti Rissanen*, Helsinki: Société Néophilologique, pp. 209–25.

(1998) 'Vernacularisation of Medical Writing in English: A Corpus-Based Study of Scholasticism', *Early Science and Medicine*, 3 (2): 157–85.

(eds.) (2004) *Medical and Scientific Writing in Late Medieval English*, Cambridge: Cambridge University Press.

Taavitsainen, Irma, Pahta, Päivi and Mäkinen, Martti (2006) 'Towards a Corpus-Based History of Specialized Languages: *Middle English Medical Texts*', in Roberta Facchinetti and Matti Rissanen (eds.), *Corpus-Based Studies of Diachronic English*, Bern: Peter Lang, pp. 79–94.

(comps.) (2005) Middle English Medical Texts, CD-ROM with *MEMT* Presenter Software, Amsterdam and Philadelphia: John Benjamins.

Thomas, Keith (1980) *Religion and the Decline of Magic: Studies in Popular Beliefs in Sixteenth- and Seventeenth-Century England*, Harmondsworth: Penguin Books.

(1986) 'The Meaning of Literacy in Early Modern England', in Gerd Baumann (ed.), *The Written Word: Literacy in Transition*, Oxford: Clarendon Press, pp. 97–131.

Thompson, Geoff and Hunston, Susan (2000) 'Evaluation: An Introduction', in Susan Hunston and Geoff Thompson (eds.), *Evaluation in Text: Authorial Stance and the Construction of Discourse*, Oxford: Oxford University Press, pp. 1–27.

Thompson, Geoff and Thetela, Puleng (1995) 'The Sound of One Hand Clapping: The Management of Interaction in Written Discourse', *Text*, 15 (1): 103–27.

Thompson, Geoff and Ye, Yiyun (1991) 'Evaluation in the Reporting Verbs Used in Academic Papers', *Applied Linguistics*, 12 (4): 365–82.

Tognini-Bonelli, Elena (2001) *Corpus Linguistics at Work*, Amsterdam: John Benjamins.

Traister, Barbara H. (2000) *The Notorious Astrological Physician of London: Works and Days of Simon Forman*, Chicago, Ill.: University of Chicago Press.

Traugott, Elizabeth Closs and Dasher, Richard B. (2005) *Regularity in Semantic Change*, Cambridge: Cambridge University Press.

Trotter, D. A. (ed.) (2000) *Multilingualism in Later Medieval Britain*, Cambridge: D. S. Brewer.

Tyrkkö, Jukka (2009) '*A Physical Dictionary* (1657): The First English Medical Dictionary', in R. W. McConchie, Alpo Honkapohja and Jukka Tyrkkö (eds.), *Selected Proceedings of the 2008 Symposium on New Approaches in English Historical Lexis (HEL-LEX 2)*, Somerville, Mass.: Cascadilla Proceedings Project, pp. 171–87.

Valle, Ellen (1999) *A Collective Intelligence: The Life Sciences in the Royal Society as a Scientific Discourse Community, 1665–1965*, Turku: University of Turku.

Van Bogaert, Julie (2009) 'A Reassessment of the Syntactic Classification of Pragmatic Expressions: The Position of *You Know* and *I Think* with Special Attention to *You Know* as a Marker of Metalinguistic Awareness', in Antoinette Renouf and Andrew Kehoe (eds.), *Corpus Linguistics: Refinements and Reassessments*, Amsterdam and New York: Rodopi, pp. 131–55.

Vickers, Brian (ed.) (1987) *English Science: Bacon to Newton*, Cambridge: Cambridge University Press.

Voigts, Linda Ehrsam (1989a) 'The Character of the *Carecter*: Ambiguous Sigils in Scientific and Medical Texts', in A. J. Minnis (ed.), *Latin and Vernacular: Studies in Late-Medieval Texts and Manuscripts*, Cambridge: D. S. Brewer, pp. 91–109.

(1989b) 'Scientific and Medical Books', in Jeremy Griffiths and Derek Pearsall (eds.), *Book Production and Publishing in Britain, 1375–1475*, Cambridge: Cambridge University Press, pp. 345–402.

(1996) 'What's the Word? Bilingualism in Late-Medieval England', *Speculum*, 71 (4): 813–26.
Wales, Katie (1996) *Personal Pronouns in Present-Day English*, Cambridge: Cambridge University Press.
Walker, J. Holland (1928) 'An Itinerary of Nottingham', *Transactions of the Thoroton Society*, 32. Available online at http://www.nottshistory.org.uk/articles/tts/tts1928/itinerary1928p3.htm (accessed 15 December 2009).
Walker, R. B. (1973) 'Advertising in London Newspapers, 1650–1750', *Business History*, 15 (2): 112–30.
Walton, Michael T. (1982) 'Thomas Forestier and the "False Lechys" of London', *Journal of the History of Medicine and Allied Sciences*, 37 (1): 71–3.
Wear, Andrew (1995a) 'Medicine in Early Modern Europe, 1500–1700', in Lawrence I. Conrad, Michael Neve, Vivian Nutton, Roy Porter and Andrew Wear (eds.), *The Western Medical Tradition: 800 BC to AD 1800*, Cambridge: Cambridge University Press, pp. 215–361.
(1995b) 'Epistemology and Learned Medicine in Early Modern England', in Don Bates (ed.), *Knowledge and the Scholarly Medical Traditions*, Cambridge: Cambridge University Press, pp. 151–67.
(1998a) 'Medical Practice in Late Seventeenth- and Early Eighteenth-Century England: Continuity and Union', in Andrew Wear, *Health and Healing in Early Modern England: Studies in Social and Intellectual History*, Aldershot: Ashgate, Chapter 10, pp. 294–320. First published in 1989.
(1998b) 'The Popularization of Medicine in Early Modern England', in Andrew Wear, *Health and Healing in Early Modern England: Studies in Social and Intellectual History*, Aldershot: Ashgate, Chapter 9, pp. 17–41. First published in 1992.
(1998c) *Health and Healing in Early Modern England: Studies in Social and Intellectual History*, Aldershot: Ashgate.
(2000) *Knowledge and Practice in English Medicine, 1550–1680*, Cambridge: Cambridge University Press.
Weber, A. S. (2003) 'Women's Early Modern Medical Almanacs in Historical Context', *English Literary Renaissance*, 33 (3): 358–402.
Webster, Charles (1975) *The Great Instauration: Science, Medicine and Reform, 1626–1660*, London: Duckworth.
(ed.) (1979) *Health, Medicine and Mortality in the Sixteenth Century*, Cambridge: Cambridge University Press.
Weijers, Olga (2007) 'The Medieval *Disputatio*', in Marcelo Dascal and Han-Liang Chang (eds.), *Traditions of Controversy*, Amsterdam and Philadelphia: John Benjamins, pp. 141–9.
Wing, Donald (1982–1994) *Short-Title Catalogue of Books Printed in England, Scotland, Ireland, Wales, and British America, and of English Books Printed in Other Countries, 1641–1700*, revised by J. J. Morrison et al., 3 vols., New York: Index Committee of the Modern Language Association of America.

# Index


addressee, 62, 184, 185, 209, 216, 219
adjective, 50, 66, 67, 90, 97, 98, 112, 113, 143, 188, 210, 221, 223, 226, 227, 228, 229, 230, 239, 240, 257
  stance, 228, 231, 239, 246
adverb, 50, 66, 67, 90, 234
adverbial, 229, 230, 255
  stance, 223, 226, 227, 228, 229, 230, 231, 234, 235, 246
advertisement, 15, 34, 35, 137, 140, 157, 171, 177, 180, 182–84, 185, 190–93, 194, 197–203
almanac, 5, 9, 15, 18, 32, 33, 35, 42, 95, 97, 103, 114, 138, 183
anatomy, 4, 13, 24, 70, 87, 107, 108, 120, 163, 206, 208, 209, 223, 224, 228, 231, 234
anonymity, 4, 15, 19, 20, 23, 35, 115, 136, 182, 192, 201, 218
apprenticeship, 46, 48
appropriation, 6, 36, 94–95, 97–98, 109, 113
argumentation, 3, 46, 96, 185, 187, 188, 190, 191, 192, 193, 195, 196, 203
Aristotle, 77, 78, 91
ascription, 88–91
attitude, 5, 8, 45, 46, 57, 72, 89, 94, 97, 113, 135, 146, 176, 208, 213, 214, 218, 221, 222, 225, 239, 245, 246, 255
audience, 2, 7, 32, 46, 48, 94–97, 107, 108, 113, 124, 126, 132, 138, 143, 147, 149, 157, 180, 181, 183, 184, 185, 189, 190–93, 197, 199, 201, 202–03, 221, 222, 223–25, 233, 235, 245
  illiterate, 33, 104, 137, 180
  involvement, 5, 7, 190, 191
  lay, 6, 55, 96, 114, 120, 125, 148, 156, 172, 181
  learned, 151, 172
  professional, 114, 125
  specialist, 46, 96, 225
  target, 9, 19, 20, 23, 62, 101, 104, 115, 117, 120, 123, 135, 137, 139, 140, 148, 149, 156, 157, 180, 185, 197, 202, 223, 241
  women, 5, 104
author, 5, 7, 8, 9, 12, 14, 15–16, 18, 19–20, 36, 38, 39, 41, 42, 43, 48, 51, 54–57, 59, 60, 61, 62, 68, 72, 73, 75, 79–82, 83, 87, 88, 90, 91, 92, 94, 95, 97, 104, 107, 108, 109, 114, 115, 116, 119, 125, 127, 131, 135, 136, 140, 141, 143, 145, 148, 149, 150, 151, 155, 156–57, 159, 161, 162, 170, 178, 182, 183, 184, 185–93, 195, 196, 197, 200, 201, 202–03, 205, 208, 212, 213, 214, 215, 216, 218, 220, 222, 224, 231, 233, 234, 237, 238, 239, 243–45, 246–47, 268, 269, 271
authority, 19–20, 37, 38, 40, 45, 47, 57, 72, 76, 79, 80, 81, 82, 88–91, 100, 136, 143, 148–51, 157, 163, 184, 187
  ancient, 4, 5, 48, 65, 163
  classical, 37, 149, 150
  definitional, 82, 87, 88
  divine, 143, 149, 150
  lay, 150
  medical, 59, 60, 62, 65, 149, 150, 157
  references, 59, 60, 89, 135, 148, 149, 150, 152, 156, 157, 161
Avicenna, 102

ballad, 32, 34, 35, 141
bilingualism, 117, 118, 205
blood transfusion, 164, 217
book, 5, 9, 17, 20, 23, 30, 32–33, 35, 36, 37, 38–43, 45, 46, 49, 104, 107, 113, 114, 116, 120, 131, 137, 138, 163, 164, 175, 187, 200, 201, 224, 228, 246
  chapbook, 34, 35
  collections, 35–38
  format, 9, 14, 115, 140–41, 180
  guidebook, 48, 55, 103
  handbook, 20, 96, 99, 108, 110, 111, 113, 115–16, 209
  history, 2, 6, 18, 33, 37, 38, 119
  hornbook, 176
  jest-book, 32, 34
  market, 35, 49, 138, 180, 183
  motto, 115, 129–31

newsbook, 180
notebook, 4, 10, 139
ownership, 36–37, 38, 40, 130
production, 4, 9–16, 32, 35, 37, 40, 206, 219
recipe, 5, 7, 15, 36, 129, 140–43, 180
remedy, 18, 36, 106, 131, 135, 136–37, 138, 160, 161, 223
review, 5, 7, 24, 108, 209, 217–18, 219, 223, 224, 225, 227, 228, 231, 233, 237, 238, 241, 243, 244, 246
surgical, 48, 51, 107
textbook, 22, 23, 51, 55, 99–104, 135, 176, 228
Boorde, Andrew, 40, 83, 206
Boyle, Robert, 18, 163
Braunschweig, Hieronymus, 86, 136
Bright, Timothy, 81, 89, 90, 104
Bullein, William, 34, 82, 92

Cambridge, 18, 34, 36, 40, 47, 116
case history, 51, 161, 169, 171, 177, 219
censorship, 14, 180
certainty, 5, 52, 99, 187, 213, 222, 226, 227, 234, 239, 241, 243, 245
adjective, 239
adverbial, 226, 234, 235
markers of, 222, 226, 235, 239, 243
verb, 226, 237, 241, 243, 244
charity, 38, 41, 137, 148
circulation
of manuscripts, 9, 10, 11, 13
of medical texts, 11, 12, 39, 114, 223, 225, 241
clause, 64, 66, 67, 120, 122, 126, 170, 226, 228, 243, 247
complement, 223, 226–27, 230–31, 237–38, 239, 241, 243, 244, 246
clergy, 30, 32, 138, 223
closet, 15, 35–36, 37, 38, 49, 115, 116, 141
Clowes, William, 39, 41, 81
code-mixing, 118
code-switching, 116, 117, 118–20, 121–22, 123, 127, 129, 131–32, 205
College of Physicians, 13, 14, 19, 20, 22, 34, 39, 40, 47, 137, 142, 187
collocate, 97, 98
commentary, 40, 89
commitment, 2, 3
markers of, 221, 226, 227, 246
commonplace, 44, 49, 94, 96, 103, 110, 113
*homo signorum*, 96, 103
communication, 1, 2, 10, 19, 22, 97, 98, 185, 205, 212, 224, 226, 244
oral, 10, 145, 148
written, 4
communicative purpose, 223, 224, 225, 241, 243, 246
comprehension aids, 7, 180, 193, 194, 196, 202, 203, 211
consumer, 7, 30, 182
context, 1, 6, 19, 23, 24, 35, 53, 57, 67, 75, 77, 94, 95, 97, 103, 110, 113, 116, 117, 119, 120, 131, 148, 160, 161, 184, 190, 199, 211, 212, 224
cultural, 1, 95, 185
disciplinary, 17, 96, 123
discourse, 1, 57, 63, 72, 116, 119, 123, 131, 144, 241
keyword in context (KWIC), 98, 229
linguistic, 1, 63, 98, 233
(non-)institutional, 4, 31
sociohistorical, 2, 25, 57, 95, 165
continental Europe, 10, 12, 37, 182, 205, 218
controversy, xii, 7, 43, 45, 57, 67, 88, 91, 172, 177, 180, 181–82, 185–90, 191, 194, 195–97, 201, 202–03, 216, 268
alkali and acid, 182, 187, 189
blood circulation, 181
Copernican, 181
tobacco, 181, 182, 195
conversation, 82, 92, 216, 221
corpus, 5, 22–25, 150, 163, 229
categories, 18, 50, 53, 71, 95, 100, 120, 125, 177, 239
*CED*, 98, 110
Corpus of Early English Medical Writing, 16, 119
definition of, 16
*EMEMT*, 2, 6, 7, 8, 16–25, 30, 33, 50, 53, 72, 75, 79, 89, 95, 97, 98–99, 109, 112, 113, 116, 120, 121, 123, 125, 126, 131, 139, 143, 162, 163, 165, 184, 222, 225, 227, 228, 230–31, 237, 241, 246, 258
HC, 118, 120
Lampeter Corpus of Early Modern English Tracts, 194, 195, 197, 199, 200
*MEMT*, 16, 18, 20, 23, 24, 79, 95, 97, 98, 119
*PCEEC*, 98, 109, 112
representativeness, 16–18
structure, 18–19
corpus linguistics, 2, 8, 17, 91, 98, 116, 119, 177, 229
correspondence, 6, 95, 98, 109, 113, 204, 209, 215
co-text, 95, 98
criticism, 42, 200, 206, 215, 216, 224
Culpeper, Nicholas, 14, 20, 48, 137, 139, 141, 142, 144, 147, 149, 150, 155, 157, 162
cultural practices, 5, 95, 113
culture, 1, 3, 6
classical, 131
high, 96, 116
literate, 95, 123

culture (*cont.*)
  medical, 5, 12, 43, 114, 118, 135
  of knowledge, 123, 131, 215
  popular, 95, 96
  print, xvii

Daffy, Anthony, 15, 35, 184, 192, 199
debate, 30, 74, 107, 138, 182, 185, 205
deixis, 195–202, *See also* discourse deixis
Dekker, Thomas, 176
description, 12, 17, 24, 48, 63, 77, 78, 83, 84, 85, 88, 98, 102, 103, 107, 110, 135, 138, 183, 196, 201, 209, 210, 213, 214, 218, 220, 225, 247
diachronic
  corpus, 118
  development, 6, 54, 60, 71, 116, 131
  linguistics, 5
  shift, 16, 49, 55, 72
diagnosis, 23, 38, 43
dialogue, 34, 99–101, 181, 185, 188, 189, 194, 205, 219, 244
dictionary, 74–79, 83, 84, 86, 87
diet, 24, 107, 115
discourse, 1, 17, 45, 46, 51, 52, 53, 63, 67, 70, 97, 98, 100, 102, 115, 117, 119, 129, 136, 143, 148, 193, 194, 196, 200, 219, 241, 243, 245, 247
  academic, 25
  analysis, 45, 53, 73, 97
  community, 3, 46, 72, 117, 123, 129, 205, 221, 225, 245
  context. *See* context
  deixis, 180, 193, 194, 197, 199, 202, 203
  discursive practices, 46, 49, 53, 63, 71, 116
  form, 67, 99, 101
  function, 49, 63, 64, 65, 119, 120
  organization, 63, 120, 233, 238
  participants, 189, 190, 191, 193, 238
  political, 39, 43, 63
  professional, 109, 119, 123, 129
  specialized, 7, 46, 109, 125, 205, 209
  strategy, 73, 118, 205, 219
  style, 25
  topoi, 46, 49, 64, 70, 71, 72
  unit of, 95
disease, 12, 13, 23, 25, 33, 34, 39, 40, 47, 66, 78, 81, 82, 84, 85, 86, 90, 100, 101, 104, 141, 151, 160, 161, 162, 169, 192, 200, 258, 260
  ague, 23, 80, 81
  fever, 23, 83, 88
  madness, 12
  plague, 12, 13, 15, 19, 23, 32, 33, 99, 260
  struma, 23
*disputationes*, 45, 181
drama, 6, 95, 97, 98, 99, 111, 222

*Edinburgh Medical Journal*, 219
efficacy, 7, 148, 157, 158, 159, 161, 162, 169, 170, 171, 177
  phrase, 36, 129, 155, 158–60, 161–62, 165–78
Elyot, Thomas, 32, 33
empiricism, 108, 113, 175, 225
enumerative text strategy, 99, 101
epidemics, 13
epistemology, 2, 7, 125
essay, 74, 182
  experimental, 5, 24, 108, 209, 211–15, 216, 217, 218–20, 224
etymology, 87, 88
evaluation, 2, 5, 148, 150, 214, 217, 218, 221, 224, 225, 228, 231, 239, 246
evidentiality, 213, 221
experiment, 5, 12, 109, 209, 212, 214, 215, 220, 237
experimental science, 149, 187, 204, 205, 210, 211, 212, 213, 215, 220, 223, 224, 227
experimenter, 212, 213, 214, 222

family, 23, 36, 137, 139, 223
Fennymore, Elizabeth, 34, 39
fiction, 95, 97, 98
Fioravanti, Leonard, 51, 99, 101
folklore, 23
Forman, Simon, 40
formulaic language, 151–56, 158–60, 161, 162, 169, 170, 174, 177, 189, 199
  set expression, 131, 151–56
  stock phrase, 159, 161, 162, 168, 170, 173–77
  tag phrase, 159, 161

Gale, Thomas, 48, 82, 92
Galen, 3, 55, 65, 80, 100, 102
Galenism, 43, 47, 70, 96, 142, 150, 157, 163, 164, 165, 172, 175, 176, 177, 178
genre, 5, 6, 7, 9, 13, 16, 18, 23, 95, 97, 111, 117, 118, 119, 120, 128, 129, 135, 136, 160, 177, 180, 182, 202, 203, 209–20
Grey, Elizabeth, 15, 20
guilds, 19

handwriting, 4, 10–11, 33, 130
Harvey, William, 4, 18, 48, 65, 164
healing, 35, 46, 119
health guide, 24, 48, 120, 223, 228
hedging, 213, 214, 221, 222
Helmontianism, 19, 43, 164, 172, 175, 177
herbal, 13, 14, 24, 105, 139, 160, 163
Hippocrates, 3
historical pragmatics, 2, 97
historical semantics, 97
hospital,4539n, 20
humoral theory, 6, 44, 94–95, 96–97, 98–114, 122

identity, 39, 118, 125, 127, 182
ideology, 2, 5, 6, 43, 131, 175, 181, 185
imperative, 62, 66, 100, 108, 160, 192, 193, 202
institution, 3, 4, 20, 22, 117, 121, 204
Church, 20, 34
institutionalization, 19
instruction, 10, 13, 20, 22, 24, 54, 70, 72, 105, 114, 128–29, 140, 145, 146, 155, 160, 162, 171, 199, 209, 246
interpersonality, 7, 119, 125, 135–36, 143, 145, 147, 148, 156, 157, 180, 184, 185, 190, 192, 193, 202
intertextuality, 123, 125–27, 129, 130, 131, 195–96, 197, 201, 202

Jones, John, 80, 81, 87, 92
Jonson, Ben, 34, 111
Jorden, Edward, 47, 82
*Journal des Sçavants*, 204, 217

knowledge, vii, 3, 4, 5, 8, 11, 17, 38, 40, 44, 45, 46, 47, 48–50, 52, 53, 55, 57, 61, 62, 65, 66, 67, 68, 70, 73, 76, 77, 89, 94, 95, 99, 104, 106, 111, 117, 118, 123, 124, 125, 131, 136, 138, 149, 150, 151, 154, 163, 184, 218, 224, 225, 227, 241
access to, 20, 41, 69
ancient, 3, 47
assertions of, 48, 49, 65, 68
assertive, 64, 68
attitude to, 5, 7, 8, 45, 46, 57, 150
base, 8, 123
claim to, 68, 70
communication of, 3, 7, 16
dissemination of, 4, 6, 7, 9–10, 12, 38, 45, 46, 48–49, 70, 114, 125, 223
epistemic, 44, 67
epistemology of, 7, 44, 45, 47, 48
lack of, 55–57
organization of, 6, 124
practical, 44, 47, 53, 66, 68, 69, 70
professional, 48, 61, 124
references to, 45–46, 48, 49, 51, 60–63, 67, 72, 150
sources of, 119, 123, 125, 127, 185
special, 1, 3, 116, 123, 142, 162, 218, 219
theoretical, 44, 47
topoi of, 62, 63, 67, 70
transmission of, 9, 121
verbs of, 6, 49, 50

Langton, Christopher, 20, 76–77, 80, 84, 90, 92, 206
language
Arabic, 7, 75, 83, 121, 151, 207
French, 39, 117, 121, 142, 204, 205, 225
German, 116, 118
Greek, 7, 75, 83, 121, 124–25, 128, 131, 136, 151–54, 207
Italian, 118, 121, 140
Latin, 3, 4, 7, 10, 12, 13, 14, 15, 16, 18, 22, 24, 37–38, 40, 41, 42, 43, 46, 47, 48, 75, 76, 80, 83, 115, 116–18, 119, 121, 122, 124–25, 126, 127, 128–29, 131, 136, 139, 141, 142, 151–56, 159, 160, 168, 174, 177, 205–06, 207, 208, 209
Middle English, 16, 22, 25, 50, 60, 77, 79, 95, 97, 119, 161, 208
language contact, 117
language-mixing, 118
lapidary, 24, 106, 160
lay
audience. *See* audience
authority, 143, 150
people, 5, 9, 36, 38, 48, 59, 60, 61, 69, 95, 98, 99, 108, 110, 114, 135, 136, 141, 142, 148, 149, 150, 156, 157, 162, 165, 223, 224, 225
readership, 19, 23, 137, 138–39, 140, 143, 144, 145, 148, 156
writing, 94, 98, 109–12, 113, 144, 145, 146, 148, 149, 150, 155, 157, 162, 165–68, 169, 171, 172, 174, 177
letter, 4, 10, 24, 35, 36, 97, 109–10, 209, 215–17, 222, 223, 224, 225, 227, 228, 231, 233, 238, 241, 243, 244
lexical borrowing, 208
lexico-grammatical features, 51, 221, 222, 223, 225, 241
lexicography, 74, 75, 76, 77, 79, 91, 92
library, 17, 18, 37–38
lifestyle, 36, 107
likelihood, markers of, 226, 227, 234, 239, 241, 243
lingua franca, 117, 121, 151, 205
literacy, 2, 6, 30–33, 34, 35, 36, 37, 38, 39, 40, 41, 42, 43, 104, 138, 154
cultural, 32, 33
functional, 31–32
practices, 6, 123, 129–30, 131, 132
subscriptional, 30–31
London, 4, 7, 13, 15, 16, 19, 20, 22, 31, 34, 39, 40, 138, 183, 204, 210

magic, 23, 106, 164
Malpighi, Marcello, 164, 205
manual, 9, 20, 36
manuscript, 4, 9–11, 13, 36, 40, 48, 117, 122, 130, 136, 137, 138, 148, 205, 209
marker, 22, 33, 155, 221
deictic, 180, 193–202, 203
stance, 7, 221, 222, 225–27, 231, 235, 237, 239, 241, 243, 244, 245, 246
*materia medica*, 23, 105, 120, 160, 161, 177, 228

meaning, 1, 8, 53, 74, 76, 78, 87, 94–95, 97–98, 99, 109, 110, 111, 112, 113, 115, 116, 117, 165, 206, 207, 208, 226, 227, 228, 233, 241, 243
media, 9, 18
medical marketplace, 39, 45, 48
medical practitioner, 6, 10, 15, 20, 23, 25, 34, 39, 40, 44, 47, 48, 57, 84, 89, 105, 108, 114, 135, 137, 139, 223, 224, 225
  apothecary, 10, 13, 14, 20, 38, 39, 43, 44, 45, 46, 47, 48, 61, 137, 139, 142, 156, 157
  barber-surgeon, 19, 38, 39, 43, 46, 70, 91
  bone-setter, 46, 48
  empiric, 20, 40, 43, 224
  healer, 44, 48, 143, 145
  herbalist, 20, 224
  midwife, 15, 20, 38, 41, 46, 48
  mountebank, 34, 224
  physician, 10, 13, 14, 19–20, 22, 34, 38, 39, 40, 43, 44, 45, 46–47, 48, 49, 67, 68, 71, 74, 76, 82, 91–92, 95, 99, 110, 114, 115, 127, 136, 137, 139, 142, 143, 149, 151, 164, 175, 176, 182, 185, 187, 210, 223
  quack, 41, 47, 140
  surgeon, 19, 20, 24, 34, 38, 41, 44, 45, 47, 48, 51, 61, 67, 91, 92, 101, 139
  unlicensed, 39, 40, 41, 137
  wise women, 20, 149
medicines, 5, 7, 13, 19, 23, 34–35, 39, 66, 90, 137, 141, 142, 164, 170, 171, 172, 176, 183, 184, 190, 191, 192, 200
  proprietary, 35, 180, 182–84, 190
  tobacco, 5, 181
merchant, 32, 37, 38, 138, 183
metatext, 7, 99, 104, 144
  metacommentary, 79, 80, 82
Middle Ages, 3, 43, 44, 96, 121, 176, 178
midwifery, 12, 15, 20, 23, 260
modality, 213, 241
  deontic, 53, 66, 70
Moore, Philip, 49, 107
multidimensional analysis, 222
multilingualism, 7, 115, 116, 117, 118, 132
  multilingual practices, 7, 116, 118, 123, 128, 131–32
  multilingual resources, 116, 117, 130, 131–32

narration, 212, 213, 214, 220
narrative, 141, 200, 210, 214, 219
news, 5, 7, 33, 180, 204, 209–11, 215, 216, 219, *See also* book
  newspaper, 182–84, 222
noun, 50, 54, 67, 79, 120, 121, 122, 124, 143, 196, 200, 223, 226, 227, 228, 229, 239
  stance, 231, 239, 246
noun phrase, 120, 122, 124

observation, 3, 5, 163, 170, 177, 206, 209, 212, 213, 215, 237
Oldenburg, Henry, 22, 204, 217
Oxford, 18, 40, 47, 142

pamphlet, 7, 14, 15, 35, 39, 45, 95, 140, 176, 180–84, 185, 187, 188, 189, 190, 191, 193, 194, 195, 196, 197–203
Paracelsianism, 43, 47, 150, 164
paraphrase, 44, 125, 127, 160, 168, 170, 177, 208, 211
paratext, 41–43
patient, 10, 38, 39, 46, 48, 49, 51, 82, 110, 143, 145–48, 149, 156, 157, 162, 164, 168, 176
patron, 34, 42, 189, 190, 202
Pepys, Samuel, 32, 210
perception, 46, 213, 221
persuasion, 7, 43, 46, 115, 131, 148, 158, 164, 170, 171, 187, 188, 189, 190, 191, 216
*Pharmacopoeia Londinensis*, 13, 14, 137, 139
*Philosophical Transactions*, 4, 7, 16, 24, 51, 53, 72, 73, 108, 120, 204, 222, 262
philosophy, 37, 44, 77, 175
  natural, 44, 47, 48
phlebotomy, 23, 107
phrase, 77, 79, 100, 111, 112, 115, 116, 122, 124, 126, 130, 131, 154, 187, 204, 228
  efficacy, 158–78
  epistemic, 187
phraseology, 63
physiognomy, 96, 108
physiology, 4, 24, 86, 96, 97, 98, 99, 103, 108, 110, 111, 113, 223
polarity, 46, 52, 54, 55, 57, 112
  negative, 55, 56, 57, 65, 113
  positive, 65
politeness, 5, 97, 216, 245
political writing, 39, 97
power, 44, 49, 106, 162
pragmatics, 2, 51, 56, 72, 94, 95, 97, 98, 113, 135, 219
prepositional phrase, 120, 122
prestige, 4, 35, 38, 83, 116
professional. *See also* audience
  communities, 5, 31, 45, 46, 47, 57, 64, 95, 109, 120, 148, 156, 219, 224
  knowledge. *See* knowledge
  readership, 6, 96, 101, 124, 128, 129, 138–39, 141, 142, 143, 146, 147, 154, 180, 202, 224, 225
  services, 42, 140, 148
  treatise. *See* treatise
  writing, 5, 94, 95, 98, 103, 105, 112, 113, 141, 143, 144, 145, 146, 148, 149, 150, 155, 156, 157
professionalism, 9, 104, 118, 123, 124, 155, 157, 210, 214
professionalization, 19, 62

prognostication, 9, 32, 33, 35, 103, 161
pronoun, 54, 60, 61, 148, 184, 185, 191, 192, 193, 202, 203
first person, 63, 64, 100, 180, 184, 185, 188, 190–92, 193, 202, 213, 216, 222
possessive, 143, 184, 187, 188, 189, 190
relative, 143
second person, 52, 63, 66, 67, 100, 143, 145, 180, 184, 185, 190, 192–93, 202, 216
third person, 184
public health, 33, 34
publishing, 4, 12, 14, 18, 182, 224

reception of texts, 1, 2, 8, 119
recipe, 7, 10, 24, 34, 36, 39, 107, 113, 120, 123, 128, 129, 131, 147, 158–78, 183, 223, 224, 231, 232, 233, 234, 241
collection, 10, 20, 23, 36, 53, 54, 55, 61, 105, 115, 125, 131, 135–57, 228
Recorde, Robert, 85, 91, 92
regimen, 12, 13, 24, 48, 50, 54, 55, 57, 62, 107, 114, 160, 223, 224, 228, 231, 241
register, 6, 16, 119, 194, 197, 200, 221–22
legal, 199
medical, 16, 180, 194
scientific, 195, 199
religion, 25, 32, 39, 96, 97, 119, 131, 138, 181, 197, 218
remedies, 10, 12, 13–14, 15, 18, 20, 24, 35–36, 39, 40, 89, 90, 106, 107, 114, 115, 135, 136, 138, 141, 142, 147, 149, 158, 160, 164, 170, 175, 176, 206
Renaissance, 44, 45, 75
report, 209, 212–13, 214, 219–20, 223, 224, 225, 227, 228, 231, 237, 241, 243
research article. *See* scientific journal
rhetoric, 46, 49, 52, 62, 220
rhetorical function, 63, 81, 125, 127, 138, 185, 222
Royal Society, xvii, 4, 5, 7, 16, 20, 22, 24, 43, 204–05, 210, 212, 216, 222, 223, 225

Salmon, William, 106, 142, 144, 147, 149, 154, 155, 171
scholasticism, xvii, 46, 47, 49, 57, 60, 70, 71, 72, 96, 99, 101, 159, 172, 175, 181, 206
scientific community, 62, 163, 205, 210, 215, 218, 219, 224, 237, 246
scientific journal, xvii, 4, 7, 22, 24, 160, 219–20, 224, 227
articles in, xvii, 17, 22, 24, 62, 209, 212, 219–20, 222, 223, 224, 225, 227
scribe, 10, 40
semantics, 58, 60, 62, 87, 94, 95, 97, 98, 99, 112, 113, 123, 127, 208, 221, 225, 226, 227, 228, 231, 233, 237, 239, 241
sentence, 52, 65, 97, 115, 116, 120, 122, 126, 130, 131, 154, 188, 189
Sharp, Jane, 15, 20
social class, 31, 89
gentry, 31, 32, 37, 38, 138
middle, 38, 48, 138
upper, 110, 138
Society of Apothecaries, 13
speech, 10, 118, 184, 188, 194, 197
stance, 5, 7, 55, 221–23, 225–27, 230–47
style, 5, 17, 23, 46, 54, 55, 57, 59, 68, 70, 71, 79, 96, 99, 101, 128, 157, 181, 185, 187, 192, 196, 203, 216
surgery, 13, 20, 24, 82, 107, 206
Sydenham, Thomas, 18, 71
synonymy, 74, 83–84, 90
syntax, 17, 45, 46, 52–53, 62, 63, 67, 70, 72, 120, 122

terminology, 35, 48, 75–76, 78, 80, 82, 83, 86, 87, 88, 98, 109, 110, 111, 112, 118, 119, 121, 123–25, 128, 129, 131, 135, 136, 151–56, 157, 162, 164, 175, 176, 202, 206, 207, 208, 211
text-organizing device, 159, 175, 177
text type, 18, 94, 95, 97, 161, 194, 209, 215, 216
theory, 1, 22, 47, 59
medical, 3, 6, 8, 13, 18, 44, 46–48, 70, 94–114, 116, 120, 122, 136, 148, 159, 164–65, 176, 177, 225
scientific, 7, 125, 182, 184, 193, 215, 220, 225, 244
thought-style, 2, 3, 5, 6, 22, 46, 49, 53, 57, 67, 70, 72, 73, 91
topos, 46, 62–72, 73
tradition, 16, 17, 20, 24, 44, 47, 70, 75, 80, 83, 84, 88, 106, 131, 136, 137, 142, 164, 176, 181, 195, 223, 224, 225, 241
learned, 116, 127, 131, 148, 151
translation, 4, 12, 14, 15, 16, 37, 81, 89, 117, 118, 127, 135, 139, 142, 155, 168, 205, 206, 207, 209
transmission, 9, 25, 48, 121, 125, 137, 148, 224
treatise, 49, 114, 205, 209, 223, 241
anatomical, 24, 107, 120, 224, 228, 231, 234
comprehensive, 22, 120
general, 22, 23, 50, 54, 55, 99, 104, 224, 228, 232
medical, 48, 50
on specific topics, 23, 104, 120, 224, 228, 231
professional, 102, 108
specialized, 18, 22, 53, 54, 55, 61, 70
surgical, 12, 24, 50, 54, 55, 107, 121, 223
theoretical, 160, 206
Tudor, 39, 45
typography, 32, 33, 140, 141

uncertainty, 187, 222, 227, 245
university, 6, 20, 34, 37, 44, 46, 47, 48, 76, 91, 95, 99, 148, 206, 223, 224

van Leeuwenhoek, Antonie, 164, 205
variation, 2, 6, 16, 31, 72, 95, 125, 148, 158, 165–71, 175, 177, 202, 227, 231, 241, 246
veracity, 47, 49, 53, 57
verb, 52, 53, 64, 73, 79, 170, 185, 188, 213, 222, 223, 226, 229, 237, 238, 239, 241, 243, 244, 246
  attitudinal, 226, 237, 245
  certainty, 226, 237, 243, 244
  communication, 226, 227, 237–38, 241, 243, 244, 246
  epistemic, 187
  knowing, 45, 46, 49–50, 53, 55, 63, 66, 67, 72
  likelihood, 226
  mental, 187
  modal, 52, 53, 54, 63, 66, 70, 185, 189, 222, 226, 228, 229, 230, 231–34, 243, 244, 246
  non-communication, 237, 246
  reporting, 60, 218
  semi-modal, 223, 226, 228, 230, 246
  speech-act, 188, 199
  stance, 223, 226, 228, 231, 237, 238, 243, 246
verb phrase, 120, 159
vernacularization, 3, 117, 206
Vesalius, Andreas, 3, 48, 163
voice
  active, 52, 53, 64, 212, 222
  passive, 52, 53, 64, 66, 160, 190, 192, 193, 202, 212, 213, 220
  textual, 39, 120, 127, 129, 191, 192, 195

Winter, Salvator, 140, 154, 155, 156, 191, 192, 199, 201
Woolley, Hannah, 20, 141, 150, 154, 155, 156
word formation, 207, 208
  borrowing, 75, 87, 207–08
  neologism, 208
world view, xvii, 9, 46, 96, 97, 164